HARTLAND'S
MEDICAL & DENTAL HYPNOSIS

DAVID WAXMAN
L.R.C.P., M.R.C.S.

Founder and First President of the section for Medical and Dental Hypnosis of the
Royal Society of Medicine; Past President of the European Society for Hypnosis in
Psychotherapy and Psychosomatic Medicine; Past President and Founder Fellow of the
British Society of Medical and Dental Hypnosis; Vice President of the British Society of
Experimental and Clinical Hypnosis; Affiliate of the Royal College of Psychiatrists;
Founder Fellow of the International Society of Psychosomatic Obstetrics and
Gynaecology; Formerly Associate Specialist in Psychiatry, Central Middlesex Hospital,
London

Third Edition

Baillière Tindall
LONDON PHILADELPHIA TORONTO SYDNEY TOKYO

Baillière Tindall   24-28 Oval Road
W.B. Saunders   London NW1 7DX, England

The Curtis Center
Independence Square West
Philadelphia, PA 19106-3399, USA

1 Goldthorne Avenue
Toronto, Ontario M8Z 5T9, Canada

Harcourt Brace & Company (Australia) Pty Ltd
32-52 Smidmore Street
Marrickville, NSW 2204, Australia

Harcourt Brace Japan Inc.
Ichibancho Central Building, 22-1 Ichbancho
Chiyoda-ku, Tokyo 102, Japan

© 1989 Baillière Tindall

Third edition 1989
Fourth printing 1995
Fifth printing 1995

British Library Cataloguing in Publication Data

Waxman, David
  Hartland's medical and dental hypnosis.—3rd ed.
  1. Medicine. Hypnotherapy
  I. Title
  615.8,512
  ISBN 0-7020-1323-4

Typeset by *The BeesNees*, Chessington, Surrey
Printed in Great Britain by T.J. Press (Padstow) Ltd,
Padstow, Cornwall.

HARTLAND'S

MEDICAL & DENTAL HYPNOSIS

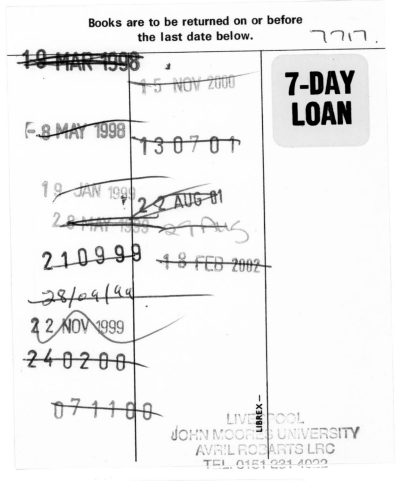

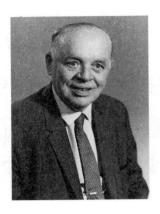

JOHN HARTLAND (1901–1977)

Most of the tributes to John Hartland on his death in 1977 bore witness to his personal qualities — warmth, energy and enthusiasms, ranging from classical music, photography, football, the detective novel to the wines of France — before describing his contribution in establishing the credentials of hypnotherapy as a branch of psychosomatic medicine and in rendering it more accessible to general medical and dental practitioners. Indeed, his personality had much to do with his own success as a therapist, together with his extraordinary care for verbal suggestion techniques: he took permanent delight in the richness and rhythms of the English language.

He thought later that he owed much to 30 years' experience in general medicine practice in West Bromwich, in the heart of the 'black country' of the English industrial midlands, among a people for whom he felt great affection.

His commitment to psychiatry came, however, from frustration in being denied the opportunity to leave general medicine. This was in 1939 when at the outbreak of war he volunteered for the Royal Navy. He was told to stay where he was. The industrial midlands were likely to be bombed. He turned his energies to the organization of an air raid post, to the raising of morale and money for military charities through the writing and production of musical revues, to the Red Cross, and — through curiosity in the phenomena of hypnosis — to psychiatry.

After the war he combined full-time general medicine with a hospital appointment as consultant psychiatrist and a growing private psychiatric practice. He began to lecture and demonstrate, first in Britain, then in the United States, France, Sweden, Australia and Singapore; was a driving force in the British Society for Medical and Dental Hypnosis; and edited the British Journal of Medical Hypnosis. The turning-point was publication of his paper on "ego-strengthening technique" in the United States in the early 1960s. One of the greatest rewards of his travels to the United States was his friendship with Milton Erickson.

Nothing would have given him greater satisfaction today than to know that his book, which first appeared in 1966, was still valued and thought worthy of a third edition.

Contents

Foreword to the Second Edition by M. H. Erickson

To write a foreword to this book is a most unusual pleasure and privilege. The book is not one primarily based upon other men's ideas with special interpretations elaborately evolved to explain the work of those others. Nor is it simply a survey of current literature on hypnosis. It is, rather, an earnest, sincere, objective account of one medical practitioner's experience over a period of twenty-five years, detailing instructively, in an orderly systematic fashion, the learnings he has derived from his day-to-day encounters with all manners of patients in his busy medical practice.

One realizes while reading this book that the author had a much greater purpose in mind than adding just another book to the literature on hypnosis, or a recounting of varied experiences solely for their interest. Each page makes clear that a long overlooked and seriously neglected need is being fulfilled, one of great importance in the furtherance of the scientific modality of hypnosis as an important adjunct in the healing arts. A methodology of the medical use of hypnosis of great value to the patient himself and to medicine as a whole is developed and adequately elucidated in this book. This is achieved by centring around a clear-cut well-ordered basic orientation which acquaints the medical practitioner with the varieties of hypnotic understandings pertinent to the clinical practice of medicine as the author himself has learned from one patient to another, from one kind of medical problem to another. Every effort is made to present clearly, comprehensively and understandably the multitude of problems and questions encountered in a busy twenty-five years, yet to do this simply, concisely, most informatively.

Wherever necessary the literature is adequately cited for content and meaning in relation to specific medical problems, not for speculative purposes; and the author does not hesitate to give full credit to others.

In brief, this book is one which the medical man, even though he may be a novice in hypnosis, can read with interest and intellectual gain. He will be inspired to improve his art of medicine, and after each trial he will return to the book to learn what more he needs to understand in order to care more adequately for his patients and to develop a better understanding of the personal values in the medical development of human welfare.

The writer of this foreword is medically trained and well experienced in hypnosis, and the manuscript of this book was read with a feeling of intense interest, of personal gain and of profound satisfaction that Dr Hartland had written so well this much-needed volume on the use of hypnosis in medicine.

MILTON H. ERICKSON, M.D.

Foreword to the Third Edition by E. R. Hilgard

The practice of hynotherapy is both an art and a science. As an *art* it is often best communicated through an apprenticeship to an experienced expert. However, such an opportunity is not always provided for students in medical and dental study, and not easy for those already in practice who wish to become familiar with hypnotherapy. For both student and qualified practitioner this book is an attractive alternative because of the detail with which appropriate practices are presented. As a *science* research on hypnotic phenomena and hypnotherapy can best be followed through attendance at scientific meetings in which hypnotic advances are presented, and through following the published research studies as in any other medical specialty. This book is helpful in suggesting where to look.

It has been over two decades since Dr Hartland's *Medical and Dental Hypnosis* appeared in 1966. The book was well received and has often been cited. Over the intervening years there have been many advances, however, both in the hypnotic research and in the clinical practice of hypnotherapy and hypnoanalysis. It is a welcome addition to the literature of hypnosis to have this revision by Dr Waxman, himself an able practitioner who has already gained respect and prominence for his own contributions to the field.

The essential qualities of the original book have been preserved — breadth of coverage of the history and theories, details of practice based on long years of practice both as physicians and psychiatrists, case materials, and a writing style suitable to qualified practitioners who may be novices to hypnosis and those already experienced who may wish to broaden their techniques to make them applicable for the benefit of a greater variety of patients. Dr Waxman has added material from his own experiences, wide reading, and thoughtfulness, resulting in a book updated throughout.

Because much of the material in the chapters of the first two parts is expository it requires somewhat less documentation; even so, about half the references are new. The third part, dealing with hypnotherapy as appropriate to a variety of problems for whose treatment hypnosis has been successful, is more fully documented. Of the many references, some three-quarters have been added by Dr Waxman as related to material that he has added to the text. The enrichment is particularly noticeable in the chapters on treatment of neuroses, problems of personality, depression, and, most extensively, on hypnosis in the alleviation of pain and in surgery.

Many controversies continue within hypnosis, both in definition and theory, and within recommended practices. While these are recognized in the book, they are played down, so that one gets the impression that, for those in practice, there may be something to be learned from each of the positions. There is no expressed intention to serve as resolvers of conflict; rather, the intention is to present those in practice with what is positive that has been learned through successful hypnotherapy with patients. Welfare of the patient is what therapy is all about. There is also an avoidance of sampling problems, control groups, and statistical tests that might be appropriate to the research literature read by investigators but of little interest to those whose attention is primarily upon treatment.

Perhaps some mention should be made of one of the initiatives made early by Dr Hartland that has been very influential upon the practices of other hypnotherapists: what he called the *ego-strengthening* technique, as contrasting with or supplementing *symptom removal*. He claimed that he had a 70% success rate with patients in brief hypnotherapy (less than 20 sessions), using ego strengthening alone, that is, without any attention to symptom removal. The details are given again in Chapter 11.

Whether one is coming new to hypnotherapy, or wishes to gain additional ideas, this book is to be recommended as a fine source for initial acquaintance or enrichment of knowledge already possessed.

Stanford University
Stanford, California,
U.S.A.

ERNEST R. HILGARD, PhD.
Professor of Psychology
Emeritus

Foreword to the Third Edition by
G. Guantieri

Reading Hartland's book on hypnosis, especially in Dr Waxman's fine, new and expanded edition, is always a source of extreme interest and satisfaction. For what is especially noticeable in this work is the author's deep and wide-ranging clinical experience and his painstaking and emotional response to that experience. It is the response not only of a serious, careful and objective researcher, but also of a therapist who is always ready to pay special attention not only to symptomatology and diagnostic and therapeutic techniques, but also to the human being with his emotions, and therefore to the interpersonal relationship running between doctor and patient. This work, which covers large areas of medicine and surgery, thus acquires great importance not only on account of the numerous and varied references to situations relieved by hypnosis, but also for the holistic vision permeating it and consequently the quality of approach for the patient, that important approach in diagnostic and therapeutic areas outside clinical hypnosis, we could call psychosomatistic. This orientation is a constant element which becomes more and more evident as one reads on. It concerns both the patient with his symptoms and the factors preceding and concurrent with the induction and deepening of the hypnosis responsible for these processes, as well as their spontaneous and induced phenomena, not to mention their therapeutic action. Here we should also note the importance given to the doctor figure, characterized by affective sensitivity, inner opening and a capacity for human contact, leading him to accept and use what the patient initially offers him, displaying trust, respect, empathy and sympathy, and forming together with the patient a unity made up of intimate responses. From this picture there derives a methodology which also leads, quite logically, to David Waxman's personal technique (called the "ego-assertive retraining"), a technique which is well founded, clearly understandable and utterly convincing. This methodology becomes the clear expression of a healthy marriage of art and science, quite distinct therefore from the exercise of pure technique, a marriage without which no *true* medical act — whether diagnostic or therapeutic — can exist. A clear example of this is the studied attention devoted not only to words but also to pauses; in other words, the weighing up and interpretation of the possible significances behind the frequency, duration and quality of both utterances and silences, and an assessment of how and when they are inserted into the thread of sound.

Hartland's book is prompted above all by the author's genuine desire to offer doctors the tangible results of his experience and to impart concrete aid as regards the real cure of patients. It ca⊓ therefore be especially recommended — both from the technical point of view and as a formative influence — to a wide circle of colleagues: to the beginner, to the expert, for the important knowledge and insights that may be gained; and finally even to those who do not — and never intend to — resort to hypnosis, both for the valuable information concerning professional practice in many specialist areas and also because it may help to spread the understanding that it is possible to be therapeutic purely *as a person*, sometimes even without the need to resort to any other remedy.

Professor of Psychosomatic Medicine and   GUALTIERO GUANTIERI
Clinical Hypnosis at the University of Verona

Preface to the Third Edition

It is a tribute to the reputation and memory of the late Dr John Hartland that although more than twenty years have elapsed since *Medical and Dental Hypnosis* was first published, it has remained in demand throughout the world as one of the most popular textbooks of hypnotherapy.

Inevitably, however, with the passage of time, the areas of its clinical application have extended and crystallized and experiment and research into the psychological and neurophysiological status of hypnosis have greatly increased knowledge of its mode of action and role in therapy.

We have learned, too, much about its limitations and the need for eclecticism.

John Hartland was a man of immense stature and charisma, who by his writings, his travels and his lectures, gained world renown as one of the premier exponents and teachers of hypnotherapy.

It was with some trepidation therefore, that the present writer faced the formidable task of "revising and updating Hartland".

Whilst undertaking this, it was obvious that the distinctive style of the original author must be retained and every effort has been made to achieve this objective, although much of the content, now outdated, has had to be amended, deleted or extended where required, in order to bring the work into line with modern thinking and developments. However, because of the increasing popularity and its effectiveness in many disciplines of general and psychological medicine, the intention has been to take hypnosis out of the somewhat limited use by the family doctor so that it may be included in the many other specialities where it would be of advantage to the patient.

The book has now been divided into four separate parts and twenty-six chapters with an appendix. The extended lists of references are intended to acquaint the reader with some of the great names and contributions to clinical and experimental hypnotherapy and for the sake of convenience are now included at the end of each chapter. The order of chapters has been re-aligned so as to bring the subject matter under the appropriate heading.

Generally speaking, the arrangement of the chapters in Part 1 is unchanged although Theories of Hypnosis is now included with The Nature of Hypnosis. Much additional material is also added as well as some of the more recent and better known induction techniques.

Part 2 now includes an enlarged chapter on post-hypnotic suggestion and the chapter on hypnoanalysis and analytical psychotherapy has been moved to this section which also contains a brief description of Ericksonian hypnosis and neurolinguistic programming.

The various treatment chapters have been reorganized and largely rewritten and have been transferred to Part 3. Also included are more up-to-date chapters on the alleviation of pain, on obstetrics and on hypnosis with children. New chapters on hypnosis in the treatment of depression and hypnotherapy in chronic and terminal illness have been added. The chapter on dental hypnosis remains largely unchanged.

Finally, Part 4 includes chapters on some additional uses as well as on some of the misuses of hypnosis.

The guidelines listed in the appendix are intended to assist the beginner in following the proper application of what will be to him an entirely new form of treatment, to help maintain the ethical status and dignity to hypnosis in therapy and for the ultimate benefit of the patient.

It is hoped that in so doing, this volume will also help perpetuate the name of John Hartland who contributed so much to the alleviation of human suffering.

London   DAVID WAXMAN

Acknowledgements

Thanks are due to the many friends and colleagues of the late Dr John Hartland and to the authors and publishers who generously supplied material for the earlier editions and granted permission to quote from their works. Acknowledgement must also be made of Mr John Hartland, who provided such invaluable help to his father in the preparation of the second edition and has given generous support to this new edition.

The late Dr Milton H. Erickson, Dr A. Spencer Paterson and Mr Eric Wookey were of considerable help in checking and advising on the original manuscript and much of the chapter entitled The Use of Hypnosis in Dental Surgery is based upon the original contribution which the late Mr Stanley Tinkler supplied for the first and second editions.

Thanks are also due to the following authors and publishers who gave permission to use some of the earlier quotations:

George Allen & Unwin for the quotation from *Psychological Healing* by Pierre Janet; Edward Arnold (Publishers) for quotations and material from *The Common Neuroses* and *Analytical Psychotherapy* by Dr T. A. Ross; The Dental Items of Interest Publishing Co. for the description of a basic picture-visualization technique from *Hypnodontics* by Aaron Moss, D.D.S.; Dr Milton H. Erickson for material derived from his numerous writings and lectures, especially from his article 'Confusion technique', in the *American Journal of Clinical Hypnosis,* and also for permission to quote the article 'The effects of hypnosis on a complicated obstetric case', written by the first author and Mr Wilfred Mills and originally published in the *American Journal of Clinical Hypnosis*; The Julian Press (Publishers) for various quotations from *The Study of Hypnosis* by Albert Moll; Dr Andre Weitzenhoffer, Grune & Stratton and John Wiley & Sons for material from *General Techniques of Hypnotism* and *Hypnotism*; Dr Lewis R Wolberg, Grune & Stratton and William Heinemann for permission to quote freely from *Medical Hypnosis* and *Hypnoanalysis*; Dr Calvert Stein and Charles C. Thomas, Illinois, for quotations from *Practical*

Psychotherapy in Non-psychiatric Specialities; Dr Michael Scott and Charles C. Thomas, Illinois, for permission to quote from *Hypnosis in Skin and Allergic Diseases*; and Dr Erika Fromm for material from 'Dissociative and integrative processes in hypnoanalysis' in the *American Journal of Clinical Hypnosis.* Thanks are also due to Dr Wm E. Edmonston, Jr, Editor of the *American Journal of Clinical Hypnosis,* for permission to draw upon these two articles; to Dr Jay Haley and Grune & Stratton for quotations from *Strategies of Psychotherapy* and *Advanced Techniques of Hypnosis and Therapy: Selected Papers of Milton Erickson*; also to Dr Dennis K. Chong for his personal advice and guidance concerning the origins and description of neurolinguistic programming and to Dr Maurice Yaffé for permission to quote from the details contained in his article 'The contribution of psychology to sport: an overview'.

Thanks are also due to the librarians of the Royal Society of Medicine for their untiring efforts in verifying countless references and supplying reprints of numerous original papers.

Particular thanks are due to Professor Ernest R. Hilgard for his support during the planning of this third edition.

PART ONE

THE HISTORY, NATURE AND TECHNIQUES OF HYPNOSIS

CHAPTER 1

The Development of Hypnosis

Hypnosis has emerged from early history to the present day as a powerful and effective technique which may readily be adapted for use in many areas of medicine in general and in psychiatry in particular. Because of the mystery and misunderstanding which has surrounded the subject for so many years, a considerable folklore has developed. The ease with which the hypnotic state may be produced has invited extensive misuse and charlatans and entertainers abound. Anecdotal reports and unvalidated claims of miraculous cures prejudice the findings of serious therapists and the inability of the medical profession to develop satisfactory instruments for scientific studies had resulted in hypnotherapy remaining in limbo for nearly two centuries.

However with the advancement of electroencephalographic and other investigatory procedures and with the development and extension of experimental laboratories worldwide, neuro-physiological and psychological research has increased and the true place for the clinical application of hypnosis has at last been found.

Healing in a trance state is one of the oldest of the medical arts. It was believed to be divinely inspired and that the miraculous cures which often resulted were religious in nature. The mysterious forces that produced the trance state were the work of the gods, who behaved in an irregular and unpredictable manner. Because of this, cures were both uncertain and capricious in nature.

But as scientific knowledge slowly progressed, men began to learn how to treat certain of the simpler ailments themselves, and handed over such elementary matters as fractures and dislocations to the surgeons. But many diseases remained for the relief of which some supernatural power still had to be invoked. One of the classical means of healing emerged from ancient Greece. It often entailed travelling long distances to one of the shrines such as the Temple of Aesculapius at Epidaurus, which contained a statue believed to be endowed with miraculous powers. The sufferers, after their long and arduous journeys, would lay valuable offerings at the gates of the Temple, after which they were cleansed in the waters of a fountain. They then spent one or two nights in prayer and supplication, and subsequently were admitted to the Temple itself. Here, advice was given by oracles, or in the form of prophetic dreams. This atmosphere of mysticism and ceremonial was highly important, and its significance will presently become clear. However, whether hypnosis was unwittingly involved in this form of sleep and dream treatment is open to some dispute and has been discussed extensively by Stam and Spanos[1] in a learned paper.

Even in the Middle Ages, miraculous cures were thought to be effected by sacred statues, healing springs, fragments of the true cross or the bones of a saint. Miracles could also be performed by virtue of the exalted rank of an individual. The kings both of England and of France were believed to have the power of curing by the 'laying-on of hands'. This practice was known as 'touching for the King's Evil'. Indeed, belief in miraculous healing has persisted into the twentieth century. Even today, the cures reported from the spring at Lourdes are hardly less remarkable than those which occurred at the Temple of Aesculapius, many centuries before Christ. The power of suggestion was certainly known in Biblical times, and it seems probable that many of the cures produced by the prophets and saints were based upon this alone. But though the phenomena of the trance state, which many recognize today as being hypnotic in character, had all been observed as isolated facts, it never occurred to anyone that they might be due to a common or natural cause. They were consequently thought to be supernatural religious manifestations, the results of magical spells or the work of evil spirits. One of the first 'scientific' theories of illness was propounded by the great physician Galen of Pergamum whose ideas dominated medicine from the second century AD until the Renaissance. He considered that there was some invisible fluid which filled the universe and flowed through the body and the mind of every person, maintaining good physical and mental health. Sickness would be caused by interference with this flow and the cure depended upon achieving a satisfactory balance once more. This idea was generally accepted and no further explanation was sought until the year 1530, when Paracelsus formulated his theory concerning the effect of the heavenly bodies upon mankind—especially on their diseases. Then, one hundred years later, Athanasius Kircher, a German priest and scholar, maintained the view that not only did the stars influence men, but that men could mutually influence each other through the agency of magnetic powers.

Franz Anton Mesmer was born in 1734 in the village of Iznang near Lake Constance and graduated in medicine in Vienna at the age of 32. Taking, as he thought, the treatment of illness to its logical conclusions, he wrote a dissertation entitled 'The Influence of the Planets on the Human Body'. All known theories were now brought together under a single therapeutic umbrella, that of magnetism. The ethereal fluid of Galen, the correct balance of which was essential for health, influenced, as it was now believed, by the heavenly bodies, could be controlled and guided through the body of the patient. Magnetized iron plates, shaped to fit various parts of the subject (an idea that Mesmer obtained from Maximilian Hell, Professor of astronomy at the university) were placed over the affected area and could then be manipulated in order to turn the flow of this 'current' in various directions. Mesmer was convinced that by this means he could alleviate the symptoms of illness and restore good health to his ailing patients. The results were often both dramatic and surprising. Patients suffering from retention of urine, toothache, earache, depression, trances, temporary blindness and attacks of paralysis, who had hitherto been considered to be incurable, lost their symptoms completely. Mesmer's eventual clash with the medical hierarchy was precipitated by his treatment of the daughter of the private secretary to the

Archduchess of Austria. Marie-Thérèse Paradis had suffered from blindness since childhood. She had become a brilliant pianist and was acclaimed throughout the concert halls of Europe. The medical experts of the day had failed to restore her sight and Dr Mesmer was consulted. His treatment was successful and one can imagine the chagrin of his professional colleagues. One can also imagine their delight when the patient subsequently relapsed, for once sighted, she also lost that sixth sense which had made her expertise on the keyboard so unique and her performances so much in demand. Poor Marie had been receiving a state pension on account of her affliction, but her parents had overlooked the fact that it would be withdrawn upon her recovery. They were furious and insisted that Mesmer release the patient from treatment. Not surprisingly, she soon became 'blind' again and the hostility amongst Mesmer's medical colleagues forced him to leave Vienna. He moved to Paris, where he set up one of the most famous clinics in Europe, in which he treated every conceivable type of illness.

Notwithstanding, the message to be learned from the case of Marie-Thérèse Paradis rings loud and clear. The blindness was a symptom of a problem which the patient did not want to look at— and which Mesmer failed to see. Today we would apply the term *conversion* to this and we know that the remedy is not by way of symptom removal but by exploration and treatment of the origin of the trouble.

At his Paris clinic, Mesmer developed a number of essential principles for his treatment of the sick. Pierre Janet, in his book entitled 'Psychological Healing'[2] gives the following description of his procedure.

Mesmer used an elaborate apparatus, and his practice was attended with a ceremonial similar to that employed at the miracle shrines of old. The patients were ushered into a hall of which all the windows were thickly curtained, so that what was to follow could be carried out in semi-darkness. The air was filled with plaintive strains of violins. In the middle of the room was a large oaken tub, Mesmer's famous 'baquet'. This was filled with a mixture of water, iron filings and powdered glass. It had a lid pierced with holes, and emerging through the holes were jointed iron rods.

The patients applied the rods to the ailing parts, linked hands and were required to remain in absolute silence. Mesmer, the great magnetizer, now appeared, wearing a silken robe of a pale lilac colour, and holding in his hand a short iron wand. He passed slowly through the ranks, fixing his eye upon the patients, passing his hand over their bodies or touching them with the wand. Many patients were unable to notice much result and declared that they could feel absolutely nothing. But some of them coughed, spat and felt as if insects were running over their skin. Finally some, especially young women, would fall down and go into convulsions, so that the hall certainly deserved the name of the 'Hall of Convulsions'. This convulsive state, attended by hiccoughs, outbursts of laughter and sometimes delirium, constituted what was known as the 'crisis', and was considered to be salutary. The patients were then carried off to a side room and further treated by one of the great man's assistants. Two or three sessions of this kind were usually sufficient to effect a cure.

Now, theatrical though this procedure may have been, it should be borne in mind that although Mesmer failed to understand the real character of the phenomena he induced, he at least perceived that they were due to a common cause. That cause he believed, was his power to alter the direction of movement of the ethereal fluid through the human body. He experimented extensively with his magnets but subsequently found them to be quite unnecessary. He believed that he could control the ebb and flow of this fluid and channel it through his patients not only with the use of magnets but with anything that he touched. Later, he maintained that he himself was the magnet. No other artificial aids were required. Thus the cures that he was able to produce were due to 'animal magnetism'. In making his 'passes' a few inches from the body surface, Mesmer believed that this invisible magnetic fluid flowed out of his fingertips into the patient's body, achieving the necessary redistribution and restoring the balance. Once this had been effected, the patient regained his health.

There is no doubt whatever that Mesmer did actually succeed in curing a great many people who had been given up as incurable, and naturally his fame spread rapidly. Patients travelled from every part of Europe to attend his clinic, much to the irritation of the medical profession which once again became exceedingly hostile. As a result, in 1784, King Louis XVI appointed a Commission to investigate mesmerism, or animal magnetism as it was now called. Amongst its members were Antoine Lavoisier, the famous chemist, Dr Guillotin, the inventor of the machine that bears his name, and Benjamin Franklin, the American scientist and statesman. Naturally enough, the Commission failed to discover any concrete evidence of animal magnetism or of the existence of the supposed invisible fluid. It consequently concluded that the phenomena embraced nothing that could not be explained by imitation and imagination, and that in the long run the effects of the treatment could not fail to be harmful.

Today, it seems unfortunate that the Commission chose to investigate the wrong aspect of Mesmer's work. Had it attempted to discover whether Mesmer's cures were in fact genuine and what part imagination had played in effecting them, much light might have been thrown upon the subject and future developments would not have been retarded, as in fact they were, for the next 60 years or so. The Commission's report severely damaged Mesmer's reputation and fashion turned against him. The final blow fell when the Medical Faculty of the University of Paris issued a decree that any physicians found guilty of practising animal magnetism would be excluded from the profession, and lose their licence to practise. This compelled Mesmer to leave France, and when subsequently he wished to return, his place had been filled. Animal magnetism had undergone changes and had entered into a new phase.

The second period of animal magnetism dates from around the year 1787. Two significant discoveries were made at this time. One of Mesmer's followers, the Marquis de Puységur, described a state which became known as artificial somnambulism. The chief characteristic of this state was a kind of sleep in which the ideas and actions of the magnetized person could be directed by the magnetizer. At the beginning of the nineteenth century, Bertrand described this as being entirely due to the working of the subject's imagination. This was put to good use by a Portuguese priest, the Abbé José Custodio di Faria, who was the first to induce somnambulism in his subjects by simply saying to them, 'I wish you to go to sleep'. Despite this, however, the unyielding opposition of the medical profession forced mesmerism to remain virtually unused for many more years. During this period it was exploited only by showmen at travelling fairs who used to demonstrate the phenomenon of the trance.

Several years later the same uncomprising opposition of the medical profession caused the physician, John Elliotson, to be dismissed from his professorial post at the University College Hospital, London, because he gave public demonstrations of mesmerism. He was a firm champion of any cause in which he believed however and was later rehabilitated and invited to give the Harveian Oration. This he did with relish, inserting a strong plea for the benefits of mesmerism to be studied and utilized. He compared the manner in which Harvey's discovery of the circulation of the blood had been initially discredited, with the fate of his own ideas of mesmerism. He had believed too that certain of his subjects were endowed with far-reaching powers which could be used for the purpose of diagnosis. However, by now, in addition to the treatment of disease, mesmerism was also being used extensively for the alleviation of the sensation of pain. James Esdaile, who was practising surgery in India, sent a report to the Medical Board of 75 operations performed painlessly under hypnotic anaesthesia, but his letter was never even acknowledged.

Then in 1841 the French magnetizer, Lafontaine, visited Manchester and gave a demonstration of magnetic experiments. James Braid, a well-known local surgeon, happened to be present with a colleague. They saw a girl apparently put into a trance, and Braid was so incensed that he went upon the stage himself to expose it as a complete fake. To his intense astonishment he found that the trance was perfectly genuine. He consequently began a series of experiments upon his relatives and friends, and found that he could soon produce a similar trance state quite easily by inducing them to fix their eyes upon a bright object, such as his lancet case. He also discovered that he obtained excellent results when he used the trance for medical and surgical purposes, and in 1842 he offered to read a paper on the subject for the British Association (for the Advancement of Science) which was meeting in Manchester. Needless to say his offer was rejected and his paper branded as ridiculous, together with his reports of cures of contractures and disorders of sensibility such as deafness through the use of mesmerism.

The importance of Braid's work lies in the fact that he was quick to realize that no mysterious magnetic fluids were involved in the production of the trance. He maintained that animal magnetism was a form of sleep brought on by the total concentration of the subject and so he called the condition hypnos, after the name of the Greek god. Braid expounded his theories in his book entitled 'Neurypnology or the Rationale of Nervous Sleep Considered in Relation with Animal Magnetism'[3]. Following this the more scientific sounding name neurypnology was substituted for animal magnetism or mesmerism. However, this too was soon to be replaced by the term hypnology from whence the name hypnotism was derived. Braid had concluded that the results were purely subjective in nature: *the phenomena were due to suggestion alone, acting upon a subject whose suggestibility had been artificially increased.*

If we examine the implications of this statement, we shall see quite clearly how Mesmer actually obtained his results. The impressive ritual, the ceremonial, Mesmer's own personality, his striking robe and above all his great reputation strongly suggested to his patients that something marvellous was going to happen, and of course it did. Bernard C. Gindes[4], summed up the situation admirably in 1953 when he suggested the following formula:

Misdirected Attention + Belief + Expectation = The Hypnotic State.

To this we can also add *Imagination,* which is the integrating factor which welds belief and expectation into an irresistible force. Indeed this same principle has to be accepted today, no matter whether recovery takes place through the agency of hypnosis, Christian Science or the miracles reported from Lourdes. This brings us face to face with a truth of the greatest importance namely that *no psychological cures have ever taken place in the absence of belief.*

Subsequent developments originated from the work of Dr Am-

broise August Liébeault, in France, who may well be considered
the real father of modern hypnotism. He was a modest country
practitioner in Nancy who became interested in the phenomena
of hypnotism and animal magnetism. Like Braid, he soon refuted
the theories of the latter and consequently became the founder of
the therapeutics of suggestion. He was certainly the first to demonstrate the curative value of hypnosis on a large scale, for he
treated thousands of patients in this way with outstanding success. He accomplished this by waiving his fees altogether if the
patient would accept hypnotic treatment in place of more orthodox procedures. In point of fact, so well known did his work
become that it attracted the attention of Professor Hippolyte-
Marie Bernheim, a famous neurologist, when he succeeded in curing a chronic case of sciatica which had been under Bernheim's
care. Bernheim was annoyed by the claims which were being
made and determined to visit Liébeault's clinic and to expose him
as a fraud. But he was so amazed at what he saw that he became
completely converted and fully accepted Liébeault's views upon
the significant part played by suggestion in hypnosis. He rapidly
became one of the greatest authorities on the subject, and such
was his reputation as a physician throughout Europe that, for the
very first time, the medical profession was unable to ignore his
opinions or to maintain its attitude of hostility. In 1886 he first
published his famous book, *De La Suggestion*[5], later published as
Suggestive Therapeutics. In it he gave many examples of the curative effects of hypnosis which he fully accepted as being entirely psychical in nature and resulting from the state of increased
suggestibility which was produced. The work of these two men,
following upon that of Braid, laid the foundation upon which the
development of modern hypnosis has been erected.

No account of the history of hypnosis, however brief, would be
complete without reference to the work of the great neurologist,
Professor Jean Martin Charcot, and his colleagues at the Salpêtrière Hospital in Paris. Despite his exceptional abilities as a clinician, Charcot seems to have had little understanding of the real
nature of hypnosis. He did his utmost to devise scientific tests for
it, as a result of which he concluded that hypnosis was a pathological phenomenon similar to hysteria, and consequently the pro-

duct of an abnormal nervous constitution. He found that he could both produce and reduce hysterical symptoms and postures through the use of hypnosis. But since Charcot used only a limited number of more or less trained subjects, his observations lacked validity and resulted in many errors. However, as a result of his findings there followed a bitter struggle between the rival schools of Charcot and Bernheim. Eventually the views of the Nancy School prevailed, the methods and conclusions of Charcot and his followers were exposed as unscientific, and hypnosis came to be considered as a normal manifestation. Nevertheless, it was through the use of hypnosis that Charcot made the all important discovery, that hysterical symptoms were not just confined to women as a result of some hypothetical displacement of the uterus as was hitherto believed, but were psychogenic in nature and could occur in either sex.

Many extravagant and unfounded claims were made for hypnosis during this period. The permanency of its results were never checked, largely due to the lack of follow-up studies on patients presumably cured. At this time nothing was known of the defensive value of symptoms and the way in which they often help the individual to adjust to his difficulties. Hypnosis was consequently used merely as a bludgeon to crush the patient's complaints, and it seems probable that failures were far more frequent than cures.

In the latter half of the last century however, there was a great upsurge of interest in psychology and in psychological theories of the hypnotic state. Pierre Janet considered the condition to be a dissociation or splitting of the unconscious from the conscious part of the mind. This could occur, he said, spontaneously in certain personalities but could also be brought about deliberately. Hysterical personalities were themselves 'split' in this way and this, he maintained, could be an explanation of the view held by Charcot. Moreover his patients could often recall events, whilst under hypnosis which they had been unable to remember whilst in the normal waking state. Perhaps, he felt, some forgotten emotional shock could even be revealed which could point to the origin of the neurosis.

Whilst Janet was engaged in his work, a Viennese general practitioner named Josef Breuer accidentally discovered that one of his patients began to speak spontaneously whilst under hypnosis. During sessions when this occurred she displayed a profound emotional reaction which was followed by the disappearance of many of her symptoms. At this point suggestive therapy was doomed. A momentous advance in the practice of hypnotherapy was henceforth to take place. When Freud's attention was drawn to this case, he joined Breuer in investigating it more fully and succeeded in confirming his results. The importance of this discovery lies in the subsequent change in emphasis in hypnotic therepy *from the direct removal of symptoms to the elimination of their apparent causes.* The patient whose name was to make hypnotherapeutic history was Bertha Pappenheim, the 21 year old daughter of a Viennese grain dealer. The latter had been ill for several months and was devotedly nursed by young Bertha. By the time he died in April 1881, Bertha herself had been ill for over six months and was attended by Dr Breuer. Her symptoms were bizarre to say the least, ranging from a persistent cough, a squint, various paralyses with visions of black snakes, and what Breuer called 'a psychosis of a peculiar kind'. Eventually, Breuer decided to use hypnosis. It was then that she regressed spontaneously and whilst in the hypnotic state, talked of her experiences and problems. It was the emotional response which often accompanied the ventilation of these problems which was considered the reason for the loss of symptoms. Appropriately enough, she called the treatment 'chimney sweeping' or 'the talking cure'.

Bertha Pappenheim was to become immortalized in the first case history written up by Breuer and Freud under the title 'Fraulein Anna O'[6]. Freud called the emotional response a catharsis or purging because he felt that the patient had purged herself of the problem which had been the cause of her symptoms and which had been repressed below the level of conscious awareness. Later however, he also discovered that his patients did not necessarily tell the truth, even under hypnosis. Perhaps they told what they believed to be the truth and that was what was important from the clinical point of view. It was also with his work with Breuer and Bertha Pappenheim, that Freud discovered the transference. The transference of the love, possibly the erotic love, which the patient felt for her father or in other cases for some important person from the past, to the person of the therapist. The possibility of counter-transference too had to be considered and of equal importance was the fact that the transference could involve positive or negative feelings in either case. All these effects had to be understood by the therapist and explained to the patient. Interpretation and insight directed psychotherapy became an integral part of hypnotherapy.

This first case and his further investigation of the fashionable illness of 'hysteria' led to Freud's discovery of the phenomenon of conversion. He maintained that early mental experiences that had produced emotional feelings which were too traumatic for the patient to tolerate could be re-interpreted in the form of physical symptoms. In this way, past memories and any unacceptable emotional response engendered, could be hidden from consciousness and satisfactorily converted and thus expressed in other symptoms without the accompanying painful emotion which might otherwise have been experienced. Thus the patient would derive some gain additionally which could be utilized for his or her own protection.

Freud experimented extensively with hypnosis but was rarely able to repeat the dramatic results that Bertha Pappenheim had obligingly produced. He considered that the unconscious was too stubbornly defended, readily to permit any intrusion. Even with the use of hypnosis he failed to penetrate this resistance and so was led to explore other techniques. He developed his ideas of free association and of dream interpretation and the foundations of the new school of psychoanalysis were firmly set. As a result, Freud abandoned hypnosis and this fact together with the disappointment aroused by the failure of hypnosis to produce a permanent cure of hysteria, nearly succeeded in dealing it a death-blow. However the grave shortage of psychiatrists during the First World War demanded a much abbreviated form of psychotherapy. Hypnotherapy was once again revived and used both for direct symptom removal and for the restoration of repressed traumatic experiences. War neuroses, in fact, provide the most dramatic examples of how valuable hypnosis can be in effecting the relief of unacceptable symptoms, through a 'reliving', whilst in the hyp-

notic state, of the events of the traumatic experience which originally produced them.

One of the pioneers of this form of treatment, which he called
'hypnoanalysis' was English psychiatrist J.A. Hadfield. But it
should be remembered that its origin lay in the work of Breuer
and Freud. The successes which were achieved were soon forgotten however and once more the use of hypnosis fell into a decline.
Once again it was abandoned to misuse by charlatans, entertainers and lay therapists, claiming the cure of an extensive variety
of ailments by direct symptom removal. In spite of this, a hard
core of medical and dental practitioners continued to use hypnosis
and psychologists, mainly in the United States of America, re-em-
barked tentatively upon research into the hypnotic condition.
Freud's claim that our neuroses lie buried in the hitherto hidden
areas of the unconscious was not easily to be relinquished. Nevertheless, although this spark of learning still remained alive, the
use of hypnosis for the treatment of the sick failed to reach its full
potential.

It was not until 50 years after Freud abandoned hypnosis that
another psychotherapeutic technique was to expand into the con-
troversial field of hypnotic treatment. As a result of the experiments of Ivan Pavlov on the conditioning of dogs, the ideas of
learning theory were eventually born. Pavlov considered that
hypnosis was a conditioned response to suggestions given by the
therapist. The words of the therapist would dampen down the cortical or higher centres of the brain allowing the more primitive
centres to take over. Since this latter area is more sensitive to
suggestion a particular response could more easily be obtained.
The renowned American psychologist J. B. Watson[7] was to exploit
the ideas of the conditioned response. He was founder of the school
of behaviourism which is based on what is known as learning theory.

Learning theory implies that we learn to behave in a certain
way. We begin to learn of course from the moment we are born.
As we know, unfortunately the behaviour that we learn may
sometimes be inappropriate and unacceptable to the subject. That
behaviour can be unlearned and a new and more acceptable response can be relearned, and this is the basis of behaviour ther-

apy.

In 1958 and again in America, Joseph Wolpe[8] finally incorporated the ideas of Pavlov concerning hypnosis, with the work of Watson and the behaviourists into the effective treatment known as desensitization. In simple terms this means that a person can be 'de-conditioned' and then 're-conditioned' to respond with calmness to situations formerly interpreted as stressful. Additionally, whilst in hypnosis, the subject is able to visualize (with varying degrees of reality) scenes or situations which may be suggested to him and to remain calm and relaxed in that situation. The advantages of this method are obvious. The subject will unlearn the unacceptable response (almost invariably related to anxiety) and relearn a more acceptable response of calmness and composure in that situation. Treatment by desensitization under hypnosis is extensively described by Wolpe in his book *Psychotherapy by Reciprocal Inhibition* and this is now an established and additional form of treatment.

Nevertheless there was still no organized teaching of hypnosis. Various theories of the nature of the hypnotic state emanated from the USA but there was as yet no meaningful research in the UK.

In 1953 the Psychological Medicine Group Committee of the British Medical Association appointed a subcommittee to consider the use of hypnosis and its report was published in 1955[9]. It recommended that a description of hypnosis and of its psychotherapeutic possibilities, limitations and dangers be given to medical undergraduates and instruction in its clinical use be given to all postgraduate psychiatric trainees and possibly also to trainee anaesthetists and obstetricians. However, this advice was largely ignored. A study by Scott in 1978[10] found that of 32 medical schools and 18 dental schools in Britain only two of each provided some very limited undergraduate training and three medical schools but no dental schools provided some official, equally limited postgraduate lectures. There has been no change in the situation to this day and instruction to students of psychiatry varies according to the whim of the teachers.

In the field of psychological training, Fellows[11] recently distributed a questionnaire to 58 university and polytechnic departments in Great Britain. He established that relatively few departments are engaged in any sort of teaching or research in hypnosis although there does exist a fairly positive attitude to both. There was anxiety about the nature of hypnosis and what it can do.

In the UK at least, the teaching of hypnosis has been largely by private enterprise. In 1952 a group of members of the British Dental Association formed the British Society of Dental Hypnosis under the chairmanship of Mr Eric Wookey. This became the Dental and Medical Society for the Study of Hypnosis in 1955. Then amalgamating in 1961 with a smaller group led by Dr Gordon Ambrose, the Society for Medical and Dental Hypnosis was born. In 1968 this was reconstituted to become the British Society of Medical and Dental Hypnosis under the presidency of the original author of this book. Ten years later, in 1978, psychologists working alongside the medical and dental professions established the British Society of Experimental and Clinical Hypnosis under the Presidency of Professor Gwynne Jones, former President of the British Psychological Society. Perhaps the most significant advance however was the formation of the Section of Medical and Dental Hypnosis of the Royal Society of Medicine. This organization hitherto had comprised 33 sections, made up of almost every other medical and surgical discipline in the country, working together under the umbrella of the one parent body. It is of interest to note that the first president of the Royal Society after its incorporation as the Royal Medical and Chirurgical Society of London in 1834 was none other than physician and mesmerist John Elliotson. Medical hypnosis had gone full circle. The objects of the latest section are as follows:

'To extend knowledge of the hypnotic state, to investigate
further its neurophysiology and to promote interest in its
clinical use.'

In addition to the advances in Great Britain the use of medical hypnosis has spread world wide. There is an International Society of Hypnosis and a European Society of Hypnosis comprising an affiliation of 27 national societies, proof enough of the advancement of hypnosis since the days of animal magnetism. Advancement in knowledge of the hypnotic state, advancement in laboratory experimentation and in the exploration of the neurophysiology of hypnosis and advancement in hypnotherapeutic techniques of treatment. In the last decade, hypnosis has taken a giant step forward in its development—and the momentum continues.

REFERENCES

1. Stam H.J. and Spanos N.P., 1982. The Asclepian dream healings and hypnosis: a critique. *Int. J. Clin. Exp. Hypnosis,* **XXX,** 9–22
2. Janet P., 1925. *Psychological Healing*, Vols. 1 and 11. George Allen and Unwin, London.
3. Braid J., 1899. *Neurypnology or the Rationale of Nervous Sleep Considered in Relation with Animal Magnetism.* Redway, London.
4. Gindes B.C., 1953. *New Concepts of Hypnosis.* George Allen and Unwin, London.
5. Bernheim, H., 1900. *Suggestive Therapeutics. A Treatise on the Nature and Uses of Hypnotism.* Translated by C.A. Herter, Putnam, New York.
6. Breuer J. and Freud S., 1955. Studies on hysteria. In: *Complete Works of Sigmund Freud* (ed. Strachey), Vol. 11, pp. 1893–1895. Hogarth Press, London.
7. Watson J.B., 1913. Psychology as the behaviourist views it. *Psychol. Rev.,* **20,** 158–177.
8. Wolpe J., 1958. *Psychotherapy by Reciprocal Inhibition.* Stanford University Press, Stanford, California.
9. British Medical Association, 1955. Psychological Medicine Group Sub-Committee *Br. Med. J. (Suppl.),* **1,** 190–193.
10. Scott D.L., 1978. University training in medical and dental hypnosis. *Proceedings of the British Society of Medical and Dental Hypnosis*, Vol. 4, No. 1, p. 13.
11. Fellows B.J., 1985. Hypnosis teaching and research in British psychology departments: current practice, attitudes and concerns. *Br. J. Exp. Clin. Hypnosis*, **2,** 151–155.

CHAPTER 2

The Nature and Theories of Hypnosis

Before studying the various techniques used for the induction of the hypnotic state it is useful to have some knowledge of the numerous theories of the nature of hypnosis which have been advanced through the years.

Serious attempts to explain the psychological changes which occur have been continuing since the rejection of the theory of magnetism. Perhaps the first unwitting contribution to this area was the finding of the Royal Commission of Louis XVI which pronounced Mesmer's cures to be the result of the imagination and imitation. Thus although the psychosomatic origin of his patients' illnesses were recognized they were not seen to be recognized! So mesmerism was laid to rest and the way was open for a harvest of other ideas in the two centuries that have passed.

These may be summarized as follows:

1. The 'suggestion' theory
2. The 'modified sleep' theory
3. Charcot's 'pathological' theory
4. The 'dissociation' theory
5. 'Psychoanalytic' theories
6. The 'conditioned response' theory
7. Theories of 'role playing'
8. The theory of 'atavistic regression'
9. The 'neurophysiological' theory
10. The theory of 'hemispheric specificity'

It may be seen therefore that numerous speculations have been advanced to explain the psychological condition of hypnosis. More scientific theories must include ideas of changes produced in the neurophysiology of the hypnotized person.

We now know that hypnosis is not sleep nor the normal state of wakefulness but a condition somewhere in between the two. It may therefore be described as an altered state of awareness, resulting in psychological, physical and neurophysiological changes in which may be produced distortion of emotion, sensation, image and time (Waxman[1]).

1. The Suggestion Theory

Hypnosis is essentially a state of mind which may be induced by one person in another. It is a state of mind in which suggestions may be given that are more readily accepted than in the waking state and will be acted upon if not beyond the capability of the hypnotized person. It is this effect which highlights one of the principal phenomena occurring in hypnosis, that of enhanced suggestibility. This idea was amongst its earliest theories and was extensively described by Bernheim in 1886[2].

The first step is to try to make clear what we mean by suggestion and suggestibility. Definitions are always awkward and seldom complete, but as they are necessary to a proper understanding of the subject a simple but viable explanation of these terms is provided.

Suggestion is the process whereby an individual accepts a proposition put to him by another, without necessarily having a logical reason for doing so. In a different sense, the term is also used to describe an idea which is presented to the individual for his uncritical acceptance.

Suggestibility is the degree to which an individual is inclined towards the uncritical acceptance of ideas and propositions. In other words, it is a measure of the extent to which an individual will react to what is said to him, without employing his critical faculties.

Perhaps few of us realize that we spend every day of our lives constantly exposed to suggestion of various kinds. Leading articles in the daily newspapers suggest what we should think about politics; attractively dressed shop windows suggest what we should buy; advertisements in magazines, on poster hoardings or on television screens suggest to us what food we should eat or what particular toothpaste we should use. No matter where we go we cannot escape entirely from this barrage of suggestion which tends to influence our daily thoughts and actions, for the most part quite unconsciously.

One of the finest examples of insidious suggestion working in this way is to be found in Shakespeare when the subtle and deadly insinuations of Iago work on the mind of Othello. And here, we discover a very significant and important truth: *the power of suggestion is tremendously enhanced when it acts upon the unconscious rather than on the conscious mind.*

The reason for this we shall presently discover. In view of these facts, it would seem that we are now justified in concluding that Mesmer's cures depended not upon iron rods or magnetic fluids, but upon the implicit belief in recovery that was instilled in the patient's mind because his suggestibility had been greatly increased by the mysterious ritual and ceremonial.

All available evidence points to the conclusion that 'suggestibility' and 'hypnotic state' are closely connected and that the more suggestible the subject the more readily can hypnosis be induced and deepened. Weitzenhoffer[3], interpreting Bernheim, clearly showed that he spoke more in terms of 'suggestion' than of suggestibility, that suggestion is the basis for all hypnotic phenomena and suggestibility is the measure of the depth or degree of hypnosis. Moreover, Bernheim believed that expectation and autosuggestion were potent factors in the achievement of hypnosis. If all hypnosis is suggestion as Bernheim was saying, this does not account for many of the phenomena of the trance state that may be produced in minor form in the waking state. That hypnosis is state of enhanced suggestibility is a different matter. In that state, suggestion may be employed deliberately and certainly in the good subject, i.e. the more suggestible subject, with greater effect than in the waking state.

Chemnitz and Feingold[4] described suggestion as 'a stimulus which induces suggestible behaviour and experience. Suggestible behaviour and experience are described as emotional, uncontrolled, uncritical and often unconscious behaviour, whilst suggestibility is understood as the tendency to react to suggestions and therefore means a personality trait.' Such a definition should satisfy the many critics of Professor Bernheim.

Pavlov considered that in hypnosis, the suggestions given by the therapist would result in changes in the cortical or higher centres of the brain in which the power of criticism is dampened down whilst the more primitive centres become dominant. We believe that it is these earlier centres which are more susceptible to suggestion.

That the tendency to react to suggestions is the 'entire modus operandi' of traditional hypnotism is the opinion of many modern researchers such as Gill and Brennan[5], Erickson *et al.*[6] and Weitzenhoffer[3].

The question now arises as to why suggestions should be accepted and acted upon more readily in the hypnotic than in the waking state. Quite briefly, the answer is to be found in the following simple fact, as Pavlov considered, namely that in the hypnotic state, the power of criticism is either fully or partially suspended

To understand how this occurs we must first accept the concept of the *unconscious mind*. This postulates that in everyone there is a portion of the mind that is constantly influencing our thoughts and behaviour, the processes of which we are normally unaware. The conscious mind is the part of the mind which thinks, feels and acts in the present. The unconscious mind is a much greater part of the mind, and normally we are quite unaware of its existence. It is the seat of our memories, our past experiences, and indeed of that which we have learned. In this respect it resembles a large filing cabinet to which we can refer in order to refresh our memory whenever we need to do so. Under certain circumstances it can also undertake most of the functions of the conscious mind, with one important exception—the power of criticism.

Let us take a simple example. Suppose that you are given a fountain-pen to hold in your hand, and as you are holding it the suggestion is made that it is gradually becoming hotter and hotter and will soon burn your fingers.

Nothing will happen.

In a fraction of a second several thoughts will have flashed through your mind, enabling it to exercise the function of conscious criticism. You will have said to yourself 'Rubbish. No fountain-pen has ever become hot before. Why should this one? Besides, it can't possibly become hot. There's nothing to make it hot.' Notice how you have drawn upon the past experience and knowledge in your unconscious mind in order to criticize the proposition made, as a result of which you have been able to reject it completely.

Let us suppose now that the same suggestions are made to a deeply hypnotized subject, who is holding the pen. In the deep hypnotic state, the conscious mind and its power of criticism will have been bypassed. It will be powerless to draw upon the information that is stored in the unconscious mind. The suggestions will consequently enter the individual's unconscious mind which, possessing no power of criticism itself, will be unable to reject them. So the individual will promptly accept the suggestions without reservation. He will believe implicitly that what you tell him is going to happen will be bound to occur. He will thus begin to feel a sensation of heat, his fingers will relax their grip, and the pen will fall to the floor.

The important conclusions to be drawn from these two experiments can be summarized in the following way.

1. The power of criticism is restricted largely to the conscious mind.

2. It is by virtue of this alone that the conscious mind possesses the ability to reject any suggestions that may be made.

3. When suggestions bypass the conscious mind, as they do under hypnosis, they penetrate directly to the unconscious mind which, being able to exercise little or no power of criticism, is quite unable to reject them, and the individual is bound to act upon them.

Suggestions are therefore not only more readily accepted, but are also realized to the fullest possible extent during the hypnotic state since direct access is gained to the unconscious part of the mind. We are now able to define certain further principles applicable to the hypnotic state.

1. The response to hypnosis will depend upon the extent to which the power of criticism is suppressed and the power of rejection normally exercised by the conscious mind is removed.

2. The depth of hypnosis in any given case will be directly related to the degree of suppression attained. Slight suppression will result in light hypnosis only: complete suppression will result in deep hypnosis or somnambulism.

3. The more the conscious mind is suppressed, the more the suggestibility of the individual will increase.

Consideration of another simple analogy may help to show more clearly what we try to achieve when we induce the hypnotic state.

If we look at an iceberg we know that we can see only one-eighth of its total bulk above the surface of the waves; seven-eighths are hidden from sight. What we try to do when we start to induce hypnosis is to cause the iceberg to topple over, so that the hidden seven-eighths rise above the surface and the visible one-eighth disappears. In other words, the unconscious mind rises to the surface, becomes more accessible, and eventually assumes temporary control. Moreover, the degree of displacement achieved will correspond roughly with the various stages of hypnosis. If the iceberg only topples over slightly the result will be light hypnosis, and the power of criticism will be somewhat impaired but not to any great extent. If it topples three-quarters of the way, the result wil be medium to deep hypnosis; the power of criticism will be much more gravely impaired, and the suggestibility of the subject greatly increased. Even so, it will not be totally abolished. But when the iceberg becomes completely reversed, the result will be very deep hypnosis or somnambulism. In this case, the conscious mind will be entirely submerged and will be completely inactive. The unconscious mind will have temporarily assumed control and the power of criticism will be removed altogether.

In trying to induce hypnosis, the main problem is to get the conscious mind out of the way so as to make use of the increased degree of suggestibility that will inevitably follow. Fortunately this is not as formidable a task as it might seem, since the secret lies in a very simple but universal fact.

Even in everyday life, whenever concentration of attention occurs, it induces a tendency towards a splitting of consciousness which renders the unconscious mind much more accessible.

2. The Modified Sleep Theory

Although the responses of the subject during the average induction process closely resemble those of the early stages of normal sleep, it is soon evident that hypnosis is not sleep. The Abbé Faria invited his patients to close their eyes and to concentrate on sleep. He replaced Mesmer's animal magnetism with the idea of intense concentration. His work 'On the Cause of Lucid Sleep' published in 1819, was the basis of Braid's theory, that it was the fixed attention of the subject which would result in the state of 'nervous sleep'[7]. In this state a person could be most readily influenced and it would invariably be followed by spontaneous amnesia for all events that transpired during that state. Other ideas were soon to follow but nevertheless Braid's contribution to research assured him of a place in history.

Some 50 years later, Freud still regarded him as the first real scientific student of hypnotism. Even the great Pavlov himself thought of hypnosis as a conditioned response into a form of sleep and the injunction 'go to sleep' remains in use by many therapists to this day.

3. Charcot's Pathological Theory

The eminent neurologist, Jean Martin Charcot[8] formed the opinion that hypnosis was a pathological condition similar to hysteria and considered it to be the product of an abnormal nervous constitution. There seems to be little truth in this since at least 90 per cent of ordinary people can be hypnotized and obviously it is absurd to suppose that most of the population is markedly hysterical. Since Freud's subsequent definition of hysteria as a conversion, that is as a symbolic representation of some psychic conflict in terms of motor or sensory manifestations, Charcot's theory can no longer be valid. More recently, Hans Eysenck devised a method of assessing hysterical personality traits and tested a random group of persons for both hysteria and hypnotizability. He failed to obtain any correlation between the two although he succeeded in establishing a close connection between hypnotizability and suggestibility. Nevertheless, perhaps Charcot was too readily maligned. He had shown that hysteria was not a symptom specifically peculiar to the female sex but that it could also occur in the male. In so doing he had paved the way for further research into hypnosis and the discoveries of Sigmund Freud.

4. The Dissociation Theory

This theory was originally formulated by Pierre Janet[9], who worked at the Salpêtrière Clinic and believed, as did Charcot, in the close association between hysteria and hypnosis. He eventually concluded that hysteria was caused by a splitting of the mind into two parts and that hypnosis represented the same splitting process, artificially induced.

This concept of splitting of consciousness has proved to be a very valuable one, and has entered into medicine under the technical term *dissociation*. For many years, this theory of dissociation was considered to be the key to hypnosis, the depth of which was held to be directly related to the degree of dissociation achieved. In many ways it is an attractive theory and as in the case of the conditioned response, there is probably a great deal of truth in it. But whilst it explains some of the phenomena of hypnosis, it fails to account for many others. Undoubtedly the tendency to dissociate can be greatly increased by suggestion, but this does not necessarily prove that hypnosis and dissociation are one and the same thing.

One of the main difficulties in accepting the dissociation theory of hypnosis lies in its dependence on the occurrence of amnesia. The recall of memories depends upon the association of ideas, and the failure to remember events is caused by a break in the chain of ideas which would restore them to consciousness. Whenever this happens, dissociation has occurred and the result is a state of amnesia (loss of recall). Amnesia consequently becomes a necessary element in the theory.

Since the unconscious mind is capable of assuming most of the functions of the conscious mind, Janet concluded that such phenomena as 'fugues' and even 'multiple personalities' were due to a splitting of consciousness which resulted in the unconscious mind becoming the dominant part for the time being. It is thus often maintained that hypnosis results from a similar splitting of consciousness during which the unconscious part of the mind becomes the dominant one. It should be remembered, however, that in a fugue state the individual has no recollection whatever of his ordinary life and when restored to normality he has a complete amnesia for the events of the fugue. Obviously the dissociation theory depends largely upon the development of amnesia following the trance and it is interesting that half a century earlier, James Braid had insisted on the need for amnesia as an essential part of the post-hypnotic state. The idea however is greatly weakened by the fact that deep trances can occur without any appreciable degree of amnesia. Even when present this amnesia is rarely spontaneous and is more often produced by direct suggestion. Moreover, post-hypnotic amnesia can be removed quite easily and the memory restored by suggestion. Ernest Hilgard[10] indicated that this fact and other post-hypnotic phenomena which could be produced and then removed by direct suggestion might indeed be accounted for by Janet's theory of hypnosis as a dissociation.

He offered a more up-to-date version which he has called 'neodissociation' and in which he states that 'some cognitive systems, even though not represented in consciousness at the time, continue to register and process incoming information and when such a system is released from inhibition it uses this information as though it had been conscious all along.'

Thus post-hypnotic amnesia will occur if it is suggested. But the memories will be rendered only temporarily unavailable although they will still be present. Or a positive challenge may be given of some motor response, e.g. that the subject will bend an arm which has previously been rendered rigid by suggestion. In this way, one control mechanism will retain the stiffness whilst another will attempt to break it.

5. Psychoanalytic Theories

Freud regarded the susceptibility of the hypnotic subject as being due to an unconscious desire for libidinal gratification on his part, and pointed out the similarity of hypnosis to the state of being in love. According to this theory there is an erotic relationship between the hypnotist and his subject which is not usually allowed to progress very far. This seems to be accompanied by the desire for unconditional subjection. Ferenczi agreed with this view and expanded it further by postulating a 'parent–child' relationship which develops between the hypnotist and his subject.

Both these attitudes, however, tend to exist to some extent between any doctor and patient in ordinary medical practice. The doctor who likes his patient will often be able to get him well more easily than a doctor who dislikes him. And the patient who likes his doctor will put so much trust and confidence in him that he will do much better than when he is treated by a doctor for whom he does not care. Moreover, patients are frequently over-awed by their doctor in exactly the same way as a child by his parent, so that these relationships are certainly not confined to hypnosis.

The pyschoanalytic theories however, fail to explain instances of hypnotization by mirrors, rotating discs or metronomes, or the fact that hypnotic states can sometimes be produced by inanimate objects. Since under such conditions no inter-personal relationships are involved, it is difficult to see how any libidinal gratification can ensue.

6. The Conditioned Response Theory

This theory is based upon the work of Pavlov and the East European scientists who have adapted and developed reflex psychology. It will be remembered that Pavlov rang a bell before each occasion on which a dog was given food, and after a number of occasions upon each of which feeding was preceded by the ringing of the bell, saliva would flow whenever the bell was rung even though no food was offered. This process was called *conditioning*. Pavlov also found that de-conditioning could be effected if a small unpleasant electric shock was administered when the bell was rung. It should be noted, however, that both conditioning and de-conditioning require the process to be repeated on many consecutive occasions.

Explained in these terms, hypnosis is considered to be a physiological state produced by a life-time of conditioning, in the course of which certain words tend to act like Pavlov's bell in causing effects due to long association. For instance, when the word *sleep* is mentioned to a subject, he immediately associates this with feelings of tiredness, heaviness and drowsiness. He will thus come to associate the word *sleep* with such words as *heavy, tired, drowsy* and *relaxed,* and the constant repetition of these words during induction produces a state which the subject has become conditioned to associate with such words.

There can be no doubt whatever that conditioning does play an important part in the induction of hypnosis, and it has been shown that people who are capable of establishing conditioned responses easily are usually good hypnotic subjects. But it is far from being the whole story. In the first place, the theory assumes that the states of hypnosis and normal sleep are similar, and as we know, this is certainly not the case. Secondly, an even more convincing argument against hypnosis being solely a conditioned process lies in the fact that de-conditioning has always involved a slow, repetitive procedure, the length of time required depending largely upon the time taken to achieve the original conditioning. In the hypnotic state, however, de-conditioning can be effected immediately upon word of command. Thirdly, to regard hypnosis as being a conditioned response takes no account of the fact that people have often been hypnotized by rotating discs, mirrors or metronomes, none of which could have been associated by previous conditioning with the idea of the hypnotic trance.

7. Theories of Role-playing

R. W. White formed the conclusion that hypnosis should be regarded as meaningful, goal-directed striving, its most general goal being to behave like a hypnotized person as this is continually defined by the operator, understood by the subject and which takes place in an altered psychological state[11]. We suggest, and make it quite clear, to the subject what we expect him to do, and because of the existing rapport he seems to strive to fulfil the role we have outlined. His dominant motive seems to be submission to the operator's demands.

This theory, however, disregards the occurrence of phenomena that are outside voluntary control. Estabrooks[12], reported on the testing of hypnotic anaesthesia by electric shocks and found that hypnotized subjects could experience without discomfort, currents nearly ten times as strong as those that could be tolerated in the waking state. This directly refutes the 'role-playing' theory for no one trying to behave as a hypnotized person could voluntarily produce such a degree of anaesthesia.

Sarbin[13] however, took White's views a stage further. The goal-directed striving in the altered psychological state is a type of behaviour in which the person is entirely orientated into that role.

Shor[14] also showed the need for motivation to be involved in the roles of hypnosis together with the striving to behave like a hypnotized person. He explained the altered psychological state of hypnosis as the generalized reality orientation fading into a state of relatively 'non-functional awareness' or trance state.

'Hypnosis', he said 'as conventionally understood, is viewed as the production of a special task-orientation with the concomitant breakdown or voluntary relinquishing of the usual reality orientation so that the former functions in relative isolation from the totality of general working experiences'.

T.X. Barber[15] maintained that hypnotic performance depends upon the attitudes, motivations and expectations of the subject in carrying out the role of the hypnotized person, that is thinking and imagining with the suggestions. Any of the responses obtained in hypnosis can be achieved without the 'trance' state but as the result of the correct training in human potentialities.

Nicholas Spanos had earlier emphasized the need for the subject to engage in 'goal-directed fantasy' (Spanos and Barber[16]). This attitude would of course assist in the experience of the responses suggested.

8. Theory of 'Atavistic Regression'

This involves the concept that suggestion is an archaic mental function that can be used to explain the nature of hypnosis. The idea was conceived by Ainslie Meares[17] and is not unrelated to the Pavlovian theory of dominance of the primitive brain centres achieved by the gradual 'switching off' of the higher centres. In clinical psychiatry, the term 'regression' is usually applied to the return to a former type of behaviour. When Ferenczi considered hypnosis to be a parent–child relationship developing between the hypnotist and his subject, he was postulating regression as a return to childhood or infantile patterns of behaviour. The atavistic theory requires that regression be applied, not in the field of behaviour, but in the field of mental function. In other words, a regression from normal adult mental function at an intellectual, logical level, to an archaic level of mental function in which the process of suggestion determines the acceptance of ideas. This type of regression is considered to be the basic mechanism in the production of hypnosis.

As Meares himself pointed out, this hypothesis does not in any way suggest that primitive man lived in a state of hypnosis. It assumes that primitive man, before he developed the ability of logically evaluating ideas, accepted them by the more primitive process of suggestion. In fact, the essence of the atavistic theory is that hypnosis is a return to a more primitive form of mental functioning in which suggestion plays a major role. This is a concept which can be of practical value to the clinician, for anything, word or act, which tends to aid this regression will assist the induction of hypnosis. In clinical practice, greater depth of hypnosis is the result of more profound atavistic regression; in lighter hypnosis the regression is less complete.

It would appear then that no single theory of hypnosis is complete enough to explain all the phenomena of the trance. White maintained that no scientific hypothesis can be formulated until it can adequately explain the following facts:

1. That a hypnotized person transcends the normal limits of voluntary control.

2. That he behaves without the experience of will or intention or self-consciousness, and without subsequent memory.

3. That these changes occur because the hypnotist says they will.

None of the theories so far advanced is capable of fulfilling these requirements. It would seem that our present knowledge of human behaviour is not yet sufficiently developed to produce a complete and satisfactory theory of hypnosis. In trying to define it accurately we are only describing an end result which is often due to a combination of several of the factors already mentioned. In most trance states, suggestion, dissociation and conditioning all play a part to some extent. It can be said that an understanding of these mechanisms does much to render trance behaviour intelligible despite the gaps which still remain to be filled before our knowledge is complete.

9. The Neurophysiological Theory

Although psychological theories of the nature of the hypnotic condition abound, there is very little hard evidence of the existence of hypnosis as a specific neurological state.

The idea generally accepted by clinical physicians in the UK is that proposed by Barry Wyke of the Royal College of Surgeons of England[18,19].

Characteristic patterns of brainwave activity in various states and pathological conditions have been well established for many years. The recordings in hypnosis had previously been investigated and had been considered unremarkable, but Wyke claimed that specific changes do in fact take place.

Hernández-Peón[20] had noted the important role played by the reticular system in the central part of the brain stem and which is involved in the state of alertness and attention. This system receives afferent connections from tracts in the spinal cord and from the cranial nerves as it ascends until it eventually reaches the limbic system. Wyke described how the voice of the therapist will travel along this particular channel and by strict concentration of attention, other sources of sensory input are blocked. The continuing and monotonous flow of calming and relaxing suggestions, diminish the patient's awareness of his environment as the activation of the reticular system is gradually reduced and there results the state known as hypnosis. Should the monotonous and calming suggestions continue, habituation will result and upon the instruction 'go to sleep' the patient will cross the brink and actually fall asleep.

Care must be taken therefore during hypnotherapy to maintain the state of hypnosis but to ensure that the patient does not drift off into sleep. Habituation may be experienced by many people, who, used to the ticking of a clock in the bedroom, maintain that they are unable to fall asleep unless they hear the sound of the clock.

In his earlier experiments, Wyke was also able to trace electroencephalographic differences between the waking state, sleep and hypnosis. He found alterations in general cerebral activity so that although in the early stages of hypnosis there appeared to be no difference in the alpha rhythm from that of the subject relaxing with his eyes closed midst quiet and peaceful surroundings, as the hypnosis was deepened, although there was little change in frequency, a marked diminution of voltage occurred. If specific suggestions of sleep were then given, the frequency diminished, the voltage increased and the EEG recordings were as those of normal sleep.

Ulett *et al.*[21], in an extensive electronic analysis of EEG measurements made on volunteers and in later experiments using certain psychotropic drugs, concluded that hypnosis is a unique behavioural state with a demonstrable neurophysiological basis.

Rozhnov[22], reported a flare up of infraslow oscillations of the potentials of the brain during the suggestion of the hallucination of the aroma of a rose whilst in hypnosis. This fact, together with other specific variations not previously discovered, led to the conclusion that hypnosis is a special psychophysiological state, differing from both sleep and wakefulness.

It is reassuring to note the remarks of Perry *et al.*[23], that although there is disagreement among the leading investigators of hypnosis as to its essential nature, there is also much consensus.

In conclusion, it can be said that many workers still maintain that no difference exists between hypnosis and the state of being awake but relaxed. Nevertheless there does appear to be emerging some electroencephalographic evidence that there is a particular neurophysiological state which we call hypnosis.

10. The Theory of Hemispheric Specificity

A further interesting theory, lately to engage the thoughts of experimental psychologists is that of hemispheric lateralization and specificity. J.G. Beaumont, in his 'Introduction to Neuropsychology'[24] describes in detail the known relationship of the brain to human behaviour. He emphasizes nevertheless that although advances in research have uncovered much in recent years, the brain 'still holds many secrets'. Hemispheric specificity is one of those secrets now in the process of revelation.

The idea of lateralization has over the past two decades stimulated notions regarding states of consciousness, cultural development and learning, together with the evolution of the specialization of each cerebral hemisphere and the balance of activities of the two sides.

Split brain studies have shown that each side has certain functions which are basically specific to that side.

It is now generally accepted that the left hemisphere in right handed people is characterized as verbal, voluntary and rational. Language, speech analysis and problem solving are mediated on this side. The right side can be classified as non-verbal, submissive and emotional (Sperry[25]; Gazzaniga and Le Doux[26]; Moscovitch[27]). Skills such as art and music are right hemispheric activities. Imagination is also a right hemisphere activity and a high level of imagination is an essential requisite of hypnotic responsiveness.

Macleod-Morgan[28], in an interesting paper given at the 8th International Congress of Hypnosis and Psychosomatic Medicine in Melbourne reported that highly hypnotizable subjects show more specific lateralization than do low hypnotizables, during right and left hemisphere tasks.

Mészáros et al.[29], in their on-going research in Budapest were able to produce positive data to support the current hypothesis that hypnosis accentuates a preference for right hemisphere use and Bányai et al.[30] were able to show that the dominance of right hemisphere EEG activity can facilitate the marked changes of conscious awareness characterizing deep hypnosis, whilst a left hemispheric dominance is more favourable in keeping the control.

It may therefore be that the induction of hypnosis is a left hemisphere activity which then switches to the right hemisphere during the imagining and deepening suggestions.

All in all some fascinating research is being carried out on a fascinating theory, yet the question as to what actually happens in hypnosis remains an enigma.

REFERENCES

1. Waxman D., 1981. *Hypnosis: A Guide for Patients and Practitioners.* George Allen and Unwin, London.
2. Bernheim H., 1900. *Suggestive Therapeutics. A Treatise on the Nature and Use of Hypnotism.* Translated by C.A. Herter, Putnam, New York.
3. Weitzenhoffer A.M., 1978. What did he (Bernheim) say? In *Hypnosis at its Bicentennial* (eds Frankel and Zamansky). Plenum, New York.
4. Chemnitz G. and Feingold E., 1980. Various conditions of suggestion and suggestibility and their significance for medical and psychotherapeutic treatment. In *Hypnosis in Psychotherapy and Psychosomatic Medicine* (eds Pajntar, Rŏskar and Lavrič). University Press, Ljubljana.
5. Gill M.M. and Brennan M., 1959. *Hypnosis and Related States.* International University Press, New York.
6. Erickson M.H., Rossi E.L. and Rossi S.I., 1976. Hypnotic realities. In *The Induction of Clinical Hypnosis and Forms of Indirect Suggestion.* Irvington, New York.
7. Braid J., 1899. *Neurypnology or the Rationale of Nervous Sleep in Relation with Animal Magnetism.* Redway, London.
8. Charcot J.M., 1890. *Oevres Completes, IX, Metallotherapie et Hypnotisme.* Bourneville et Brissand, Paris.
9. Janet P., 1925. *Psychological Healing.* George Allen and Unwin, London.
10. Hilgard E.R., 1978. States of consciousness in hypnosis: divisions or levels? In *Hypnosis at its Bicentennial* (eds Frankel and Zamansky). Plenum, New York.
11. White R.W., 1941. A preface to the theory of hypnotism. *J. Abnorm. Soc. Psychol.*, **36,** 477–505.
12. Estabrooks G.H., 1957. *Hypnotism.* Dutton, New York.
13. Sarbin T., 1950. Contributions to role-taking theory: 1. Hypnotic behaviour. *Psychol. Rev.*, **57,** 255–270.
14. Shor R.E., 1969. Hypnosis and the concept of the generalized reality-orientation. In *Altered States of Consciousness* (ed Tart). Anchor Doubleday, New York.
15. Barber T.X., 1975. Responding to 'hypnotic' suggestions: an introspective report. *Am. J. Clin. Hypnosis*, **18,** 6–22.
16. Spanos N.P. and Barber T.X., 1974. Towards a convergence in hypnosis research. *Am. Psychol.*, **29,** 500–511.

17. Meares A., 1960. *A System of Medical Hypnosis*. Saunders, Philadelphia.
18. Wyke B.D., 1957. Neurological aspects of hypnosis. *Proceedings of the Dental and Medical Society for the Study of Hypnosis*. Royal College of Surgeons, London.
19. Wyke B.D., 1960. Neurological mechanisms in hypnosis. *Proceedings of the Dental and Medical Society for the Study of Hypnosis*. Royal Society of Medicine, London.
20. Hernández-Peón R., 1959. Sensory perception and centrifugal control of sensory input to the brain. *Electroenceph. Clin. Neurophysiol.*, **11,**373–374.
21. Ulett G.A., Akpinar S. and Itil T.M., 1972. Hypnosis: physiological, pharmacological reality. *Am. J. Psychiat.*, 128, 799–805.
22. Rozhov V.E., 1978. Towards understanding the nature of hypnosis. In *Hypnosis at its Bicentennial* (eds Frankel and Zamansky). Plenum, New York.
23. Perry C., Laurence J.R., Nadon R. *et al.*, 1986. Past lives regression. In *Hypnosis Questions and Answers* (eds Zilbergeld, Edelstein and Araoz). Norton, New York.
24. Beaumont J.G., 1983. *Introduction to Neuropsychology*. Blackwell, Oxford.
25. Sperry R.W., 1974. Lateral specialization in the surgically separated hemispheres. In *The Neurosciences: Third Study programme* (eds Schmitt and Worden). MIT Press, Cambridge, Mass.
26. Gazzaniga M.S. and Le Doux J.E., 1978. *The Integrated Mind*. Plenum, New York.
27. Moscovitch M., 1979. Information processing and the cerebral hemispheres. In *Handbook of Behavioural Neurobiology 2* (ed Gazzaniga). Plenum, New York.
28. Macleod-Morgan C., 1985. Hemispheric specificity and hypnotizability: an overview of ongoing EEG research in South Australia. In *Modern Trends in Hypnosis* (eds Waxman, Misra, Gibson and Basker). Plenum, New York.
29. Mészáros I., Bányai E.I. and Greguss A.C., 1985. Evoked potential correlates of verbal versus imagery coding in hypnosis. In *Modern Trends in Hypnosis* (eds Waxman, Misra, Gibson and Basker). Plenum, New York.
30. Bányai E.I., Mészáros I. and Csókay L., 1985. Interaction between hypnotist and subject: a social psychophysiological approach (preliminary report). In *Modern Trends in Hypnosis* (eds Waxman, Misra, Gibson and Basker). Plenum, New York.

CHAPTER 3

General Principles Underlying the Induction of Hypnosis

We have already discovered that a willingness to co-operate, confidence and the ability to concentrate are amongst the basic needs for the successful production of hypnosis. As the induction commences and the field of awareness becomes narrowed it is considered that the part of the mind which is known as the unconscious becomes more accessible. Suggestions appear to bypass consciousness and if not unacceptable may be acted upon without criticism. Moreover every suggestion that is accepted and acted upon, reinforces the suggestibility of the subject and facilitates the deepening of the hypnosis. The initial requirements which are essential for the achievement of the hypnotic state are therefore:

1. Positive motivation.
2. Removal of doubts and fears.
3. Fixation of attention.
4. Limitation of the field of consciousness.
5. Relaxation and limitation of voluntary movements.
6. Monotony.
7. Suppression of all ideas except those upon which attention is to be concentrated.

We must begin by examining the first two in some detail, since they will often be the determining factors between success and failure.

POSITIVE MOTIVATION

It is normally quite impossible to hypnotize a person against his will, for in order to succeed, he must be neither unwilling nor afraid. He must either want to comply with the suggestions of the hypnotist or must feel sufficiently confident not to oppose them. Indeed the more one can increase the desire of a person to be hypnotized, the more successful the induction is likely to be. Nevertheless enthusiasm must be tempered with patience, and subjects should be warned against trying too hard to 'make' themselves relax. Consequently, the most important of all the preliminary steps in the induction of hypnosis is the preparation of the patient's mind to accept it—to fertilize the soil as it were. This is not a difficult task, provided that it is approached systematically. It must be known whether the subject is really willing to undergo hypnosis, whether the proposed treatment is understood and trusted and how much inconvenience or discomfort the symptoms are causing. Provided the case has been properly assessed and is suitable for hypnotherapy the patient should be reassured of a postitive response and a successful outcome. It is most important that there is complete faith in the method before commencing an induction.

THE REMOVAL OF DOUBTS AND FEARS

This is another vitally important preliminary step *which must never be omitted* if one is to ensure a successful induction. Many patients are understandably timid, anxious and apprehensive, and will certainly never be able to enter the hypnotic state until their fears have been removed. These fears and anxieties, which can often prove serious obstacles to trance induction, usually fall into two categories:

1. *Fear of failure and over-anxiety to succeed.*
The one almost invariably leads to the other, and jointly they can be a source of considerable difficulty. It must be understood that many patients who attend for hypnosis have often tried other methods of treatment without success. They may consequently be convinced that hypnosis can offer them a last chance of recovery.

Now this might seem to be a great asset, but because the patient feels that much is at stake the mere possibility of failure will result in an increase in the level of anxiety and thus be counterproductive. Or the patient may be so keen to help that the act of trying to be successful engenders even more anxiety and will interfere with the induction process. Unless prompt steps are taken to deal with these problems by offering the strongest reassurances, all attempts at induction will be bound to end in failure.

Quiet confidence must always be the attitude of the therapist, not only to inspire hope and encourage motivation but also to show the patient that hypnosis is a state into which one may allow oneself to enter without doubt or fear and with complete trust.

2. *Fear of the hypnotic state itself.*

This particular difficulty is much more commonly met. Indeed there are a surprisingly large number of patients who are both afraid and suspicious of what is involved in hypnosis, and who are under the mistaken belief that they will be giving up control. Such doubts and fears as these are almost always due to a complete misconception on the patient's part regarding what is likely to take place in the hypnotic state.

Sometimes the patient will be entirely unaware of any difficulty. Many people are both anxious and willing to submit to hypnosis yet quite unconsciously their minds will entertain these fears. Under these circumstances, the mind will conjure up any excuse or reason for failing to enter into hypnosis. Unconscious resistance such as this may show inself in many different ways. During the actual induction, the patient may seem to be highly amused and even laugh or may complain of physical discomfort. Both reactions are evidences of an unconscious resistance to hypnosis and are merely rationalizations, and so it is important that reassurance be given that nothing unnatural will transpire which could result in the loss of control.

Occasionally the reverse situation can occur, which emphasizes even more strongly the significance of unconscious attitudes, for an unconscious desire to be hypnotizable may sometimes be stronger than the conscious desire to resist. Under these circumstances, many people who fight against succumbing to a trance are quite unable to stay awake once the induction process is started.

In order to succeed with inductions, all difficulties such as these must be adequately dealt with before commencing. Indeed, the preparation of the patient's mind is a most important stage in the successful induction of hypnosis. *Many failures to induce the hypnotic state are due to lack of adequate preparation of the subject, and lack of adequate discussion before induction is attempted.*

This problem presents more difficulties for the dental surgeon than the doctor, since the dentist who wishes to use hypnosis to secure relaxation or analgesia must necessarily achieve the trance state quickly. He is consequently not able to spend as much time in preparation as is the doctor. Fortunately, in many cases it is not so essential since dental patients, knowing that they are to be relieved of pain and discomfort are likely to prove more susceptible and less difficult than many of the cases with which the doctor has to deal. But whilst the motivation of such patients for hypnosis is certainly strong, it must not be forgotten that the dentist has other problems to overcome such as fear of visiting the dentist and fear of the hypodermic needle. Effective preparation of the patient, however, need not necessarily be a very lengthy procedure, but none the less time spent upon it is never wasted, and will pay handsome dividends. For this reason, this aspect will now be considered in some detail.

THE PREPARATION OF THE PATIENT'S MIND

There are certain difficulties which occur from time to time, any one of which can seriously interfere with the successful induction of hypnosis. Some of these are as follows.

   1. A complete misunderstanding of what is likely to happen during the hypnotic state.
   2. Confusion of hypnotic 'sleep' with ordinary sleep.
   3. The expectation of amnesia following the trance.
   4. The part played by 'will-power' in inducing the trance.
   5. The fear of being dominated by the hypnotist.
   6. The fear of loss of control.

One or more of these arise frequently in patients' minds and it is most important that every one of these points should be dealt with adequately in the preliminary talk, so that the patient knows exactly what to expect. Once this has been accomplished successfully, the induction of hypnosis will offer much less difficulty. Possibly the easiest way is to describe the procedure that should be adopted in the preparation of a patient never previously hypnotized. Let us take as an example the hypothetical case of a young and otherwise healthy man who has been referred for treatment.

1. *Begin by asking him what he knows or what he has heard about hypnosis, and what he expects to happen during and after the hypnotic state.*   If he knows anything at all, his ideas will invariably have been derived from newspaper articles, sensational magazine stories, stage performances or television. More often than not patients expect to be completely unconscious during the period of the trance, and to remember nothing at all of what has happened until wide awake again. Explain that medical hypnosis is not at all like this, and that hardly any of the things that he believes, will, in fact, occur.

2. *Tell him that there is no real resemblance between hypnotic sleep and ordinary sleep.*   Although during the induction his eyes will begin to feel more and more tired and will close just as they do when he goes to sleep, yet all the while they are closed he will remain just as wide awake and alert as when they were open. Describe this to him in the following words:

> When you go to sleep at night and put your head on the pillow, your eyes begin to feel more and more tired until eventually they close. And the moment you fall asleep, you become completely unaware of your surroundings until you awaken.
> If I were to come into your bedroom and speak quietly to you without waking you, you would not know I was there and you would not hear a single word I said.
> When you go into hypnotic sleep your eyes begin to feel tired and will close exactly as they do when you go to bed at night. But there will be one important difference.
> You will remain just as alert and wide awake as you were before your eyes closed. You will still know that you are in this room with me. You will be able to hear everything that I say to you. If

I ask you a question, you will be able to answer me without waking.

If you were to drift into ordinary sleep, you would not be able to hear me at all, and *if you couldn't hear what I said, how could I possibly help you?*

Even if you go into the deepest trance, you will always hear everything I say, and remain fully aware of everything that is going on.

Then drive this point home by telling the patient that you are going to show him exactly how he can expect to feel when he is in the hypnotic state and proceed as follows:

I want you to lie back in the chair and close your eyes for a few moments.

Don't open them until I tell you to. Just listen to what I am saying.

Now, you're lying back comfortably in the chair with your eyes closed, and if anyone came into the room they would think that you were fast asleep.

But you know that you're not asleep. You are just as wide awake as you were before you closed your eyes.

You can hear everything that I am saying to you.

If the telephone bell rang, you would hear it. And if I answered it, you would not be able to help taking a mild interest in what I was saying.

Now tell the patient to open his eyes, and explain the purpose of what he has just done.

No matter how deeply you go into the hypnotic state, you will always feel much the same as you did then. Except for one slight difference. If you went into a very deep trance state, you would still remain fully aware of everything that was going on, but you would feel so remote from them that they wouldn't seem to concern you at all. You would still hear the telephone bell and what I said when I answered it, but it would seem so far away that you wouldn't be the least bit interested in what I was saying. In fact you would be oblivious to the world around, whilst concentrating entirely on my words.

The reason why it is necessary to go into this matter in so much detail is both simple and highly important.

Most people seem to start with the wrong impression in their minds. When they are hypnotized they expect to experience a sort of 'black-out' during the trance, and after awakening to remember nothing of what has taken place. Although this may not be serious enough to prevent the induction of light hypnosis with spontaneous closure of the eyes, it will often be extremely difficult, if not impossible, to deepen the hypnosis any further. The patient's eyes will close. He will enter the light hypnotic state and he will not try to open them until he is told to do so. But he will fail to respond to any deepening technique. Once he is awakened, he will very often say 'I don't think I've been hypnotized. Nothing actually happened to me. I knew everything that was going on.' And as long as the patient entertains a doubt in his mind as to whether he has actually been hypnotized or not, there will be difficulty in inducing him into any deeper stage. Indeed, when you try, and fail, he is quite likely to say, 'Just give me some proof that something has happened. If only you can convince me that I have really been hypnotized, I know I shall be able to go deeper.'

Unfortunately he is asking the impossible during these early stages, for only when considerable depth has been achieved can satisfactory proof be afforded. So the awkward situation will probably arise when the patient says, 'Give me some proof that I've been hypnotized, and I'll be able to go deeper.' To which the reply must be, 'You go deeply first, and then I'll be able to give you plenty of proof.' This will result in the loss of that confidence which is essential for successful treatment. Indeed the odds are that you will never be able to make much further headway with this particular patient.

If, before attempting induction, the patient has been given a full explanation of what he must expect and what he is likely to feel, this particular difficulty will not occur. Occasionally such a patient will still find it hard to believe that he has really been hypnotized despite all your explanations, but curiously enough if these have been made, his doubts no longer seem to be strong enough to prevent further deepening.

3. *Tell the patient that he need not necessarily expect to forget what has happened during the trance once he is wide awake again.* Since the patient has probably seen demonstrations of hypnotic experiments on television, in which specially trained subjects are

often used, he may get the idea that exactly the same things are going to happen to him if he allows himself to be hypnotized. Most important is the fact that he will certainly expect to have a complete loss of memory for what has occurred during the trance state, and when he finds that he remembers everything that has happened he will be convinced that he has never actually been hypnotized at all. Consequently if you fail to correct his views upon these points, particularly regarding his anticipated loss of memory, you will encounter exactly the same scepticism that we have just discussed and a similar result will be inevitable.

Tell the patient that few people are able to achieve such depths, and that for ordinary medical purposes it is certainly not necessary and very seldom desirable. Explain that the subjects he has seen have been specially trained to achieve great depth, in order to be able to take part in experimental work and research or are especially selected deep trance subjects. Point out that in routine medical hypnosis, 'loss of memory' only rarely occurs, and that it is hardly ever essential for ordinary treatment purposes. If by chance, however, he should spontaneously forget what has happened during the trance there would still be nothing for him to worry about. It would simply mean that he was an exceptionally good subject, and he would still be able to recollect anything that he particularly wanted to. Nevertheless it had originally been maintained by Braid that amnesia always followed for all events transpiring during hypnosis, and was an essential part of that state, but this has long been known not to be the case.

4. *Explain to the patient that whilst will-power is most important in the induction of hypnosis, it is in fact his own will-power that plays a significant part and not that of the hypnotist.* There is a widespread impression amongst the general public that if you allow yourself to be hypnotized, you have no choice but to obey implicitly all the hypnotist's commands. That it is his greater will-power that causes you to surrender yours completely with the result that you are bound to carry out his orders quite automatically. This, of course, links up the next difficulty on our list—the fear of being dominated—with the fear of losing control which has already been mentioned.

Tell the patient that if we really believed this to be true, many of us would not be willing to allow ourselves to be hypnotized.

If hypnosis could only be produced through the stronger will-power of the hypnotist, it would naturally follow that the easiest people to hypnotize would be very weak-willed people. This is certainly not the case, for in actual fact the reverse happens to be true. It is always difficult and sometimes impossible to hypnotize very weak-willed individuals. This is because the weak-willed person cannot concentrate sufficiently and his attention cannot be held long enough to permit him to enter the hypnotic state. On the other hand, amongst the most difficult people in the world to hypnotize are those powerful and matter-of-fact business men who are accustomed to giving orders and unaccustomed to obeying others. But provided that they really are willing subjects, anxious to succeed and can accept the fact that they can utilize their own will-power to get rid of their problem, then this greatly increases their susceptibility.

5. *Assure the patient that he need have no fear whatever of being dominated by the hypnotist, and that he can never be compelled to do or say anything to which he strongly objects* Explain that if one were to try to compel him to do such a thing it would arouse so much mental conflict in his mind (I must, but I can't), that he would either wake up spontaneously or would display so much mental distress and anxiety that there would be no alternative but to awaken him immediately.

It is always essential to be honest with your patient and tell him that if he allows you to induce a really deep trance state, there is no doubt that he will follow your suggestions but only in so far as he is prepared to do so. Assure him that he could never be compelled to do anything to which he had a rooted objection. He must be satisfied that apart from the usual steps necessary to induce and deepen hypnosis, nothing further will be done and no questioning undertaken without having previously obtained his consent. Tell the patient that he will never lose control. That the object of all treatment is to give back to him that control which he has already lost and which therefore has resulted in his symptoms.

It may seem to you that we have considered this subject of the preparation of the patient's mind prior to induction, at unnecessary length. This is far from being the case. Indeed this is the main key to success. More failures result from too hasty and inadequate preparation than from any other cause. The time spent in removing misconceptions, doubts and fears is never wasted. It will not only ensure more rapid and successful inductions, but failure will become much less frequent.

When these explanations are completed always ask the patient whether he has any other questions he would like to put. If so, by answering them, one is usually able to dispel any last lingering doubts and fears, and thus secure full co-operation and trust.

The patient should understand quite clearly that hypnosis is essentially a matter of teamwork. That the part he plays, however passive it may be, is every bit as important as the doctor's and that without his co-operation and willingness nothing can be achieved.

Many of these preliminary explanations, however, can be dispensed with in the case of children who, unless excessively timid and nervous, are generally speaking much more easily hypnotized than adults. Children are less critical and are usually much more amenable to suggestion. Here one can rely almost entirely on a sympathetic and understanding approach. Indeed, in most cases, the simplest of explanations calculated to inspire confidence will be found to suffice.

Young children may be told, quite truthfully, that they will be shown how to go into a special kind of sleep. That although their eyes will begin to feel tired and will close exactly as they do when they go to sleep at night, it will be quite different because they will be able to hear everything that is said and will even be able to talk without waking. Provided that the child's confidence is gained and interest is aroused, then this is usually all that is required.

CHAPTER 4

Some Preliminaries to Trance Induction

DEPTH OF TRANCE AND SUSCEPTIBILITY TO HYPNOSIS

It is now generally accepted that 90 per cent of the population can be induced into the hypnotic state by any individual hypnotist, provided that the subject is willing and not afraid. The fact, however, that the remaining 10 per cent will probably fail to respond does not mean that they are unhypnotizable. Some other hypnotist may succeed quite easily with them, although he in turn may encounter another 10 per cent with whom he will be unsuccessful. So it is possibly true to say that most people are hypnotizable by someone or other.

Analytically minded people, who almost invariably try to work out the why and wherefores of what is happening to them, are not likely to be easy subjects. Yet even in these cases, sufficient depth for successful treatment can usually be obtained with adequate preparation, gradual training, patience and perseverance.

Different authorities have described over 20 stages of the hypnotic trance, but for practical clinical purposes, these may be conveniently reduced to four:

1. Light stage.
2. Medium-depth stage.
3. Deep stage.
4. Somnambulistic stage.

These will now be described in detail.

1. Light Stage

Many therapists will maintain that once the eyes are closed, the subject is in hypnosis and this is sufficient depth for simple treatment to commence. This may be true, and indeed one may occasionally have to accept that further deepening cannot be achieved. Certainly this is the threshold of the hypnotic state. Electroencephalographic studies will reveal that the subject is in that relaxed condition which can be achieved, simply by resting quietly in a comfortable position and thinking pleasing thoughts whilst undisturbed by external influences. Indeed the electroencephalographic recordings are the same in the latter case as they are when gentle suggestions of eye closure and relaxation are given by the therapist, viz. the alpha rhythm of approximately 8–12 cycles per second. Nevertheless it was claimed by London, Hart and Leibovitz[1] that measurable differences occurred even in the early stages and that these differences depended upon hypnotic susceptibility. Be that as it may, the answer must inevitably depend upon the results of further research into the neurophysiology of the hypnotic state and whatever the finer points, hypnosis does *begin* at this stage. This may therefore be considered a hypnoidal state which will imperceptibly drift into the light stage of hypnosis. The differences, if any, at this point between the EEG recordings of the subject who is awake and the subject who is in hypnosis are certainly too subtle to be picked up by instruments in present day use.

2. Medium Stage

There is no absolute dividing line between the stages of hypnosis. Rather are they classifications arbitrarily made for the convenience of therapy. The medium stage trance begins to develop as the deepening proceeds. The patient begins to look more relaxed. The respiration rate slowly decreases and it becomes evident that simple suggestions given are being acted upon. Images and awareness of altered sensations may be offered and the patient may be asked to confirm these experiences by an ideomotor signal (e.g. raising the right index finger). The patient will be fully aware of what transpires and no amnesia can be achieved for the session. Many patients remain too defended to allow further depth to occur but nevertheless treatment may be commenced.

3. Deep Stage

Where further suggestions of deepening are acted upon, the state of relaxation becomes visibly more apparent. Deepening by 'pacing' is a particularly satisfactory method and may be achieved for example by slowing down the rate of speech using emphasis on words, in order to slow down the rate of respiration. As the facial expression becomes one of obvious repose, the simultaneous reduction of the respiration rate and flaccidity of the limbs will indicate that a deep state of hypnosis has been reached.

Arm catalepsy, analgesia and amnesia can all be achieved and post-hypnotic suggestion may be acted upon.

4. Somnambulistic Stage

The word somnambule is derived from the Latin *somnus,* sleep and *ambulare,* to walk. This stage (see Chapter 1) is said to be attainable by 5 per cent of the hypnotizable population. The patient will open his eyes, talk, move about and obey other instructions and generally act as if he were awake and yet remain in hypnosis. Obviously it is most valuable from the point of view of hypnotherapy and is an assurance of potential success in treatment, as anything could be.

If we adopt these four stages, then the average susceptibility of the general public can be expressed in the following figures.

Ten per cent will probably fail to respond at all. These, however, might still do so in the hands of a different hypnotist.

Ninety per cent will probably achieve the light trance state. Even in this state, anxiety and nervousness can be considerably diminished.

Seventy per cent of these subjects will probably achieve the medium depth trance. At this stage, much more passivity and relaxation can be secured. Some degree of analgesia can often be obtained: dental fillings can sometimes be carried out with diminished discomfort, and burns dressed with less pain and inconvenience to the patient.

Twenty per cent of these subjects will be able to achieve the deep trance. At this depth, considerable degrees of analgesia can usually be secured.

Five per cent of these will be somnambules.

Now, you must not expect to be able to obtain these figures when you first start using hypnosis. If you do, you are likely to be disappointed. You will probably find that a higher percentage of your cases will appear to be unhypnotizable, and that most of the trances you succeed in inducing will be either light or medium. You must not become discouraged by this, however, for practice makes perfect and the percentage of successes will improve rapidly with experience. Having said this however, with practice and with the correct diagnosis and assessment of the patient, one hundred per cent of patients *properly selected for treatment* by hypnosis should be hypnotizable in spite of the figures. The therapist should be able to rely upon his clinical judgement, thus entirely obviating the need for the hit or miss attempt or for the elaborate assortment of hypnotizability tests which have emerged from the experimental laboratories. There is nothing likely to impair the doctor–patient relationship more than the 'I'll see if it works' attitude.

As in any other speciality, the therapist new to the techniques may feel somewhat anxious and unsure and this impression will transmit itself to the patient, who in turn will lack confidence in the procedure and may fail to respond. This will not happen in the case of the experienced hypnotherapist whose manner and attitude will ensure a good rapport and feeling of security on the part of the patient.

But even belief in oneself and one's clinical judgement will be useless unless it is based upon real skill, ability and mastery of techniques, and these can only be acquired by constant practice, even in the face of early setbacks. If you happen to be a person who is normally full of self-confidence, you may achieve tremendous initial success. But once one or two failures have dampened this early enthusiasm, the loss of confidence that will inevitably follow will seriously affect your figures.

Remember that medical and dental hypnosis is nothing more than another useful therapeutic instrument, and one should try to adopt the same attitude towards it as when using any other medical or dental technique for the first time. Only when able to do this will percentage figures of success fall into the proportions already quoted.

So far, in discussing this question of susceptibility, the figures given are those which are generally published. But with patience, and the gradual training of the patient to enter the deeper stages over a period of several sessions, these results can be greatly improved upon. Indeed, there are relatively few patients who cannot be trained to achieve sufficient depth to enter the hypnotic state immediately upon a given signal, verbal or otherwise. Such depth will be found to be quite sufficient for most clinical purposes. Only when extensive analgesias or hypnoanalytical techniques are required is greater depth likely to be necessary.

THE GENERAL PRINCIPLES OF TRANCE INDUCTION

During the induction of hypnosis the following sequence of events usually occurs:

1. Fixation of attention.
2. Limitation of the field of awareness.
3. Physical relaxation with limitation of voluntary movements.
4. Suspension of all ideas other than those upon which concentration is suggested.

The hypnotic state is produced by the constant repetition of a series of monotonous, rhythmical sensory stimuli, which may be visual, auditory or sometimes even tactile.

Visual stimuli. Staring at a fixed point, particularly if the eyes are held in a somewhat strained positon, rapidly causes retinal fatigue, blurring of vision, and a feeling of tiredness in the eyes. At the same time it induces concentration and a narrowing of attention.

Other visual stimuli such as a swinging pendulum, or rotating, flickering discs and mirrors have also been used to produce the same result. Even a metronome can be employed for the same purpose, and this will simultaneously provide the advantages of both visual and auditory stimulation. However the use of such contrivances does introduce an unnecessary element of mysticism which must always be avoided and the good therapist should be able to rely upon his own verbal suggestions rather than upon any extraneous or theatrical device.

Auditory stimuli. Talking to the subject in a monotonous, rhythmical and persuasive manner also tends to produce the desired state of mind, particularly when repeated suggestions of relaxation are made. The incorporation of certain key words such as *tiredness, heaviness* and *drowsiness* will greatly accelerate the process.

Tactile stimuli. Suggestions may be given of lying back in a comfortable armchair or a soft couch. Resting in a deckchair or lying on the warm sand according to the verbal picture which is drawn, and of *feeling* the comfort of the armchair or the couch or the deckchair or the sand etc.

Suggestions of relaxation are continued to eye closure. Other deepening techniques are described in a later chapter. The use of soft lighting, background music or touching or stroking of the skin is to be strongly discouraged. Patients are often highly anxious and such methods may invoke fantasies which could prove compromising and difficult to explain. Without doubt, the therapist's place is behind his desk where he may maintain a position of benign authority.

Only occasionally should it be necessary to touch the patient, such as when checking for analgesia and in surgery or for certain specific deepening techniques.

Most methods of hypnotic induction depend upon the use of one or more of these forms of stimuli to produce sensory fatigue. We need hardly be surprised at their effect when we realize how often people drop off to sleep whilst listening to monotonous lectures or sermons, or even whilst watching television. Indeed, the hypnoidal state can sometimes be produced with fatal ease, and can rapidly merge almost imperceptibly into natural sleep. In the past, some motorists experienced a dangerous feeling of drowsiness while driving along roads in France, for the lines of tall trees flanking some roads for miles, cast ladder-like shadows across the highway which could induce a feeling of increasing drowsiness.

Now, before commencing the induction of hypnosis, there are certain important decisions that have to be made, which may well decide the precise method of induction that is used.

THE TYPE OF APPROACH TO ADOPT

Basically, there are two ways in which the induction of hypnosis may be approached and the one which is selected must be largely determined by the personality of the patient who is undergoing treatment.

1. *Active participation with attention.* The subject is encouraged to pay the closest attention to what is actually taking place, to concentrate his attention upon everything that is being said, everything that is happening, and upon all the feelings that he experiences during the induction.

2. *Passivity of mind with distraction.* This involves the encouragement of a lethargic attitude in the subject, with a suspension of organized mental activity. *The subject is told to try not to listen to what the hypnotist says.* At the same time, he is given some mental task to perform which will occupy his mind, and distract attention away from the actual process of induction. In this way his unconscious mind will be rendered much more accessible and the hypnotic state will be more readily entered.

It may be compared with a mother trying to spoon-feed her baby for the first time. She carries the spoonful of food to the baby's mouth but he will have none of it, and pushes the spoon away, spilling the food all over the place. Now the wise mother will never try to force the issue. She will pick up the baby's rattle and shake it, and the moment the baby looks up and his attention is distracted to the rattle, into his mouth goes the spoon and down goes the food. Similarly during this type of induction, whilst the subject's mind is distracted from the actual induction process, the suggestions which consequently produce the desired result are fed into his unconscious mind.

Each of these methods naturally has its own advantages, and in comparing them, the following facts should be noted.

1. It is much easier to concentrate upon what is happening than it is to make the mind passive, unless some efficient form of distraction technique is simultaneously employed.

2. There is little doubt that passivity combined with distraction not only favours a quicker induction, but also tends to facilitate the further deepening of the trance since the response tends to be more unconscious.

Distraction is a far more difficult technique to apply and the decision as to which method to use should have regard to the therapist's assessment of the potential responses of the patient. In any case, one should be prepared to be versatile, using participation with attention at one time, yet turning to passivity with distraction at another should this seem to be advisable, particularly if hypnosis is not achieved at the first attempt. In other words, one must always be prepared to vary the method to suit the requirements of the individual subject.

THE MANNER OF GIVING AND PHRASING SUGGESTIONS

It is not very difficult to induce some degree of hypnosis in most patients who are willing to undergo treatment. As has already been indicated, the hypnotic induction must commence with an attitude of quiet confidence which will be reflected in the voice and demeanour of the therapist. This will go a long way towards ensuring success. If, on the other hand, the manner is hesitant or faltering as it certainly will be if failure is anticipated, then it will be difficult to induce even the lightest trance state.

Although suggestions delivered in a flat, monotonous voice will often prove successful, there is no doubt that their effectiveness can be greatly increased by the proper use of vocal expression which can be varied in many different ways:

1. Alterations in the volume of the voice.
2. Changes in the rate of delivery.
3. The stressing of particular words.
4. Changes in the inflection and modulation of the voice.
5. The insertion of suitable pauses between successive ideas.

Generally speaking, loud tones are best avoided and it is best to speak quietly and monotonously but with definite emphasis. Indeed, in most cases, a slow deliberate rhythmical delivery in an even tone of voice will often prove effective. Sometimes, however, it may be advisable to speak more quickly in order to keep the subject's mind fully occupied. This will forestall criticism by preventing him from concentrating too much upon his own feelings. On other occasions, particularly when suggestions of heaviness, drowsiness or sleepiness are being made, it is better to speak even more slowly and deliberately than usual, prolonging the key words sufficiently to heighten the impression which is conveyed.

In some instances, a more thorough and effective response is obtained if, in addition to quickening the delivery, increased stress is placed upon critical words. But as soon as the response is obtained, the voice should once again revert to its former flat monotonous tone. This variation seems to call the subject's attention to what is happening, and exercises a powerful effect in reinforcing the idea.

Great care must be exercised however, in the selection of the correct words to be stressed. The importance of this is illustrated in trance induction, where the hypnosis may either be deepened or even accidentally terminated by the tone of voice and emphasis adopted by the hypnotist. If one should say to a subject: 'Try to open your eyes. They are tightly closed. You cannot possibly open them' the effect produced by this suggestion may depend entirely upon the kind of emphasis used, and where it is placed. By accidentally laying emphasis upon the word try—'*Try* to open your eyes'—the last part of the suggestion is bound to be more easily resisted, and the subject will probably succeed in forcing his eyes open and waking up. If, on the other hand, emphasis is upon the word cannot — 'You *cannot* possibly open them' — the subject will probably fail to open his eyes despite the most strenuous efforts to do so, and the hypnosis will deepen. However, it should here be emphasized that a statement such as this, made as a test of successful deepening, is a direct challenge to the patient and one which he could act upon with success and thus ruin the therapeutic session.

The acceptance of a suggestion can often be facilitated by raising the voice towards the end of a sentence, thereby conveying increased emphasis and carrying more conviction. Conversely, the lowering of the voice at the end of such phrases as 'deeper and deeper asleep' seems to heighten their effect considerably. Also, when giving suggestions, it is wise to pause for at least 15 to 20 seconds between successive phrases or ideas. This not only helps to enhance their effect but also tends to avoid confusion in the subject's mind. In fact, whenever time permits the further lengthening of such pauses it will be found to increase their effectiveness to an even greater extent.

During therapeutic sessions, the effect of a suggestion can often be greatly increased if the hypnotist uses his voice in such a way as to express an emotion in keeping with the idea he is trying to convey. The suggestion of disgust, for instance, can be given much more effectively when the hypnotist adopts a tone of voice in keeping with this, although he is not actually experiencing this emotion at the time.

The Permissive Method of Giving Suggestions

In this case, the suggestions are given almost unobtrusively in a quiet persuasive tone of voice. It cannot be denied that this is a much slower method, but it is much more certain, and possesses certain definite advantages. Instead of losing their force, suggestions given in this way actually gain strength through repetition. And since they become persuasions rather than commands they tend to arouse little conscious resistance.

The fact has already been stressed that many subjects dislike the idea of being dominated and are afraid of yielding up control. Thus there can be no doubt at all that, if failures are to be kept to a minimum, this is by far the wisest method to adopt. Nevertheless, the personality of the subject must first be carefully considered before deciding upon the technique to be adopted in each individual case.

Whilst in hypnosis the suggestibility of the subject is always increased; the degree to which this occurs will vary with the depth of the trance, and this has to be taken into account when putting the suggestions into words.

The Authoritarian Method of Giving Suggestions

In this method, suggestions are always given in a commanding and assertive tone of voice. Some therapists, wishing to assert their personality, in inducing hypnosis have to give suggestions as if they were orders. There is no doubt that occasionally this may succeed despite some resistance on the part of the subject. When it does so, it certainly gives more far-reaching and dramatically successful results than any of the milder forms of suggestion.

Only too frequently, however, it awakens a deliberate conflict of will which ultimately defeats the whole object. It also has the grave disadvantage that suggestions cannot be continuously repeated without losing all their force. Once a suggestion is given, success or failure must follow immediately, and unfortunately failure is much more likely to occur.

In Light Hypnosis

Suggestions should be phrased less positively and with less emphasis than in the deeper stages. Indeed, the approach should be entirely permissive in character.

In Deep Hypnosis

Suggestions can be given more positively and forcefully, but never to the extent that they would appear to the subject as commands. These would not only be resented but would often be followed by a refusal to comply. It is not a difficult matter to phrase positive, direct suggestion in such a way that the subject will not feel that he is being dominated, yet at the same time convey to him the confidence that it will be accepted.

It should also be remembered that, since any suggestions are always more likely to succeed when they convince the subject that you, the therapist, have a firm belief in the idea advanced, then such ideas should not only be logical, but should be accompanied whenever possible by sound reasons for their acceptance.

The Personality of the Subject

This must always be taken into account. The inadequate, dependent individual who is vainly seeking some authority figure upon whom he can rely, will both expect and respond to a positive approach. In this case, suggestions should be given authoritatively, emphatically and with conviction, but even so must never appear in the nature of commands. Such patients may incorrectly interpret the intentions and strong negative feeling could result. As a consequence considerable difficulties could arise in any further attempt at therapy.

Others will resent the slightest semblance of dominance and will fear losing control. They will require a great deal of reassurance, and consequently your delivery should almost resemble a lullaby, slow and deliberate, monotonous, yet with a marked rhythmical beat. Assurance must be given once again, that the object of treatment is not to take over control but to restore that control which has already been lost.

THE LAWS AND GENERAL PRINCIPLES OF SUGGESTION

Before proceeding to study the various methods of trance induction, it is necessary that we should become fully acquainted with certain laws and principles which govern the action of suggestion. These are not only important to our understanding of the techniques of trance induction and deepening, but will also be found to be equally applicable and significant when we come to consider the question of the treatment which is to follow.

There are three important laws that govern the effectiveness of suggestion.

1. *The law of concentrated attention.* Whenever attention becomes concentrated upon an idea, that idea spontaneously tends to become realized. In the hypnotic state, it is the attention of the unconscious mind that we are trying to enlist, and this is most easily achieved when no conscious attention is aroused. Suggestions that are made too forcefully or issued as commands tend to defeat this object.

2. *The law of reversed effect.* Whenever the state of mind is such that the subject thinks 'I should like to do this — but I cannot', despite the fact that he may really wish to do so, the harder he tries, the less he is able. We often come across this in everyday life. The patient who suffers from insomnia goes to bed convinced that he is going to be unable to sleep, and thus the harder he tries, the more wide awake he remains. The same difficulty often hinders trance induction. The more actively the subject tries to cooperate, the less he will be able to do so. But the more passive he remains, the more easily he will enter the trance.

This law may be employed to great advantage in phrasing suggestion during the induction and deepening of the trance.

> Your arm has become so stiff and straight that it is impossible
> to bend it. *The harder you try to bend it—the stiffer and
> straighter it will become.*

3. *The law of dominant effect.* This is based upon the fact that a strong emotion always tends to replace a weaker one. The attachment of a strong emotion to a suggestion will always tend to make that suggestion more effective. Notice how the threat of danger will immediately suppress any feelings of pleasure or comfort. The induced emotion of disgust can nullify the pleasure a child gains from biting its nails.

Naturally, great latitude is permissible in the precise wording of suggestions, but the laws must always be observed if satisfactory results are to be obtained. Some ideas of the principles which should be adopted are given below.

1. *Always couple an effect that is intended with one that the subject is actually experiencing at the moment.* This principle should be employed throughout all trance induction and trance deepening procedures.

For example:

> Be aware of your body seated comfortably in the chair and allow
> yourself to sink deeper and deeper into the cushions.

The subject relates sitting comfortably in the chair with his recollection of this feeling of relaxation suggested to him. This will reinforce subsequent inductions.

Pain if often caused and is always aggravated by tension.

As you become more relaxed and less tense...you are beginning to feel more comfortable.
And as you allow yourself to relax even more...*your pain will slowly become less and less...and presently it will disappear completely.*

In this case, the subject will be feeling more and more relaxed as his hypnosis deepens, and this will certainly produce a greater feeling of comfort. By relating the suggested disappearance of the pain to these two established facts, he becomes much more readily convinced that this also will occur.

2. *It is always much easier to secure the acceptance of a positive suggestion than a purely negative one.* For example it is never very profitable to suggest to a patient suffering from headache that his pain is going to disappear. In most cases, it is much easier to produce a feeling of warmth by direct suggestion. If the positive suggestion of this increasing warmth is then coupled to the desired negative suggestion of the gradual disappearance of the pain, this is much more likely to occur.

As you concentrate upon your forehead...you become aware of a feeling of warmth spreading all over this area. And as I continue to talk to you...the warmth is increasing and your head is beginning to feel more and more comfortable. All pain and aching is gradually disappearing...and in a few moments, your head will feel so warm and comfortable that the headache will have disappeared completely.

3. *It is sometimes easier to secure the acceptance of a suggestion if it is coupled with an appropriate emotion.* In some subjects it is possible to cause the heart to beat more rapidly by direct suggestion alone. If however the subject has the capacity for visual imagery and is induced to picture himself in a terrifying situation that arouses the emotion of fear, this suggestion is much more likely to succeed. In a similar way the feeling of calmness and deepening of the hypnotic state can be enhanced by emphasizing the reduction of the rate of respiration and the slow and silent yet powerful and healthy beat of the heart. Additionally in the treatment of alcoholism for example, the suggestion of the loss of desire

for drink will be strengthened if the patient is also told that in-dulgence will arouse strong feelings of nausea and disgust.

4. *Suggestions should always be worded in such a way that they are both clear and unambiguous.* The subject must be left in no doubt as to the intention conveyed. Only one interpretation must be possible. Failure to achieve this could possibly be followed by the most disconcerting and unexpected results. A patient who was terrified to go into the street because of the traffic was once told by a hypnotist that when she left his rooms she would no longer bother about the traffic, and would be able to cross the road with-out the slightest fear. She obeyed his instructions so literally that she ignored an oncoming vehicle and awoke in hospital. However this is an extreme example. Patients would not usually accede to any suggestions which would invite such behaviour.

5. *Over-complication should be avoided at all costs. Simplicity is essential.* Other than when using some specific confusional tech-nique of induction, every effort should be made to avoid confusion in the subject's mind. The more complicated a suggestion is, the more difficult it will be for him to carry it out.

6. *The word 'must' should never be employed.* There should never be the slightest suspicion of domination of any kind.

7. *In phrasing suggestions a definite rhythmical pattern should be aimed at, and repetition is essential.* The same ideas should be re-stated and constantly repeated, over and over again. In framing suggestions, both rhythm and repetition can best be achieved by using successively several different words or phrases, each with exactly the same meaning. Certain words are repeated with particular stress in order to emphasize the rhythm.

> And these same things will continue to happen to you every
> day...and you will continue to experience these same feelings,
> every day...*just* as strongly...*just* as surely...*just* as powerfully
> when you are back home again...as when you are with me in this
> room.

If you repeat these suggestions aloud, you will notice that the stressing of a word 'just' serves to accentuate the rhythm, like the beat of a metronome. You will also notice that the choice of the three words—strongly, surely, powerfully is quite deliberate. The phrases not only ensure repetition, but also express the same basic idea in three different ways.

Too little attention is often paid to this question of repetition. Post-hypnotic suggestions should be repeated at least once before awakening the subject. In some instances it is even wise to ask him whether he fully understands what has been said, and to ask him to repeat the exact suggestions that have been given.

8. *No matter how deep the trance, no suggestion should ever be given that the subject might find distasteful or objectionable.* The temperament of each individual subject should be taken into account. What one person may readily accept, another may strongly resent and reject. Even during instructional courses, where post-hypnotic suggestions are given to demonstrate the phenomena of hypnosis, the utmost care should be taken to avoid suggesting any action that might cause the subject to feel embarrassed or to appear ridiculous in the eyes of other people.

Whilst it is true that even in deep hypnosis some subjects may still be able to resist suggestions of this type, others will feel compelled to carry them out despite their dislike. In such cases they will quite justifiably consider that the trust they have placed in the hypnotist has been grossly abused. After all, the deeper the trance, the more likely will suggestions be accepted and acted upon. The less the conscious mind is aware of what has been said, the less interference there will be. Additionally the most effective results will occur when post-hypnotic amnesia for the events of the trance can be suggested.

9. *The most important and crucial therapeutic suggestions should always be left until the end.* Treatment should commence with suggestions of minor importance, followed by those of increased importance and conclude with those of greatest consequence. The last suggestions of all are likely to be most readily accepted.

10. *Suggestions should be worded as far as possible to conform with the known habits and thought of the individual.* If this is done, they will more readily be complied with and will be much less likely to arouse conscious criticism.

To sum up, then, it is of primary importance that suggestions should always be given in a tone of quiet conviction, with the utmost self-assurance and confidence in their effectiveness. There is no doubt that they are always more likely to be acted upon if the therapist is able to convey his feelings in a positive way.

SUGGESTIBILITY TESTS

As research into the hypnotic state increases worldwide, so more sophisticated tests of hypnotizability and suggestibility emerge from the laboratory.

At the beginning of the century, Janet[2] taught that those subjects in whom hypnosis could be induced more easily, suffered from a hysterical illness and that as the symptoms decreased so the hypnotizability diminished. We now know that this is not the case. Hysteria is not an illness but a symptom of a much wider neurosis.

The literature abounds with reports of the considerable research by Eysenck, Furneaux and many others, on hypnotizability, susceptibility and hysteria. It was also at one time considered that patients suffering from a psychotic illness were not hypnotizable and hypnosis was even used in the differential diagnosis of neurosis and psychosis.

In clinical practice any decision as to hypnotizability or otherwise must be made on clinical grounds after a thorough exploration of the patient's problem. Nevertheless, although the patient may be assessed as susceptible to hypnosis it is not always easy to predict the degree of hypnotizability that will result. Numerous attempts at measurement of susceptibility to hypnosis have been devised over the past 50 years. Basically they all make use of specific responses obtained to suggestions of behaviour given under hypnosis. Of these the most popular are the Stanford Hypnotic Susceptibility Scales (SHSS) developed by Weitzenhoffer and Hilgard in 1959. One of these scales was later adapted by Shor and Orne in 1962 for testing hypnotic responsivity. This is called the Harvard Group Scale (HGS).

It is interesting to note, as Frankel[3] pointed out, that the term used is responsivity, not susceptibility, which implies a weakness.

Both of these scales, as well as various modifications of them, are in use in the experimental laboratory today.

The advantage of the HGS is that it can be used for testing a group of subjects at a single sitting but careful and highly skilled administration is essential.

However since there is a relationship between some kinds of suggestibility and susceptibility to hypnosis, various simplified 'suggestibility tests' have also been described which can be applied before attempting trance induction. If successful, they will help to convince the subject that he will be easily hypnotized, and when markedly positive it is likely that the individual will prove to be a good subject. It should be noted, however, that this is not necessarily the case, but it is probably true to say that the subject who resists these suggestions will not prove very susceptible to hypnosis. Although testing is without doubt of the greatest importance in the experimental laboratory, so far as the use of hypnosis in the clinical field is concerned, as has already been stated it should be the decision of the therapist based on sound experience, a thorough assessment of the patient and good clinical judgement which should finally influence the choice of treatment. Many such tests have been described from time to time. The four that are most commonly employed are described below.

The Postural Sway Test

The subject is asked to stand erect, with his feet together, and his body held perfectly rigid. He is told to fix his eyes upon a spot on the ceiling directly overhead. The hypnotist stands behind the subject with his hands on the subject's shoulders, and tells him to remain perfectly rigid. He then gently rocks the subject backwards and forwards to disturb his balance in the way that suggestion will presently disturb it. The subject is then asked to close his eyes whilst still trying to look at the spot on the ceiling. He is then given the following instructions:

> Try to imagine yourself becoming as stiff as a board...your knees stiff...and your body perfectly rigid.
> Although your eyes are closed, hold your head up...and keep your eyes still looking up through the closed lids.
> You will begin to feel that you are falling backwards...that you

will feel a force pulling you backwards towards me.
Don't resist...you won't fall to the ground for I shall catch
you...but you will begin to fall backwards.
You are falling...falling...falling.
Falling backwards...falling...falling...falling.

Usually the subject will start swaying, and as soon as he does so, the suggestions of falling are repeated with increased emphasis and the pressure of the hands removed from the shoulders. Always watch carefully in order to be sure of catching the subject when he falls, for this can occasionally happen with surprising rapidity.

This test is the one that is most commonly used by stage performers, and can sometimes be usefully employed by lecturers in hypnosis to select suitable subjects from the audience for demonstration purposes.

The Hand Clasp Test

The subject is told to sit in a chair and to hold his arms straight out in front of him at shoulder level. He is to make them as stiff and rigid as possible, and to clasp his hands tightly together. It is useful here for the hypnotist to demonstrate this to him by momentarily pressing his clasped hands firmly together. He is then told:

Clasp your hands tighter and tighter together...and you will feel
your fingers gripping more and more firmly.
And as you do so...I want you to picture a heavy metal vice and
imagine the jaws becoming screwed tighter and tighter together.
Now, picture that vice in your mind and concentrate on it...and
as you do so, you will imagine that your hands are just like the
jaws of that vice...becoming screwed up...tighter and tighter
together.
As I count up to five...your hands will become locked
together...tighter and tighter...and when I reach the count of five,
they will be so tightly locked together that they will feel just like a
solid block of metal...and it will be difficult or impossible for you to
separate them. *One*...tightly locked...*Two*...tighter and
tighter...*Three*...very, very tight...your hands feel as if they are
glued together...*Four...the palms of your hands are locked tightly
together...Five...they are so tightly locked that it will be impossible*

for you to separate them until I count up to three...the harder you
try to separate the palms of your hands...the tighter your fingers
will press upon the back of your hands...and the tighter your hands
will become locked together.

An adaptation of this devise is also commonly used by stage hypnotists to test the hypnotizability of members of the audience.

The Hand Levitation Test

The subject sits at a table with his elbow and forearm resting
upon the surface of the table, palm downwards. The hypnotist
places his own hand on top of the subject's, and tells him:

As I place my hand on yours, I want you to concentrate upon all
the feelings you experience in your hand.

(Here, the hypnotist presses lightly, almost imperceptibly upon
the subject's hand.)

And as you do so...you will gradually get the feeling that your hand
is becoming lighter and lighter...as if it has no weight in it at all.
It's growing lighter and lighter...lighter and lighter...very, very
light indeed.

The subject is then asked if he can feel this sensation of lightness. If he says 'No', the suggestions are repeated over and over
again. If, on the other hand he says 'Yes', the hypnotist slightly
relaxes the pressure of his own hand and says:

Your hand is now feeling so light that it feels as though there is no
weight in it at all.
It is getting lighter and lighter...so light, in fact, that it is
beginning to rise up from the table.
It is coming right up from the table...as if it has no weight in it
at all.
Lighter and lighter...up...and up...and up.
Rising up into the air...higher...and higher...and higher.

(As the hand starts to rise, the hypnotist gradually relaxes the
pressure of his own hand and then removes it entirely.)

The Pendulum Test (Chevreul's Pendulum)

An 8-inch circle is drawn on a card with four radii at right angles to each other. A ring is tied to the end of a thread about 12 inches long. The subject to be tested is seated at a table with the card immediately in front of him. He holds the thread with his arm extended so that the ring dangles at the other end of the thread about 3 to 4 inches above the centre of the circle. He is told to allow his eyes to travel round and round the circumference of the circle. He is to pay no attention whatever to the ring, which will begin to swing round and round the circle, gaining speed as it does so. The subject is then told to let his eyes travel up and down one of the radii, and as he does so, the ring will change direction and will swing along the line his eyes are traversing.

Details of these suggestibility tests have been included because no account of hypnosis would be complete without them. However they are of little practical value and few clinicians ever use them. If a patient really requires hypnotic treatment, an attempt to induce hypnosis may be made no matter how great or little his susceptibility may be, and since this can usually be increased sufficiently by adequate preparation and motivation the need for preliminary testing does not arise.

FINAL INSTRUCTIONS BEFORE TRANCE INDUCTION

The induction of hypnosis can easily be carried out in an ordinary consulting room. Either a couch or a comfortable chair may be used. Each has its advantages and disadvantages. Lying upon a couch may become associated in the patient's mind with the act of going to bed, and thus conjure up and encourage the idea of sleep. On the other hand, the nervous and apprehensive patient may feel much happier in a chair. He may feel less helpless and less threatened. It is purely a matter of individual choice. If a chair is used it should be comfortable and sufficiently deep to afford support to the patient's head. The room should be free from glaring lights and steps should be taken to avoid the intrusion of sudden and unexpected noises. Otherwise no attempt should be made to disguise the fact that it is a perfectly normal consulting room. As has earlier been stated, the use of any device which might add an air of mystery to the surroundings is ill-advised. Should the patient need to go to the toilet, this should be attended to before the induction begins.

First of all, make your patient as comfortable as possible and see that he is warm. A full explanation of the procedure should be given to him in the following way:

> I am going to begin by telling you three things.
> First, exactly what *you* have to do.
> Secondly, exactly what I shall be doing.
> And finally, exactly what you may expect to happen and how you will feel.
> Because of this, nothing will take you by surprise, and you will know exactly how you are going on.

Now what you actually describe will, of course, vary according to the particular method of induction you propose to use. But never omit this step, for it will make your task very much easier. Finally, remember to remove any doubts concerning the only remaining thing that may possibly cause uncertainty as to what has happened.

> As soon as your eyes have closed on their own, you will be in the lightest form of hypnotic sleep.
> You will have not the slightest desire to open them, and will not do so until you hear me give the necessary signal.
> At this stage you could open them if you wanted to, and what is more I couldn't stop you. Even if I were to tell you that you couldn't, you would be able to open them.
> In actual fact, you won't open them until I ask you to, for the simple reason that you won't want to do so if you want to get better.

There are many people who cannot believe that they have been hypnotized, just because they felt convinced that they could have opened their eyes at any moment. And once this doubt has been allowed to enter their minds, difficulty will arise in deepening the hypnosis.

Before we proceed to consider the various methods of trance induction, let us remind ourselves of the sequence of events through which this, and trance deepening are achieved.

1. All trance-induction methods aim at a gradual restriction of awareness of the surrounding environment by limiting sensory impressions.

2. This is achieved by fixation of attention, either on a material

object or upon a group of limited ideas.

3. This sensory restriction is reinforced by a rhythmic, monotonous repetition of suggestions.

4. With each suggestion that is accepted and acted upon, the suggestibility of the subject becomes progressively increased, sometimes to an enormous extent. Conversely, each suggestion that is rejected markedly diminishes the subject's suggestibility.

Most of the methods of induction used nowadays depend upon verbal suggestion which is usually, but not invariably, combined with some form of eye fixation. The latter is certainly not essential but has the great advantage of producing increasing fatigue of the eyelids. When eye fixation is used and suggestions are given to the subject that his eyes are gradually becoming tired and his eyelids heavier and heavier, this is actually true. The eyes become tired partly because they are being held in a strained position and the suggestions given reinforce the feeling of tiredness. Expectation at that point will be high, the patient will be in a condition of heightened suggestibility and the eyes will close at the given signal.

REFERENCES

1. London P., Hart J.T. and Leibovitz M.P., 1968. EEG alpha rhythms and susceptibility to hypnosis. *Nature*, **219,** 71–72.
2. Janet P., 1925. *Psychological Healing,* Vols. 1 and 11. George Allen and Unwin, London.
3. Frankel F.H., 1976. *Hypnosis: Trance as a Coping Mechanism.* Plenum, New York.

CHAPTER 5

Methods of Trance Induction and Deepening

It has already been emphasized that any doubts or fears regarding the hypnotic state must first be removed, that the method of induction to be used is explained to the patient and that reassurance is given that no loss of control will ensue.

It must be pointed out that although the word 'sleep' is used throughout the text in descriptions of induction techniques, the subject must be given to understand that hypnosis is not a normal state of sleep but a particular form of relaxation, which, for want of a better word, is called 'sleep'.

So many different techniques have been described for the induction of hypnosis that it would be impossible to discuss them all, nor is it necessary to do so. Inevitably any method practised becomes adapted to the personality of the therapist. It must additionally be tailored to meet the problems and the needs of the individual patient. New methods of induction are constantly being evolved, depending upon the ingenuity and inventiveness of the hypnotizer. The beginner however is strongly advised to learn and to practise one of the standard techniques taught before attempting anything more adventurous. For our purposes, only a relatively small number need consideration. These may be divided into permissive, intermediate and authoritarian techniques.

Permissive Techniques
  1. Eye fixation with progressive relaxation.
  2. Eye fixation with verbal suggestion.
  3. Progressive relaxation by verbal suggestion.
  4. Thumb nail technique.

Intermediate Techniques
  1. Eye fixation with distraction.
  2. Erickson's head levitation method.

Authoritarian Techniques
  1. Modified Elman technique.
  2. Erickson's confusional technique.
  3. Direct eye gaze method.

PERMISSIVE TECHNIQUES

1. Eye Fixation with Progressive Relaxation

This is a most useful method of inducing hypnosis, and one of the first that should be mastered thoroughly before attempting any of the more advanced techniques. It is a method that depends upon concentration of attention since the subject listens intently, throughout the induction, to what the hypnotist is saying.

The subject either lies on a couch or sits in a comfortable chair, and is told to select a spot on the ceiling, slightly to the rear, so that he is looking upwards and backwards at it. He fixes his eyes upon this spot, and must not allow them to wander from it for a single moment. If they do, his attention must immediately be called to the fact.

Summary of method. The subject is asked to allow himself to relax completely...It is suggested that he can experience a feeling of heaviness in his feet and ankles...in his legs and thighs...that his feet, ankles, legs and thighs are beginning to feel completely and utterly relaxed...that this feeling of relaxation is extending through his abdomen and chest and upwards through the entire length of his back, through his fingers and hands and arms and shoulders and through the muscles of his neck, over his chin and jaw muscles and face and over his eyes and eyelids...and that his eyelids are becoming so very, very heavy and tired that they are wanting to close.

These suggestions are repeated monotonously, over and over again, until the subject's eyes are seen to flicker and close, and he sinks into a light hypnotic sleep. The hypnosis is then deepened by the induction of arm levitation.

Deepening by arm levitation. The subject is asked to concentrate upon the sensations he will experience in his right or left arm...that this arm is beginning to feel lighter and lighter...as if there is no weight in it at all...that it feels as if it wants to rise up in the air...entirely of its own accord...that it feels lighter and lighter...and that as it does so, his sleep is becoming deeper and deeper...That it feels as though a balloon were tied to his wrist...causing it to float up into the air...light as a feather...and that as it floats up into the air...his sleep is becoming deeper and deeper. The moment the slightest upward movement of the fingers is observed, the subject's attention must immediately be called to the fact, and the suggestions repeated with increased emphasis. As the arm rises higher and higher in the air, he should be told that his sleep is becoming deeper and deeper. These suggestions must be made gently but given with complete confidence. If the subject perceives any hesitation or doubt on the part of the therapist then the induction is doomed to failure. Should the arm fail to rise an attempt must be made to deepen this stage by repetition of the suggestions of weightlessness.

Once a satisfactory result has been obtained, suggestions of gradually increasing heaviness are made until the arm sinks down again. The suggestions of increasing heaviness and downward movement of the arm are constantly related to the further deepening of the sleep. By this time, the subject has probably entered a medium-depth trance. Should the arm fail to rise and no upward movement occur then the suggestions should be repeated and more clearly phrased. It often happens that patients experience subjectively, the arm rising etc., although no physical movement may occur. If no visible response can be elicited, then pass on to other deepening techniques.

No attempt should be made to establish the depth of trance by testing for the degree of analgesia at this stage.

A Typical Induction Routine

Lie back comfortably in the chair.
Choose a spot on the ceiling, slightly behind you...and look
upwards and backwards at it.
Keep your eyes fixed on that spot on the ceiling.
Let yourself go...limp and slack.
Let all the muscles of your body relax completely.
Breathe quietly...in...and out.
Now I want you to concentrate upon your feet and ankles.
Let them relax...let them go...limp and slack.
And you will begin to note a feeling of heaviness in your feet.
As though they are becoming just as heavy as lead.
As if they are wanting to sink down into the carpet.
Keep your eyes fixed on that spot on the ceiling.
And as you stare at it...you will find that your eyelids are
becoming heavier and heavier...so that presently they will want
to close.
As soon as they feel they want to close...just let them close.
Let yourself go completely.
Let the muscles of your calves and thighs go quite limp and
relaxed.
Let them relax...let them go...limp and slack.
And as they do so...your eyes are beginning to feel more and
more tired.
They are becoming a bit watery.
Soon, they will feel so heavy that they will want to close.
As soon as they feel they want to close...just let them
close...entirely on their own.
Let the tension go completely.
Give yourself up totally to this very
pleasant...relaxed...drowsy...comfortable feeling.
Let your whole body go limp and slack...heavy as lead.
Now, the muscles of your stomach...let them relax...let them
go...limp and slack.
Now, the muscles of your chest...and your back.
Let them go...limp and slack...let them relax completely.
And you can experience a feeling of heaviness in your body.
As though your whole body is becoming just as heavy as lead.
As if it is wanting to press down...deeper and deeper...into the

chair.
Just let your body go...heavy as lead.
Let it sink back comfortably...deeper and deeper into the chair.
And as it does so...your eyelids are feeling even heavier and heavier.
So very, very heavy...that they are wanting to close.
As soon as they feel they want to close...just let them close.
And now, that feeling of relaxation is spreading into the muscles of your hands and arms, your shoulders and neck.
Let your neck muscles relax...let them go...limp and slack.
...Allow them to relax completely.
And as they do so...you will note a feeling of heaviness in your hands and arms.
As though they are becoming just as heavy as lead.
Let them go...heavy as lead.
Let them relax completely.
And the heaviness spreads pleasantly and comfortably through your neck and facial muscles to your eyes and eyelids.
And as it does so...your eyelids are feeling very, very heavy...your eyes so very, very tired...that they are wanting to close.
Wanting to close, now...closing...closing tighter amd tighter.
Go to sleep!

The subject has now entered the light hypnotic state. Should his eyes close, as they may well do, at an earlier stage, it is important to carry on with the relaxation suggestions until they are complete, relating these to further deepening of the hypnotic sleep.

Deepening by arm levitation.

Let yourself relax completely...and breathe quietly...in...and out.
And as you do so...you will gradually sink into a deeper, deeper sleep.
And as you sink into this deeper, deeper sleep...I want you to concentrate upon the sensations you can feel in your left hand and arm.
You will feel that your left hand is gradually becoming lighter and lighter.
It feels just as though your wrist were tied to a balloon...as if it is gradually becoming pulled up...higher and higher...away from the chair.
It is wanting to rise up...into the air...towards the ceiling.

Let it rise...higher and higher.
Just like a cork...floating on water.
And, as it floats up...into the air...your whole body is feeling
more and more relaxed...heavier and heavier...and you are
slowly sinking into a deeper, deeper sleep.
Your left hand is feeling even lighter and lighter.
Rising up into the air...as if it were being pulled up towards the
ceiling.
Lighter and lighter...light as a feather.
Breathe deeply...and let yourself relax completely.
And as your hand feels lighter and lighter...and rises higher and
higher into the air...your body is feeling heavier and
heavier...and you are drifting into a deeper, deeper sleep.
Now, your whole arm, from the shoulder to the wrist, is
becoming lighter and lighter.
It is leaving the chair...and floating upwards...into the air.
Up it comes...into the air...higher and higher.
Let it rise...higher and higher...higher and higher.
It is slowly floating up...into the air...and as it does so...you are
drifting into a deeper, deeper sleep.

Further deepening by arm heaviness.

And now feel that your arm is becoming heavier and heavier again.
Heavier and heavier...just like a lead weight.
It is slowly sinking downwards...on to the chair again.
Let it go...heavy as lead...let it sink down...further and further.
And as it does so...you are falling into an even deeper sleep.
Deeper and deeper...deeper and deeper sleep.
Your arm is feeling heavier and heavier...heavy as lead.
It is sinking down, now...on to the chair.
And as it does so...you are falling into a deeper, deeper sleep.

The moment your arm touches the chair...you will be in a very,
very deep sleep indeed.
At this point, the subject would at least have entered a medium-
depth trance. Since, even in medium depth some degree of analgesia can often be obtained, the next step in determining whether
he is actually deeper than this is to test for analgesia and the extent to which this can be secured.

Determination of depth by testing for analgesia. A sterile hypodermic needle is produced and if he is not already in that posi-

tion the subject is asked to rest both hands, palm downwards on
his lap.

> I want you to concentrate upon the back of your left hand.
> Just notice the sensations that you feel in the back of your left
> hand.
> As you do so...it is beginning to feel cold and numb...as if it is
> surrounded with ice.
> Just picture your left hand...being packed round with ice.
> It is gradually becoming more and more cold and numb...as if
> the feeling is going out of it completely.
> Colder and colder...more and more numb and insensitive.
> So cold, in fact...so completely numb and insensitive...that all
> the feeling has gone out of it...and you will be able to feel no
> pain whatever.
> Your left hand is now so cold, numb and insensitive...so cold,
> numb and insensitive...that you will not be able to feel any pain
> in it at all.

After a warning, the back of the right hand (the one upon which
the subject has *not* been told to concentrate) is pricked with the
needle and the subject will flinch slightly. The left side is then
pricked. If the subject neither moves nor flinches and shows no
response, then some degree of analgesia has been produced and
a medium trance at least has been achieved. In this case, firmer
pricking without eliciting any further response will establish the
extent of the analgesia.

If the analgesia is complete, it will be possible to push the needle
deliberately right through the skin, without the slightest evidence of pain being felt. In this case, a fairly deep trance has been
secured.

If, on the other hand, the subject shows that he has felt pain,
either the suggestions of analgesia must be continued, or should
these fail to produce any result, an attempt will have to be made
to deepen the trance by other means.

If, despite these measures, pain is still obviously felt, then no
analgesia has been produced and the subject may have achieved
no more than a light trance. It should be remembered however,
that the production of analgesia is not a test for hypnosis but
rather of the depth of hypnosis.

Once testing has been completed then *never* forget to remove the analgesia before waking the subject.

> Your left hand is now becoming quite normal again.
> It is feeling warmer...the numbness is passing off...and the
> feeling is coming back into your hand and arm.
> The sensation is returning...you will be able to feel all
> sensations quite normally again.
> Your left hand is now quite normal and feels perfectly comfortable.

2. Eye Fixation with Verbal Suggestion

The subject either lies on a couch with his head supported by a pillow, or sits back comfortably in an armchair. He is instructed to look upwards and backwards and to fix his eyes upon a spot on the ceiling of his own choice. Alternatively, he can be told to stare at the tip of a pencil held about 8 inches above his eyes. No matter what fixation point is selected, he must stare at it continuously. Should his eyes wander, his attention must immediately be called to the fact. This fixation of attention tends to diminish all other interests and external stimulations. Whilst he is staring at the selected spot or object, verbal suggestions are made to him quietly and monotonously.

Summary of method. The subject is told to let himself relax completely...to breathe quietly, in and out...that as he does so, he will feel that his eyelids are becoming heavier and heavier...that as they do so, he will want to blink...that he will let them blink as much as they like...that his eyes are becoming very, very tired...that the blinks are becoming slower and bigger...that as they do so, his eyes will feel that they want to close...that presently they will close on their own, and he will go to sleep. These suggestions are continued slowly, rhythmically and monotonously until the eyes are observed to flicker and close, and the subject sinks into a light hypnotic sleep.

A Typical Induction Routine

> Let yourself relax...as much as possible.
> Breathe quietly and normally...in and out.
> Let yourself go...quite limp and slack.
> And gradually, you will feel that your eyes are becoming very,

very tired.
Your eyelids are feeling heavier and heavier.
So heavy...that presently they will want to blink.
As soon as they want to blink...just let them blink as much as
they like.
Let everything happen...just as it wants to happen.
Don't try to make anything happen...don't try to stop it
happening.
Just let everything please itself.
Now...your eyelids are beginning to blink.
Very soon...those blinks will become slower and bigger.
And your eyelids will feel so very, very heavy and tired...that
they will want to close.
Already, your eyes are becoming a bit watery...you're feeling
very, very drowsy...and your eyes are feeling so very, very heavy
and tired...that they are wanting to close.
As soon as your eyes feel that they want to close...just let them
close, on their own...and you will drift into a deep, deep sleep.

(Should the subject's eyes begin to water a little, you should immediately call his attention to the fact, and the moment the blinks become slower and bigger, your suggestions should be given much more positively and emphatically.)

Now...your eyes are wanting to close...
Just let them go...they're closing now...closing...closing tighter
and tighter...tighter and tighter.
Go to sleep!

The moment this suggestion is made, the subject's eyes usually close immediately, and remain closed. He has then entered the light hypnotic state and deepening may commence.

3. Progressive Relaxation by Verbal Suggestion

This method depends upon the induction of passivity of mind, without employing any accompanying distraction technique. The subject should be lying on a couch, or resting comfortably in an armchair. Note that no fixation point is specifically used. In this case, fixation of attention is directed towards a limited group of ideas.

He should be asked if he ever relaxes, for example by lying on the beach in the sunshine or perhaps in the shade of a tree in the garden, or simply by sitting in his armchair at home. Occasionally one meets the patient who must not admit that he has time to relax, or at the other extreme who claims to relax by climbing mountains or sailing a boat. Such visual imagery is not particularly conducive to relaxing in hypnosis and unless the ingenuity of the therapist is such that he can work around this problem and adapt to the patient's needs, it is best to suggest some less active occupation.

Summary of method. For example, having first ascertained that this is acceptable, he is told to imagine himself lying on the sea-shore, sun-bathing...that as he does so, he is to let all his muscles go limp and slack...first, his feet and his calf muscles...then his thighs...that as they relax, he will feel...that he is becoming drowsier and drowsier...that the relaxation is spreading over his whole body...his stomach, his chest and his back...his arms...his shoulders...his neck and his facial muscles...that as it does so, he is feeling drowsier and drowsier...that his eyelids are becoming heavier and heavier...that his eyes are wanting to close...that presently they will close, and he will go to sleep.

A Typical Induction Routine

As you are lying on the couch...I want you to think of a pleasant, peaceful scene.

Just picture yourself lying on a deck chair by the sea-shore...and with the sun-shade adjusted so that it's just right for you.
You can feel the soft, warm sand...you can see the blue sky...and you can feel the warmth of the sun on your body not too hot, but just right for you.
I want you to let all the muscles of your body go quite limp and slack.
First, the muscles of your feet, and ankles.
Let them relax...let them go...limp and slack.
Now, the muscles of your calves.
Let them go...limp and slack...allow them to relax.
Now, the muscles of your thighs.
Let them relax...let them go...limp and slack.
And, already you can note a feeling of heaviness in your legs and

thighs.
Your legs and thighs are beginning to feel as heavy as lead.
Let your legs and thighs go...heavy as lead...let them relax completely.
And as you do so...you are becoming drowsier and drowsier.
You feel completely at peace...your mind is calm and contented.
You are really enjoying this very pleasant, relaxed, drowsy feeling.
And now, that feeling of relaxation is spreading upwards over your entire body.
Let your stomach muscles relax...let them go...limp and slack.
Now, the muscles of your chest...and your back.
Let them go limp and slack...allow them to relax.
And you can note a feeling of heaviness in your body...as though your body is feeling just as heavy as lead...as if it is wanting to press down...deeper and deeper onto the chair.
Just let your body go...heavy as lead.
Let it sink comfortably...onto the chair...and as it does so...you are feeling drowsier and drowsier.
Your eyelids are becoming heavier and heavier...and your eyes, more and more tired.
Presently, they will want to close.
As soon as you feel they are wanting to close...just let them go...and they will close, entirely on their own.
Just let yourself relax...more and more completely.
You can feel the heat of the sun on your body.
You are feeling warm and comfortable...completely at peace.
And that pleasant feeling of relaxation is now spreading into your hands...and your arms, your shoulders and your neck...
Now, the muscles of your hands and arms...let them relax...let them go limp and slack.
And you can note a feeling of heaviness in your arms.
As if your arms are becoming just as heavy as lead.
Just let your arms go...heavy as lead...let them relax completely.
Now the muscles of your shoulders...let them go limp and slack...allow them to relax.
Now your neck muscles relax...let them go...limp and slack.
Let all the muscles of your face relax.
And as you do so...your eyes are becoming more and more tired.
So tired that they are wanting to close.
Just let them close...on their own.

Closing now...closing...closing tighter and tighter.
Go to sleep!

As the relaxation gradually spreads over the subject's body, you will see his eyelids beginning to flutter, first spasmodically and then more rapidly, and as soon as his eyes have closed, he has entered into a light trance state. Should his eyes close, as they sometimes will, before you have completed the full relaxation suggestions, call his attention to the fact and carry on with the routine suggestions until the relaxation of the whole body is complete. Next continue with deepening as described.

4. Thumb Nail Technique

The subject may lie on a couch or sit in a comfortable armchair. With one arm raised above his head, the thumb nail is used as the focus for eye fixation.

Summary of method. The subject is asked to raise an arm slightly above the head and to concentrate upon the thumb nail. Suggestions are given of feelings of fatigue in the raised limb until it begins slowly to drop. When the fingers touch the face the eyes close and hypnosis is induced as the arm falls heavily to the side.

A Typical Induction Routine

Now as you are relaxing comfortably would you please raise
your arm slightly above your head and gaze at your thumb nail.

(In the case of right handed people it is preferable to use the left hand which will tire somewhat more easily and the right hand is used in left handed people).

Now keep your eyes fixed on your thumb nail.
Concentrate on your thumb nail and nothing else.
As you do so be aware of the fact that your arm is raised above your head.
The rest of your body is relaxed and comfortable but your arm is above your head.
As I talk to you allow your body to sink into the chair (or couch) but your arm is raised above your head.
As your body relaxes more and more, your arm is becoming tired...more and more tired.

Your eyes becoming heavier as you stare at your thumb, your
body more and more relaxed, but your arm is more amd more
tired.
Your fingers are beginning to twitch a little with fatigue...your
arm heavier and more tired...now beginning to drop a little with
fatigue...a little heavier, a little more tired, dropping...your
fingers now touch your face, your eyes close, your hand drops
heavily to your side.
Go to sleep!

At this point the patient is usually visibly more relaxed, the eyes
are closed, the respiration rate is slowed and suggestions of
deepening may commence.

INTERMEDIATE TECHNIQUES

1. Eye Fixation with Distraction

This is a method of induction that is both reliable and quick,
and provided that the subject's mind has been adequately prepared, it rarely takes more than 2 to 3 minutes to secure spontaneous eye closure.

The principle upon which it depends is the exact reverse of that
which is involved in the last method that we considered, since
passivity of mind is aimed at through the distraction of the subject's mind from the actual process of induction. This is achieved
by giving him a simple mental task to perform which will fully occupy his conscious mind, thereby rendering his unconscious mind
more accessible. Whilst he is occupied with this task, verbal suggestions of increasing tiredness and heaviness of his eyelids are
quietly made, but he is instructed to try *not* to listen to what the
hypnotist is saying. He will still hear what is said, but will do his
best to ignore it and concentrate entirely upon the mental task
that has been imposed.

One of the most effective mental tasks is a modification of the
counting method first used by Loewenfeld towards the end of the
last century. He used to ask his subjects to start counting from 1
to 100, slowly and rhythmically. He preceded this by a short period of eye fixation, but although he followed it with verbal suggestions, he never attempted to induce either tiredness or closure of

the eyes. He aimed solely at a general feeling of restfulness and drowsiness.

The same principle may be applied but in a somewhat different way. The subject is asked to count backwards, silently, slowly and rythmically until asked to stop. Accuracy is unimportant and if a mistake is made it need not be corrected but the count should be continued regularly and monotonously as the beat of a metronome. With the starting point fixed at 300 and the count reversed, a good deal more concentration is required than if the count is commenced at number one. The latter method may be of more use however in the case of young children.

In order to test the purpose achieved by this count, just close your eyes and start counting slowly backward to yourself, and go on counting backward from 300 for a minute or two. Then ask yourself this simple question: 'Whilst you were counting, how many other different things were you thinking about?' Not many, to be sure. And even if you did happen to be one of those rare individuals who could simultaneously think of other things as well, the solution would still be quite easy. Simply start at 300 and subtract 7s consecutively from it until told to stop. You will agree that it would be most exceptional if you were able to pay attention to many other things whilst you were doing that. Whenever the conscious mind is distracted in this way, the unconscious mind always becomes more accessible. Suggestion is accepted more readily and is consequently acted upon more quickly and more effectively.

Summary of method.   The subject lies back comfortably in a suitable armchair with his head supported, and is told to relax as much as possible. The therapist should sit on his left-hand side, slightly to the rear and almost out of his sight. A pencil or pen should be held about 8 inches above his line of vision, in such a way that he is compelled to stare upwards and slightly backwards at it. This is just sufficient to hold his eyes in a somewhat strained position. Whilst gazing at the tip of the pencil or pen, he is instructed to start counting backward, silently, from 300, and to continue until he is told to stop. Whilst he is occupied with the count he is quietly told that his eyes are beginning to feel very, very tired...that his eyelids are becoming heavier and heavier...that presently they will want to blink...that he will let them blink as much as they like...and that as they do so...his eyes will become heavier and heavier...and that they will want to close...entirely on their own.

Watch his eyes very closely, and the moment that they respond to these suggestions and start to show signs of closing, tell him to go to sleep. Upon receiving this suggestion, which is given firmly and emphatically, the eyes usually close immediately and remain closed, and the subject enters the light hypnotic state.

Deepening by arm heaviness. Commence the deepening process with a sequence of progressive relaxation. This, however, is not an essential feature of this particular technique and can easily be omitted if so desired. It is however a valuable addition. But, instead of attempting arm levitation as the first stage in deepening the hypnosis, this may be effected by inducing a feeling of arm heaviness. Ask the subject to place his left arm upon the arm of the chair.

He is then told that his arm is becoming heavier and heavier...that he can feel it pressing down more heavily on the arm of the chair...that this feeling of heaviness is increasing with every moment that passes, with every word that you say, heavier and heavier, heavier and heavier...that, in a few moments, his arm will feel so very, very heavy that if he tries to lift it...it will drop limply back into his lap...just like a heavy weight...and that as it drops limply back on to his lap...he will fall into a deeper, deeper sleep.

As suggestions of heaviness continue, impress upon him that he is trying to lift his arm but it is so heavy that he no longer can be bothered to do so. Finally, tell him to imagine his arm lifting ever so slightly but that it is so heavy that it just drops down onto the chair and as it does so he falls into a very deep sleep.

The feeling of heaviness must then be removed by suggestion that the arm is becoming quite normal and his sleep simultaneously deeper and deeper.

A Typical Induction Routine

I want you to lie back comfortably in the chair.

Look upwards and backwards at the tip of the pencil.
Can you see it? Good!
Don't let your eyes wander from it for a single moment.
Now start counting slowly backwards from 300.
Mentally, to yourself...not out loud.
Keep on counting...slowly and rhythmically...and go on counting
until I tell you to stop.
Try not to listen to me...any more than you can help.
You'll still hear everything that I say...but try not to listen.
Just stick to your counting.
Let yourself go, completely...limp and slack.
Breathe quietly...in...and out.
And, whilst your're breathing quietly...in...and out...you can feel
that your eyes are becoming very, very tired.
They may feel a little watery...the pencil may begin to look a
little blurred.
Already your eyelids are beginning to feel very, very heavy and
tired.
Presently they will want to blink.
As soon as they start to blink...just let them blink as much as
they like.
You see! They're starting to blink, now.
Just let everything happen...exactly as it wants to happen.
Don't try to make it happen...don't try to stop it happening.
Just let everything please itself.
And presently, your blinks will become slower...and bigger.
As they do so...your eyes will become more and more tired.
So tired that you feel they are wanting to close.
As soon as they feel they want to close...let them go...just let them
close...entirely on their own.

You must watch the subject's eyes carefully, throughout this induction. Timing is of the greatest possible importance. For instance, as soon as you notice that the individual blinks are almost shutting the eyes, you should call the subject's attention to it immediately, and continue your induction in a more authoritative tone:

Your eyelids are becoming heavier and heavier.
They're wanting to close, now.
Let them close...closing tighter and tighter...tighter and tighter.
Go to sleep!

If this last suggestion has been timed correctly, the subject's eyes will close immediately, and will remain closed.

> Sleep very, very deeply...relax completely...give yourself up
> completely to this very pleasant, relaxed, drowsy feeling.
> Stop counting, now.
> Just sleep...very, very deeply indeed.

Occasionally, it seems to be almost impossible to induce anything more than the faintest flickering of the eyelids which obstinately decline to blink. It seems that no downward movement whatever can be initiated in them to facilitate their final closure.

In such cases, continue with the suggestions for about a couple of minutes and watch for a fixed, rather distant 'far-away' look to appear in the subject's eyes. As soon as this is detected, bring the left hand gently in front of the subject's eyes, watch for the blink and immediately as it happens say to him firmly 'Go to sleep!' and his eyes will invariably close and remain closed until he is instructed otherwise.

Now produce complete relaxation of the whole body, stage by stage, continually relating each set of suggestions to the gradual deepening of the sleep. Not only is this relaxation more easily and thoroughly obtained in the light hypnotic than in the waking state, but there is no doubt that as it becomes progressively more complete, the subject does tend to sink into a deeper sleep.

Deepening by progressive relaxation.

> Now a feeling of complete relaxation is passing pleasantly through
> your entire body.
> Let the muscles of your feet and ankles relax completely.
> Let them go...limp and slack.
> Now, your calf muscles.
> Let them go limp and slack...allow them to relax.
> Now, the muscles of your thighs.
> Let them relax...let them go...limp and slack.
> And as the muscles of your legs and thighs become completely
> limp and relaxed...you can note a feeling of heaviness in your
> legs.
> As though your legs are becoming just as heavy as lead.
> Just let your legs go...heavy as lead.
> Let them relax completely.

And as they do so...your sleep is becoming deeper and deeper,
That feeling of relaxation is now spreading upwards...over your
thighs and stomach muscles.
Let your stomach muscles relax...let them go...limp and slack.
Now, the muscles of your chest...and your back.
Let them all go...limp and slack...allow them to relax.
And as you do so...you can experience a feeling of heaviness in
your body...as though your body is becoming just as heavy as
lead.
As if it is wanting to press down...deeper and deeper...into the
chair.
Just let your body go...heavy as lead.
Let it sink back comfortably...deeper and deeper...into the chair.
And as it does so...you are gradually falling into a deeper,
deeper sleep.
Just give yourself up completely...to this very
pleasant...relaxed...drowsy feeling.
And now, this feeling of relaxation is spreading into the muscles
of your arms...your shoulders...your neck and face.
Let your arm muscles relax...
Let them relax...let them go...limp and slack.
Now, your shoulder muscles.
Let them go limp and slack...allow them to relax.
Now, the muscles of your neck, particularly the back of your
neck.
Let them relax...let them go limp and slack.
And as you do so...you can now experience a feeling of heaviness
in your facial muscles and eyes.
Your eyes close and your eyelids are becoming as heavy as lead.
Let your entire body go...heavy as lead.
And as you do so...your sleep is becoming
deeper...deeper...deeper.
And as this feeling of complete relaxation spreads...and deepens
over your entire body...you have fallen into a very, very deep
sleep indeed.
You are so deeply asleep...*that everything I tell you that is going
to happen...will happen...exactly as I tell you.*
And every feeling that I tell you that you will experience...you
will experience...exactly as I tell you.
Now, sleep very, very deeply.
Deeper and deeper asleep...deeper and deeper asleep.

By now, the subject should be firmly established in the hypnotic state and further deepening techniques can be employed.

Deepening by induction of arm heaviness. Now ask the subject to place his arm on the arm of the chair.

> And as you rest your arm on the arm of the chair you will feel it getting heavier and heavier...from the shoulder to the wrist.
> And as I talk to you...you will feel the heaviness in your arm increasing.
> That feeling of heaviness is increasing...with every word that I say.
> Your arm is beginning to feel heavier...and heavier...just as heavy as lead.
> *You can feel it pressing down more firmly on the arm of the chair as if a heavy load is pressing it down.*
> And in a few moments...your arm will feel so very, very heavy...*that, if I would lift it up and then release it,...it would drop limply back on to the arm of the chair...just like a lead weight. Just imagine it happening. Lifting up...up...up...now let go....*
> And as it drops limply back...on to your lap...you fall into a deeper, deeper sleep.

Proceed to restore it to normal by removing the induced feeling of heaviness. This emphasizes a most important rule which you must never fail to observe when you are practising hypnosis: *during hypnosis, no matter what effect you produce, whether it be limb heaviness, limb rigidity or analgesia—particularly the latter—never forget to remove it again and restore normality before you awaken the subject.*

> You have now fallen into a much deeper sleep.
> And, as I talk to you...you will notice that all feelings of heaviness are leaving your arm.
> It is coming back to normal...and now feels just the same as your other arm. Back to normal...NOW.
> And as it returns to normal so...your sleep is becoming even deeper...and deeper.

This concludes the first stage of the deepening process.

If you consider the prospects are favourable you can now proceed to deepen the hypnosis further, or you may find it best to defer this until the next session. This decision may be aided by watching carefully the extent and ease with which the subject has complied with these suggestions. If the results have been easily obtained then proceed with further deepening techniques, such as the induction of graded responses, which will be described in a later chapter. On the other hand, if any difficulty has been experienced, the subject should be awakened, having been given the post-hypnotic suggestion that on the next occasion he will be able to go into a hypnotic sleep even more quickly and deeply.

The Advantages and Disadvantages of the Eye Fixation with Progressive Relaxation and the Eye Fixation with Distraction Methods of Trance Induction

Although many different methods of trance induction have been described, you will probably find that when you first start using hypnosis, the methods of eye fixation are likely to be the most useful to adopt as standardized procedures. Indeed, you should make yourself competent in as many techniques as possible, since it is always a mistake to become restricted to one particular method. Each has its advantages and disadvantages, and the choice of which you decide to use as your standard method must ultimately depend upon your own individual preference and experience. No single method can ever be described or even recommended as the best method of inducing hypnosis since results will vary considerably in the hands of different operators. The most important thing is to understand the principles underlying the various methods of trance induction and to make your choice in any individual case with due regard to the two following considerations:

1. The method must suit your own personality.
2. It must also suit the personality of your subject.

But remember, no matter what method you finally evolve as your favourite technique, you must still be prepared to vary it when occasion demands. You will certainly fail with many of your patients if, so to speak, hypnosis is 'bought off the peg', ready-made. On the other hand, few patients will present great difficulty provided that the hypnosis is tailored to suit their individual requirements.

When dealing with a very nervous, anxious and apprehensive

patient, the eye fixation–progressive relaxation method is a much better approach to the initial induction of hypnosis. However, the eye fixation–distraction method offers certain material advantages in many cases. These can be briefly summarized as follows:

1. It saves time. It is a rapid and efficient method of induction, spontaneous eye closure usually being obtained within 2 to 3 minutes. The subject enters the hypnotic state almost before he is aware of the fact. Light hypnosis always seems to be induced more quickly and easily when the subject does not have to concentrate his attention upon the suggestions that are being made. His conscious mind is distracted away from the actual induction process by the counting technique. He is consequently much less critical towards what is being said, and is thus prone to accept suggestion much more rapidly and readily.

2. In the first stage of deepening the hypnosis, it is much easier to induce a feeling of arm heaviness since the natural tendency for the arm to fall, owing to the force of gravity, greatly augments the strength of the suggestion. Arm levitation is not as certain to succeed and sometimes cannot be produced at all. Failure is always a set-back, and temporarily at least diminishes the subject's susceptibility to alternative deepening procedures. Even when it succeeds, since the arm has to rise in opposition to the force of gravity, it is only natural that the effect should take longer to occur. It must be admitted, however, that when arm levitation does succeed it certainly goes a long way towards convincing the subject that he has actually been hypnotized, since something has occurred that is quite out of keeping with his normal experience, and the increase in depth that follows is usually greater. Despite this obvious advantage, it seems that since an equivalent depth can generally be achieved without difficulty as a result of subsequent techniques, the induction of arm heaviness, which is not only more likely to succeed but is also more quickly and more readily secured, has much to commend it.

3. The complete unpredictability of the occurrence and extent of induced analgesia, renders it unsuitable as a test of depth in the course of routine inductions. Sometimes considerable degrees of analgesia can be obtained in medium-depth hypnosis, on other occasions no analgesia at all can be produced until deep hypnosis

or even somnambulism has occurred. Consequently, there is always the danger that, if this particular test fails, the subsceptibility of many subjects will become diminished to such an extent that they will find it difficult, if not impossible to achieve the depth which otherwise they might have attained.

2. Erickson's Hand Levitation Method

This procedure was originally devised by Milton Erickson in 1923, whilst experimenting with suggestions conducive to automatic writing as an indirect technique of trance induction for naïve subjects. Although successful, it proved to be too slow and laborious an induction technique in most instances. It was consequently suggested to the subject that, instead of writing, the pencil-point would merely move up and down on the paper, or from side to side. Erickson quickly realized that the pencil and paper were superfluous and that the ideo-motor activity was the primary consideration. Subsequently he succeeded in inducing a somnambulistic trance by substituting a simple 'hand-levitation' technique.

The following full description and analysis of hypnosis by means of hand levitation is that given by Wolberg in his book, *Medical Hypnosis*[1]. It is probably one of the best of the induction techniques, since it not only permits the subject himself to play a greater part in the actual induction, but also allows him to take his own time in entering the hypnotic state.

Summary of method. The subject is asked to sit back comfortably in a chair and to rest his hands, palms downwards, upon his thighs. He is then asked to gaze fixedly at his hands and to concentrate his attention upon the sensations he can feel in them. He is told that although his hand seems to be motionless some movement is still present. Very soon, therefore, one of his fingers or his thumbs will twitch; as soon as this occurs his attention is drawn to the fact, and he is told that the spaces between his fingers will gradually widen and that his fingers will slowly but surely begin to separate. When this is seen to occur the suggestions are changed to those of gradually increasing lightness in the fingers and hand. As a result his fingers are beginning to rise up from his thigh—they are slowly floating upwards—his hand and arm are floating up into the air—upwards—upwards—upwards. Then, when his hand and arm have risen to the level of his face, the suggestion is given that his hand is changing direction and that it is now being attracted towards his face. As his hand approaches his face he is told that he is beginning to feel very, very drowsy, that his eyelids are becoming very, very tired—heavier and heavier—and that as soon as his hand touches his face his eyes will close and he will fall into a deep, deep sleep.

His hypnosis can then be further deepened by any of the standard techniques.

A Typical Induction Routine

I want you to sit comfortably in the chair.
Let yourself relax.
Place your hands, palms downward, upon your thighs.
Fix your eyes upon your hands...and keep watching them...very, very closely
And whilst you are relaxing like this...you will notice that
certain things are happening...that you had not noticed before.
I will point them out to you.
Now, I want you to concentrate upon all the sensations and
feelings that you notice in your hands...no matter what they
may be.
It may be that you will feel the texture of the material of your
trousers...as your hands rest upon your thighs.
You may feel the warmth of your hands on your thighs...or you
may feel a certain amount of tingling in your hands.
No matter what your sensations may be...I want you to observe
them closely.
Keep watching your hands.
They seem to be quite still...and resting in one position.
Yet some movement is there...although it is not yet noticeable.
Keep watching your hands.
Don't let your attention wander from them.
Just wait to see what movement is going to show itself.

The subject's attention is now firmly fixed upon his hands and he is curious about what is going to happen. Sensations such as anyone might normally feel have been suggested to him as possibilities. No attempt has been made to force any suggestion on him. What he observes he considers to be a product of his own experience.

The idea is to induce him to respond to the suggestions of the hypnotist as if they, too, are parts of his own experience. A subtle attempt is being made to establish a link in his mind between his own sensations and the words spoken to him. In this way, at a later stage, this linkage will cause words or commands to tend to produce further sensations or actions.

Unless there is any conscious resistance on the subject's part, a slight twitching or jerking will occur in one of the fingers, or in one hand. As soon as this happens, the subject's attention must be drawn to the fact and he must be told that the movement will probably increase. Any other movement of the legs or body, or any alteration in the breathing should also be commented upon. This linking of the subject's reactions with the remarks of the hypnotist causes an association between the two to be formed in the subject's mind.

> It will be interesting to see which of your fingers moves first.
> It may be any finger...or it may even be your thumb.
> But one of the fingers is going to twitch or move.
> You don't know what one...or even in which hand.
> Neither do I...but keep watching...and you will find that one of them will move.
> Possibly in your right hand.
> See! The thumb twitched and moved...just as I said.
> And now you will notice that a very interesting thing is beginning to happen.
> You will notice that the spaces between your fingers are gradually beginning to widen.
> The fingers will move slowly apart...and you'll see that the spaces will become wider and wider.
> Your fingers are slowly moving apart...wider...wider...wider.
> The spaces are slowly becoming wider...wider...wider.

This is the first suggestion to which the subject is expected to respond. If the fingers do move apart, it is because the subject is beginning to respond to suggestion. The hypnotist continues to talk, however, as if it were something that had taken place in the natural course of events.

Now, I want you to watch carefully what is taking place.
Your fingers will want to rise up slowly from off your thigh.
As if they want to lift up...higher...higher...higher.

(The subject's forefinger starts to move upward slightly.)

You see!
Already your forefinger is beginning to lift up.
As it does so...all the other fingers will want to follow.
Up...and up......and up.
Rising up slowly into the air.

(The other fingers begin to rise.)

As the other fingers lift...your entire hand is beginning to feel
lighter and lighter.
So light...that your whole hand will slowly rise into the air.
As if it feels just as light as a feather...just like a feather.
As if a balloon is slowly lifting it up in the air.
Lifting...lifting...up...and up...and up.
Pulling it up...higher...higher...higher.
Your hand is becoming lighter and lighter.
Very, very light indeed.

(The hand starts to rise.)

As you watch your hand rise...you will note that your entire arm is
beginning to feel lighter and lighter.
It is wanting to rise up in the air.
Notice how your arm is lifting up into the air...up...and up...and
up...a little higher...and higher...and higher.

**(The arm has now lifted about 6 inches above the thigh, and the
subject is gazing at it intently.)**

Keep watching your hand and arm...as it rises into the air.
And as it does so...you will begin to feel drowsy and tired.
Notice how drowsy and tired your eyes are becoming.
As your arm continues to rise...you will feel more and more tired
and relaxed...very, very sleepy...very, very sleepy indeed.
Your eyes will become heavier and heavier...and your eyelids
will want to close.
As your arm rises...higher and higher...you will want to feel
more and more relaxed.
You will want to enjoy this very, very pleasant...relaxed...sleepy

feeling.
Just let yourself go.
Give yourself up entirely to this very, very
comfortable...relaxed...drowsy feeling.

Notice how as the subject carries out one suggestion, his response is used to reinforce and facilitate the next suggestion. As his arm rises, it is suggested by inference that he will become drowsy because his arm is rising. This is yet another example of the important principle of coupling, which we have already considered.

Your arm is lifting up...and up...and up.
Higher...and higher...and higher.
And you are feeling very, very drowsy indeed.
Your eyelids are becoming heavier...and heavier.
Your breathing is becoming slower...and deeper.
Breathe slowly and deeply...in...and out...in...and out.

(The subject's arm is now stretched out straight in front of him. His eyes are beginning to blink, and his breathing is deep and regular.)

As you keep watching your hand and arm...you are feeling more
and more drowsy...and relaxed.
And now you will notice that your hand is changing its direction.
The elbow is beginning to bend...and your hand is beginning to
move...closer and closer to your face.
Your hand feels as though it were being strongly attracted to
your face.
Your hand is moving...slowly but surely...towards your face.
And as it becomes closer and closer...your are feeling drowsier
and drowsier...and you will fall into a very deep sleep.
Closer and closer...drowsier and drowsier...sleepier and sleepier.
Although you are becoming sleepier and sleepier...you must not
go to sleep until your hand touches your face.
But when your hand touches your face...you will fall immediately
into a deep, deep sleep.

The subject is being asked to choose his own pace in falling asleep, consequently when his hand touches his face and his eyes do close, he is perfectly satisfied that he is, in fact, asleep. Constant coupling of the hand levitation and sleepiness techniques causes them to continue to reinforce each other.

When the subject does finally close his eyes, he will have entered a trance in the production of which he, himself, will have participated. He will thus be much less likely to deny that he has been in a trance.

> Your hand is now changing its direction.
> It is moving closer and closer to your face.
> Your eyelids are feeling heavier and heavier.
> You are becoming sleepier...and sleepier...and sleepier.

(The subject's hand is now approaching his face, and his eyelids are blinking more rapidly.)

> Your eyes are becoming heavier...and heavier.
> Your hand is moving closer and closer towards your face.
> You are becoming drowsier...and drowsier...more and more tired.
> Your eyes are wanting to close now...closing...closing.
> When your hand touches your face...they will close immediately.
> You will fall into a very, very deep sleep.
> Drowsier...and drowsier...very, very sleepy...very, very tired.
> Your eyelids are beginning to feel just as heavy as lead.
> Your hand is moving closer and closer to your face.
> Closer...and closer...closer to your face.
> The moment it touches your face...you will fall into a very. very deep sleep.

(The subject's hand touches his face, and his eyes close.)

> *Go to to sleep! Go to sleep! Sleep very, very deeply!*
> And as you sleep...you will feel very, very tired...and relaxed.
> Let yourself go...Let yourself relax completely.
> Think of nothing but sleep...*deep, deep sleep!*

Notes on the hand levitation method. No attempt whatever should be made in the early stages to force any suggestions upon the subject. Sensations that almost anyone might experience are suggested to him as possibilities. Consequently, as he observes them, he looks upon them as a product of his own experience, and this renders him much more likely to respond to the suggestions of the hypnotist as if they, too, are parts of his own experience.

The first real suggestion is made when he is told that his fingers are beginning to separate, and if they do, then he is definitely responding to suggestion. When he is told that as his hand approaches his face he will become drowsier and drowsier, he is actually being requested to choose his own pace in falling asleep. Thus when his hand eventually touches his face, he will feel himself to be asleep to his own complete satisfaction, and will then be much less likely to deny the fact that he has been hypnotized.

There is little doubt that the subject hypnotized for the first time by this method will usually achieve deep hypnosis much more easily than he would, had any other method of induction been used. The method, however, has the grave disadvantage of being much more difficult and time consuming than any of the usual methods. Once started, it must be persevered with until the arm eventually rises, even if this takes an hour or more to achieve. Moreover, it is likely to fail unless the hypnotist has had wide technical experience. It is definitely a method for the expert, and in his hands it can prove to be one of the most valuable of all methods, since when successful it lends itself admirably to the more advanced analytical techniques. The serious student of hypnosis, however, would be well advised to avoid it until he has gained considerable experience and confidence, for failure would almost inevitably render the subject much more difficult to hypnotize by any alternative procedure.

AUTHORITARIAN TECHNIQUES

1. Modified Elman Technique

An American hypnotist Dave Elman[2] devised a technique which has become a popular method of induction used by many therapists in the UK. The attraction of this technique is that in experienced hands it can be particularly economical in time.

Summary of method. The subject is asked to rest comfortably on a couch or chair, to close his eyes and to breathe deeply. As he does so, suggestions of relaxation are given from head to toe with emphasis on the musculature around the eyes to the extent that on suggestion the eyes will fail to open. He is then instructed to open them again and then to close them when the feeling of relaxation will double. Should he have opened his eyes however in spite of the suggestion that he is unable to do so then he is simply asked to close them again and the feeling of relaxation is emphasized. The exercise is repeated with feelings of relaxation compounded each time the eyes are closed. This is followed by very positive suggestions of generalized physical relaxation.

Additional deepening is achieved by instructing the patient to count aloud and backwards say from 100 when the feeling of relaxation will double with each number. Further strong suggestions may then be given of the numbers just fading away and the patient being too tired even to bother to count.

A Typical Induction Routine

Now just rest back comfortably and take a deep breath.
As you breathe out, close your eyes.
Now let your entire body relax from your head to your toes and as you do so your eyes close tighter and tighter.
As your eyes close tighter your body relaxes more and more.
As you relax more and more your eyes close tighter and tighter.
As all the muscles of your eyes relax more and more, your body relaxes more and more.
The muscles of your eyes are so relaxed you just can't be bothered to use them.
Let them relax more and more so that you just can't be bothered to use them.
Don't use them.
Let them relax more and more...more and more.
You can't be bothered to use them.
Just try them...try to open your eyes.
Good...very good.
Now I will count from one to three and they will open and then from three to one and they will close again and you will double the feeling of relaxation...one, two, three—eyes open—three, two, one—eyes closed and deeply relaxed, deep, deep, deeply relaxed.

Should the eyes open in fact when the suggestions is given that they will not, then adopt the following procedure.

Good...good...good...now let them close again and double the feeling of relaxation.

Very, very relaxed...all the way around your eyes.
Your eyelids, your eyeballs, and every single muscle that
controls the movements of your eyes.
Just let go of any remaining tension...completely relaxed.
Relax more and more, relax your eyes more and more.
So much so that the muscles will not want to work.
Let them relax more and more so that you put them out of
action temporarily and they won't work, they just don't want to.
Open your eyes.
Good...good...good...now really open them and close them again and
double the feeling of relaxation.

This process may be repeated over again until the patient eventually will follow your instructions.

Now your entire body relaxes...all your facial muscles, your chin
and jaw muscles...down through the muscles of your neck to your
shoulders and shoulder joints. Your shoulder blades and every
bone and joint in your spine, every muscle and nerve in your back.
From your shoulders down each arm and hand to your fingertips
and from your shoulders through your chest and stomach muscles
and down to the tips of your toes completely relaxed.
I want to see the number 100 in your imagination...see it in
front of you.
Now count backwards from 100—count aloud as far as you can
go.
With each number that you count your feelings of relaxation will
double...deeper and deeper into relaxation.
Count now...deeper and deeper...
Ninety nine...deeper and deeper...
Ninety eight...deeper and deeper...
Let the numbers just fade away...and deeper...deeper...
Ninety seven...deep...deep, deep...
Can't be bothered to count any more...
The numbers fading away...let the numbers fade away...
Can't be bothered...deeply, deeply deeply relaxed...
Go to sleep!

2. Erickson's Confusional Technique

This procedure can be extremely useful in circumventing unconscious resistance in a subject who consciously wishes to be hypnotized. It can also be used to induce hypnosis when the subject is unaware that hypnosis is even contemplated and therefore *should never be practised without very careful consideration*. The method was originally designed and employed for the purposes of 'age regression', but was later found to be applicable to the induction of hypnosis and other hypnotic phenomena. Its main object is to establish a situation in which the subject is never sure whether he is actually co-operating or not, and under these circumstances his defences become ineffective. It is primarily a verbal technique which is based upon three main devices:

1. *A play upon words.* The following example is quoted by Erickson: 'Write right right, not rite or write.' This can be easily understood by the reader but not by the listener, who consequently struggles in vain to find some meaning in it. Before he can reject it, a further statement is made to engage his attention. Similarly, two words with opposite meanings can be correctly used to describe the same object—'If your left hand is tied behind your back, your right [hand] is left.'

2. *Alterations in the tenses.* This keeps the subject constantly trying to discover the intended meaning. For example—'Today *is* today, but it *was* yesterday's future, even as it *will be* tomorrow's *was*.'

Here, it will be noticed that the past, the present and the future are all used in connection with the reality of today.

3. The employment of irrelevancies. Each of these, taken out of context, appears to be a sound and sensible communication. Taken in context, they are confusing, distracting and inhibiting, and lead to a growing desire and need on the part of the subject to receive some communication which he can easily understand, and to which he can respond.

When using confusional techniques, the operator must maintain a casual but interested attitude and must speak seriously and intently, as if he expects the subject to understand exactly what is being said. The tenses must be carefully and constantly shifted, and a ready flow of language maintained. The subject should be given a little time to respond, but never quite sufficient for him to react fully before the next idea is presented. He consequently becomes so confused and frustrated that he feels a growing need for a clear-cut communication to which he can respond. Confusion techniques are prolonged and highly complex procedures, but once mastered they can lead to easy and rapid trance induction under the most unfavourable circumstances. A great deal of skill and experience is required, and they are not to be recommended to the beginner. If they are used in conjunction with hand levitation, the operator makes a series of contradictory statements in such a way that the subject feels that something meaningful and precise is being said. But he is still given insufficient time to realize how illogical the suggestions are:

> Your right hand is rising into the air...and your left hand is pressing down on the arm of the chair.
> Let your left hand rise into the air...and your right hand press down on the arm of the chair.
> Both hands are pressing down on the arms of the chair.
> One hand is now lifting up into the air...and the other is pressing down on the arm of the chair.
> Your right hand is rising into the air...and your left hand is pressing down on the arm of the chair...(Erickson[3]).

Confused by these rapidly conflicting instructions, in sheer desperation the subject is likely to accept and carry out the first positive suggestion that will enable him to escape from his dilemma.

3. The Direct Eye Gaze Method

This is a method of induction which may be useful only under certain special circumstances. Whilst it undoubtedly tends to produce a rather deeper form of hypnosis which facilitates further deepening, it is far too authoritative, and for this reason alone it should never be recommended as a routine procedure. It relies far too much upon personality and the subject is bound to feel that he is being dominated by the hypnotist, an undesirable feature which is best avoided.

It should be reserved for the rare occasions when the subject's reactions to other methods of induction indicate clearly that his personality is only likely to respond to a dominant approach. On the other hand, if a subject finds it impossible to accept the fact that he has really been hypnotized, which fortunately seldom happens, it may occasionally be resorted to in the form of a challenge, the subject being told to resist the sleep suggestions for as long as he can, and that the harder he tries to keep his eyes open — the more quickly they will close. Whilst this never fails to carry conviction, it is not advisable to attempt this method until a great deal of confidence and experience has been attained.

Summary of method. The hypnotist sits in front of the subject and leans slightly forward. He holds the subject's hands, and tells him to gaze into his eyes from a distance of approximately 2 feet. Since this involves the slight risk that the hypnotist, if unduly susceptible himself, might be the first to succumb, it is usually advisable not to stare directly into the subject's eyes, but to gaze at the bridge of his nose. He will be quite unable to detect the difference.

During the induction, should the hypnotist's own eyes become tired, or should he feel the least bit drowsy himself, he should deliberately close the subject's eyes with his fingers whilst simultaneously closing his own, in order to give them a brief rest. It is quite safe to do this because the subject will never realize that it is not an essential part of the technique. After a few moments, the hypnotist can open the subject's eyes again and resume his fixed state. Whilst the subject's eyes are held unwaveringly in this manner, the same type of verbal suggestions of relaxation, drowsiness, heaviness of the eyelids and eye closure are made, as in the techniques already described.

This is not a particularly difficult method of induction, but its success depends upon one's ability to maintain an unblinking stare long enough to cause the subject's eyes to close. The eyes can be trained for this technique by gazing fixedly at the tip of a pencil held about 18 inches in front of the eyes. Practice will greatly increase the length of time they can be kept open before they start to water or blink.

AWAKENING THE SUBJECT

In a few moments...when I count up to *seven*...you will open your eyes and be wide awake again.
You will wake up feeling wonderfully better for this deep, refreshing sleep.

You will feel completely relaxed...both mentally and
physically...quite calm and composed...without the slightest
feeling of drowsiness or tiredness.
And next time...you will not only be able to go into this sleep
much more quickly and easily...but you will also be able to relax
very much deeper.
Each time, in fact...your sleep will become deeper and deeper.
One...two...three...four...five...six...seven! Eyes open...wide awake.

After waking the subject, allow him to discuss the sensations
that he has actually experienced during the induction should he
so wish. This not only enables you to set his mind at rest concerning any doubts he may have entertained, but also informs you of
any feelings he may have experienced other than those that had
been suggested. These should be carefully noted in order to incorporate them as additional suggestions during his next induction.
This can often greatly facilitate the induction and deepening of
hypnosis.

REFERENCES

1. Wolberg L.R., 1948, *Medical Hypnosis,* Vol. 1. Grune and Stratton, New York.
2. Elman D., 1964. *Hypnotherapy*. Westwood, Glendale, CA.
3. Erickson M.H., 1964. The confusion technique in hypnosis. *Am. J. Clin. Hypnosis,* **6,** 183.

CHAPTER 6

Further Methods of Deepening the Trance State

The precise depth of trance which any individual subject attains after three or four successive inductions, and after all methods of deepening have been attempted, is likely to remain fairly constant. Once having reached this depth the subject does not tend to vary or fluctuate much unless he becomes emotionally disturbed. Consequently, if after several sessions the subject has only succeeded in entering a light trance state, it is most unlikely that further training in hypnosis will convert him into a deep-trance subject. There are, of course, exceptions to this rule and the use of an alternative method of induction may sometimes result in a deeper trance. In any event, no suggestion should be made to the patient that he is only able to achieve a light state as he may interpret this as failure on his part and this would be most undesirable. A light trance state will suffice for therapy in many uncomplicated cases.

After the first successful induction, when the subject's eyes have closed and he has entered a light hypnotic state, the next objective is gradually to deepen the trance as much as possible. There are many ways of achieving this, and some which are likely to prove most useful in routine clinical practice will be described.

METHODS OF DEEPENING THE TRANCE

1. By direct suggestion.
2. By relation of depth to performance.
3. By counting and breathing techniques.
4. By the induction of graded responses.
5. By 'visualization' techniques.
6. By Vogt's 'fractionation' method.
7. By the 'dissociation' method.

Of these methods, only the first five will normally need to be employed as routine procedures. Vogt's method can occasionally prove extremely useful in refractory cases, but the dissociation method is not altogether devoid of risk and is probably best left to the psychiatrist. The first two methods particularly have already been incorporated in most of the typical trance inductions that have been described.

1. Deepening by Direct Suggestion

During the course of trance induction it is continually suggested to the subject over and over again, that he is relaxing into a deeper and deeper sleep. Indeed, the repetition at intervals of the words 'Deeper and deeper asleep' and 'Very, very deeply asleep' have a strong influence in eliciting the desired response. Post-hypnotic suggestion, with which the subject will comply after being awakened, can also be made to play an important part.

Next time...you will not only fall asleep more quickly...but you will also relax into a deeper, deeper sleep...much deeper than this time.

It is always wise to give this particular suggestion at the end of each session, before waking the subject.

2. Deepening by the Relation of Depth to Performance

The subject is repeatedly told to relate the performance of something that is actually happening to him during the hypnotic state to further deepening of the trance. Similarly, any feeling that he is experiencing can be similarly related to an increase in depth.

As your arm falls limply back on to your lap...you are falling into a

deeper, deeper sleep.
As your hand floats upwards into the air...your sleep is
becoming deeper and deeper.
As you feel more and more relaxed...so you are relaxing into a
deeper, deeper sleep.

As has already been indicated, it is important to couple in this
way, the suggestion of something that is required to happen with
something that is actually happening at the time.

3. Deepening by the Use of Counting and Breathing Techniques

The efficiency of these particular methods of deepening can be
greatly heightened if it is first explained to the subject the reason
why his depth is going to increase.

Although none of us normally realize it, each time we breathe out
in everyday life, we tend to relax. Perhaps you would like to try
this for yourself. Take a deep breath...fill your chest...and hold it
until I tell you to '*Let go*'.
Now I want you to notice the tension in your chest muscles...the
tension in your shoulders and upper arms. And I want you to
pay particular attention to how...the moment I say '*Let go*'...all
the tension disappears immediately...and you allow yourself to
sag limply down into the chair.
Now...'*Let go*'.

The subject invariably finds this simple demonstration most
convincing and it greatly facilitates the procedures that it is intended to employ.

There are a number of variations in the use of counting and breathing techniques and although a simple count alone is often considered to be sufficient, as a routine procedure a combination of
the two is preferable. The subject is told that as the hypnotist
counts slowly from one to five, he will take five deep breaths, and
that each time he breathes out—slowly and deliberately—he will
feel himself becoming more and more deeply relaxed and falling
into a deeper, deeper sleep.

I am going to count slowly up to *five*...and as I do so...you will take
five deep breaths.
And with each deep breath that you take...each time you

breathe out...you will become more and more relaxed...and your
sleep will become deeper and deeper.
One...Deep breath...let go...more and more deeply
relaxed...deeper and deeper asleep.
Two...Deep breath...let go...deeper and deeper relaxed...sleep
becoming deeper and deeper.
Three...Deeper breath...let go...more and more deeply
relaxed...more and more deeply asleep.
Four...Very deep breath...let go...deeper and deeper
relaxed...sleep becoming even deeper and deeper.
Five...Very, very deep breath...let go...very, very deeply
relaxed...very, very deeply asleep and breathing quietly and
normally now.

Not only is this an efficient method of deepening the trance, but
the extent to which the subject's respiratory efforts are increased
affords a useful guide to the extent to which he is responding to
suggestion.

This procedure can often be followed most effectively by a modification of the suggestions given to the subject in the first place,
as follows:

Once again...I want you to take one deep breath...fill your chest
and hold it until I say...'*Let go*'.
Then...let your breath out *as quickly as possible*...and as you do
so...you will feel yourself sagging limply back into the
chair...and you will become twice as deeply relaxed as you are
now...twice as deeply asleep.
Now, take that deep breath...fill your chest...*Hold it*...(five seconds
pause)...*Let go*...

The instruction to inhale deeply is repeated two or three times,
on each occasion asking the patient to retain the breath for a few
seconds longer, then to 'let go' into a deeper and deeper sleep.
Hardly ever does this fail to achieve a significant deepening of the
trance, and in many cases the subject will slump into the chair
with his head sagging either sideways or forwards, indicating a
considerable increase in relaxation and consequent deepening of
the trance. The subject who has been instructed in self-hypnosis
should not be taught to deepen his self-induced trance by employing this technique, but may be shown how to synchronize relaxation with the normal action of exhalation.

4. Deepening by the Induction of Graded Responses

This method involves deepening the hypnosis by the application of a series of graduated tests, each being a little more difficult than the last. A successful response to each of these in turn will progressively increase the subject's suggestibility and pave the way for the next.

There are seven main responses that can be suggested consecutively, each of which is rather more complicated and difficult to elicit than the preceding one, and the subject who responds successively to each of these has certainly achieved a medium trance state, and often a deep or even somnambulistic trance. It has proved to be one of the most valuable and satisfactory methods of progressively deepening the trance. Of these seven tests, however, it is preferable not to employ any which involve a direct challenge, which may tend to re-awaken conscious activity and unconscious fears.

    i.   The induction of limb heaviness.
    ii. The induction of limb catalepsy.
    iii. The inductionof limb rigidity.
    iv. The inhibition of voluntary movements.
    v. The induction of automatic movements.
    vi. Dream induction.
    vii. The induction of lid catalepsy.

i. *The Induction of Limb Heaviness*

The subject is asked to place his arm upon the arm of the chair and is told that it is gradually feeling heavier and heavier, and that presently, if he attempts to lift it, it will drop back on to the chair just like a lead weight.

> Now place your arm on the arm of the chair.
> And as it rests on the chair...you will begin to experience a
> feeling of heaviness in your arm.
> That feeling of heaviness is increasing...every time that you
> breathe out, your body sags into the chair and your arm feels
> heavier...and heavier...just as heavy as lead.
> *You can feel it pressing down more firmly on the arm of the chair.*

And in a few moments...your arm will feel so very, very
heavy...*that if you try to lift it...it will drop back limply on to
your chair...just like a lead weight.*
And as it drops back...on to your chair...you will fall into a
deeper, deeper sleep.
You have now fallen into a much deeper sleep.
And as you do so...you will notice that all feelings of heaviness
are now leaving your arm.
It is coming back to normal...and feels just the same as your
other arm.
And as it does so...your sleep is becoming even deeper, and deeper.

This restoration to normality is an important step which must
never, under any circumstances, be forgotten.

ii. *The Induction of Limb Catalepsy*

The subject is asked to raise his arm above his head and he is
told that all sensations of heaviness are leaving it and that it is
becoming lighter and lighter as if there were no weight in it at all.
He is told that as he concentrates more and more upon his arm it
will become lighter and lighter with a pleasant feeling as if floating on air. It will no longer want to drop on to his chair, but will
remain just where it is without him having to make the slightest
effort to keep it there.

Your arm no longer feels heavy.
In fact...it is beginning to feel lighter and lighter.
Just as light as a feather...as if there is no weight in it at all.
And as this happens,...your arm will no longer want to drop
down...on to your chair.
It will want to remain just where it is...exactly where it is.
*It will no longer want to fall...it will remain just where it
is...without your having to make the slightest effort to keep it
there.*
But now gradually as I speak to you, the arm is returning to
normal. As I talk to you the normal weight is returning to the arm.
The arm is slowly descending and as it touches the chair so you fall
into a much deeper sleep.

These suggestions are continued until the arm is seen to sink
on to the arm of the chair.

iii. *The Induction of Limb Rigidity*

The subject is asked to extend his arm horizontally at shoulder level. He is told to hold it out, stiffly and rigidly, with the palm facing the ceiling and he is told that it is becoming stiffer and straighter and more and more rigid, that it is feeling just as stiff and rigid as a steel poker, so that it cannot possibly be bent at the elbow, until the count of three.

> As you extend your arm...you will feel that it is becoming much stiffer and straighter.
> The stiffness is increasing...with every word that I say, stiffer and stiffer.
> You can feel all the muscles tightening up...pulling your arm out...stiffer and straighter...with every word that I say...until it is beginning to feel just as stiff and rigid as a steel poker...from the shoulder to the wrist.
> Now, I want you to concentrate on a steel poker.
> Picture a steel poker in your mind.
> And as you do so...you will feel that your arm has become just as stiff and rigid as that steel poker.
> As if the elbow joint is firmly locked.
> As if there is no elbow joint there at all.
> *So that it will be impossible for you to bend your arm at the elbow...until I count up to 'three'.*
> The harder you try to bend it...the stiffer, and more rigid it will become.
> But, the moment I count 'three'...all the stiffness will pass away immediately...your arm will bend quite easily...and, as it does so...you will fall immediately into a deeper, deeper sleep.

At this point, you will usually find that the arm is so stiff and rigid that the patient will apparently be quite unable to bend it, even if he seems to be trying hard to do so. Having tested it, count up to three, and you will notice that the stiffness passes off quite suddenly, sometimes with a distinct jerk. You can do a great deal to ensure the success of this response by seeing that the arm is being held absolutely stiff and rigid in the first place, before you begin to suggest increased stiffness and rigidity. It is also important to see that the palm of the hand faces upwards towards the ceiling. Some authorities, Weitzenhoffer[1,2] for example, always use a direct challenge to the subject after inducing arm rigidity, on the grounds that if the trance is not deep enough to make this suggestion effective it would be better to start all over again, preferably using a different method. However, there should be no necessity for this. Possibly the precise wording of the suggestion— 'It will be impossible for you to bend it'—acts as a disguised challenge, for subsequent testing certainly convinces the subject that it cannot be bent, and further deepening techniques are usually successful, sometimes to the extent of producing somnambulism. Avoiding a direct challenge in this way not only diminishes the risk of failure, but also prevents unnecessary re-activation of the subject's conscious mind.

iv. *The Inhibition of Voluntary Movements*

The success of this response in deepening hypnosis is dependent upon a direct challenge to the subject. It is therefore as well to avoid its use as a routine deepening procedure, and to reserve it for special circumstances only.

As the state of hypnosis becomes deeper, the subject becomes more and more susceptible to suggestions that he will lose control over various groups of voluntary muscles. Small isolated groups will tend to be affected at first, but eventually the whole body may become involved.

Many different tests have been devised of which the hand clasp test is probably the most useful and convenient.

> I want you to hold your arms straight out in front of you.
> Hold them as stiff and rigid as you can, and clasp your hands together.
> Interlock your fingers, and keep them tightly locked together.
> Tighter and tighter.
> As you clasp your hands tighter and tighter together...you will feel your fingers gripping more and more firmly.
> And as they do so...I want you to picture a heavy vice.
> Imagine you can see the jaws of that vice...being screwed tighter and tighter together.
> Now, picture that vice clearly in your mind...and concentrate on it.
> And as you do so...just imagine that your hands represent the jaws of that vice...that they are slowly becoming locked

together...tighter and tighter together.
As I count up to *five*...your hands are becoming locked
together...tighter and tighter...and when I reach the count of
five...they will be so tightly locked...that they will feel just like a
solid block of metal...and it will be quite impossible for you to
separate them.
One...tightly locked...*two*...tighter and tighter...*three*...very, very
tight...*four*...the palms of your hands are locked tightly
together...*five*...*they are so tightly locked that it will be impossible
for you to separate them until I count up to 'three'...the harder you
try to separate the palms of your hands...the tighter your fingers
will press upon the back of your hands...and the tighter your hands
will become locked together.*

When this process has been successfully completed be sure to
remove the suggestion and to restore the hands to complete normality, using even this suggestion to increase the depth of hypnosis.

Various other suggestions can be made. The subject may be
given something to hold in his hand and told that he will be unable to drop it. He may be told that he will be unable to pronounce
certain words, or that his body muscles have become so limp and
relaxed that he will find it impossible to get out of his chair. Tests
of this kind have been extremely popular with stage hypnotists.

v. *The Induction of Automatic Movements*

The production of automatic movements always signifies a
rather deeper stage of hypnosis. The subject is asked to place his
arm upon the arm of the chair, and to raise the fore-arm into a
vertical position, the elbow remaining supported by the arm of
the chair. Then to move the hand and fore-arm slowly, backwards
and forwards.

Imagine your arm moving slowly...backwards and
forwards...backwards and forwards...I want you to imagine that
the centre of a piece of cord is tied around your wrist...and that
each end of the cord is pulling your arm...first backwards...then
forwards.
Picture that piece of cord, tied round your wrist...pulling your
arm slowly...backwards...and forwards...backwards and
forwards.

And your arm will go on moving...entirely on its
own...backwards and forwards...backwards and forwards...until
I tell you to stop.
You won't try to make it move!
You won't try to stop it moving!
You will just let it please itself...and it will go on moving on its
own...quite automatically...backwards and forwards...backwards
and forwards...until I tell you to stop.
*Backwards and forwards...backwards and forwards...backwards
and forwards.*

(At this point, his arm continues to move automatically, backwards and forwards until he is told to stop.)

Now stop!
Put your arm back...on to the arm of your chair...and as you do
so...you are falling into an even deeper, deeper sleep.
Sleep...very, very deeply!

As the subject's arm moves backwards and forwards, tell him
that his sleep is becoming 'deeper, deeper, deeper'—timing this
so that the word deeper is repeated on each alternate forward
movement of his arm.

vi. *Dream Induction*

In this particular technique, the subject is told that presently
he is going to dream, and that he will dream that he is performing
whatever action he is instructed to dream about but this will be
a pleasant and relaxing experience. The particular action that is
suggested should always be made as simple and natural as
possible. For instance a woman can be told that she will be able
to picture herself tidying her hair, or removing an ear-ring. A man
can be told that he is straightening his tie, brushing his hair or
buttoning his coat or jacket.

When these instructions have been given and the suggestion
made to the subject that he will dream, he is told to *show* the hypnotist exactly what he is dreaming about. If a successful response
is obtained, the subject's hands will move slowly upwards and he
will actually carry out the suggested action.

You are now so deeply asleep...that everything that I tell you that is going to happen...*will* happen...*exactly* as I tell you.
And every feeling I tell you that you will experience...you will experience...*exactly* as I tell you.
Moreover, every single instruction that I give you...you will carry out faithfully.
Just as your arm felt heavy...when I told you it would feel heavy.
Just as your arm felt stiff...when I told you it would feel stiff.
Just as your arm moved on its own...when I told you it would move on its own.
So...everything else I tell you that is going to happen...*will* happen...*exactly* as I tell you.
Every feeling I tell you that you will experience...you *will* experience...*exactly* as I tell you.
And every single instruction that I give you...you will follow carefully.
You are now so deeply asleep...that, in a few moments...when I tell you to dream...*you will dream!*
And you will dream that you are performing whatever simple action I tell you to dream about but this will be a pleasant and relaxing experience.
You will be able to picture yourself...quite clearly...and see yourself...quite vividly...in your own mind...carrying out whatever action I have told you to dream about.
Just as you pictured that steel poker...in your mind...when your arm went stiff.
Just as you pictured that piece of cord, tied round your wrist...when your arm moved on its own.
So...you will be able to picture yourself in your dream...equally vividly and clearly...performing whatever simple action that I tell you to dream about.
Now...you are going to dream...that you are straightening your tie.
You are going to dream...that you are straightening your tie.
Now dream! Dream! Dream!

(Pause)

Now...show me what you are dreaming!
Show me, now!
Show me what you are dreaming!

When this test succeeds the subject's hands will be seen to move slowly upwards and he will actually carry out the suggested action. Sometimes there is a delay, and if so, just watch his hands carefully. The slightest movement of them betrays an impulse to comply with the suggestion, in which case the repetition, once or twice in a more authoritative tone, of the instruction to show what he is dreaming, will usually secure the desired response. If he still fails to comply, he should be asked whether he is dreaming, and if not, why he thinks he is unable to dream.

A female subject had responded extremely well to all the previous deepening routines, yet dream induction seemed to fail completely. She was told to dream that she was in the bathroom at home, washing her hands. When she failed to respond, she was asked whether she was dreaming, and she said no. She was then asked why she wasn't dreaming, and replied that she hadn't a bathroom at home. A subsequent suggestion that she would dream that she was knitting elicited an immediate response, and she knitted away furiously. Obviously, one has to be careful not to impose impossible conditions unwittingly.

The value of this particular deepening technique lies in the fact that, whenever it succeeds, the subject will never fail to accept the post-hypnotic suggestions that, in future, he will always enter the hypnotic state immediately upon word of command. This is known as post-hypnotic conditioning. However, it must be emphasized, throughout the suggestions given, that the dream is a pleasant and relaxing experience. It must be added also that this is not a technique for the amateur to attempt.

vii. *The Induction of Lid Catalepsy*

Whilst the success of this response will usually facilitate further deepening procedures, failure, which is quite likely to occur, will undoubtedly make these much more difficult. Lid catalepsy is most unpredictable. In good subjects, it can be one of the earliest and most convincing signs of hypnosis to be elicited, and can often be successfully induced immediately after eye closure. The subject naturally accepts this as proof that something has actually occurred, his susceptibility consequently increases and he will much more readily accept suggestions of further deepening of his hypnosis. It should be pointed out, however, that in subjects of this calibre, the phenomenon is rarely likely to be essential to the successful induction of greater depth. In other cases it will be found impossible to secure this response until the subject has already entered a deep trance, and failure to do so at an earlier stage will inevitably diminish the subject's suggestibility and render further deepening difficult, if not impossible. This is a grave disadvantage which renders it quite unsuitable as a routine procedure since the direct challenge that is involved invariably reawakens some degree of conscious activity. It should be used when satisfied that further depth will only be obtained after the subject is convinced of the genuineness of his hypnosis. This, of course, can only be done by successfully challenging his ability to perform a certain action in defiance of the instruction. The reason for any resistance to this suggestion is not difficult to understand. Inability to open the eyes may suggest to the subject—even in hypnosis—something much more threatening than merely depth of trance. It may mean the surrender of his last vestige of control, something more than even hypnotic 'sleep', even death. The failure of this suggestion will also mean considerable loss of prestige for the therapist and could well contribute to failure of treatment.

However, if it is used, the subject is told that his eyes are so tightly closed that the eyelids feel that they are glued together...and it will be impossible for him to open them...no matter how hard he tries, until he is told to do so...and that the harder he tries to open them—the tighter they will close. Notice how this last statement turns the efforts of the subject to resist the suggestion against himself, and helps to defeat any attempts that he may make.

> Your eyes are now so tightly closed...that the eyelids feel as though they are firmly glued together.
> So tightly closed...so firmly glued together...that it will be impossible for you to open them, until I tell you to do so.
> *The harder you try to open them...the tighter they will close!*
> It is impossible for you to open your eyes!
> You cannot possibly open them!
> The harder you try...the harder they will close!
> Now try to open your eyes.
> You see! You *cannot* possibly open them!

Should the subject show signs of being able to open his eyes, say to him quickly, 'Open them, now! You notice how difficult it was. Next time, it will be even more difficult.' Always try to get him to admit that he did feel some difficulty. You may say to him:

> I want you to imagine that you have a sore spot...at the top of your forehead.
> With your eyes still closed...I want you to roll them upwards behind the closed lids...and look firmly, upwards and backwards at that sore spot. Don't let your eyes wander from it for a moment...and you will find that your eyes are now so tightly closed...etc.

If you try this for yourself in the waking state, you will find how difficult it is for you to open your eyes as long as you keep look-ing upward and backward. That is because the eye muscles are being held in such a position that it is practically impossible for them to lift the lids. The subject, of course, attributes his inability solely to the effect of hypnotic suggestion.

As an alternative and more 'permissive' method of securing lid catalepsy, you can instruct the subject to *pretend* that his eye lids are so tightly closed that as long as he continues to pretend, he will allow them to become so completely relaxed that he will find it quite impossible to open them.

> I want you to pretend that your eyes are so tightly closed that you cannot possibly open them.
> And as long as you continue to pretend...you will keep relaxing your eye muscles more and more...deeper and deeper.
> Let all those muscles around your eyes relax more...and more...and more...until they are so completely relaxed that as long as you keep on pretending that you cannot open them...*it will be impossible for you to do so.*
> When you try...you'll find that they just won't respond.
> They just *won't* open.
> If you do manage to open them...it will simply mean that you have stopped pretending...and have not allowed those muscles of your eyes to relax completely. What I want you to do...is to get them so relaxed that they just won't open. After all...a relaxed muscle cannot contract...so, as long as you keep on pretending ...and really have those eye muscles relaxed...they just can't open. So, go on pretending...and relax them more and more.

And the moment you're sure that you have them so relaxed that
they won't open...I want you to test them for yourself.
You see...you can wrinkle your forehead...you can lift your eye
brows...*but you just cannot open your eyes.*

More often than not, these suggestions will act in the waking
state, so one need hardly be surprised that they are frequently effective under hypnosis and facilitate deepening of the trance.

5. Deepening by the Use of 'Visualization' Techniques

These are simple and can prove extremely effective, but before
using them it is always wise to test your subject's capacity for visual imagery. People vary in this respect, and if they do not possess this ability it is a waste of time attempting such procedures.
Testing can be done quite quickly and easily in the following manner:

I am going to test your powers of imagination, so whilst you are
lying comfortably relaxed in the chair, I want you to imagine that
you can see a pair of shoes. Just visualize them...and try to picture
them quite clearly in your mind's eye.
Tell me...what colour are those shoes?
What are they made of?
What kind of heels have they?
Do they fasten up at all...and if so...how?

Notice that you do not ask the subject whether he can visualize
the shoes. You ask him *'What colour are they?'* so that if he responds, there is no doubt that he is picturing them. Otherwise,
he would be unable to answer this question. If he has little or no
difficulty in describing these shoes, you can feel confident that he
possesses a sufficient capacity for visual imagery for you to proceed with one or other of the visualization techniques.

Many and varied visualization methods exist and equally as
many can be invented by the therapist, largely depending upon
his own imaginative powers. Holiday scenes, the garden, the
beach or countryside are favourite venues. Activities such as
mountain climbing or sailing should be avoided as also should descending stairs or escalators. The idea of going down and down
may arouse hidden fears so that words must be chosen with great

care. All possible adverse effects and misinterpretations should be anticipated and avoided. For example in depicting a garden or country scene an exclusion clause must be inserted such as...'and if you suffer from hay fever or any allergy on this occasion there is no pollen or substance around to which you may be sensitive.' Or in a description of a beach scene, make certain of the subject's response to sunshine or indeed that the type of holiday is to his liking, since many prefer a more active form of 'relaxing' and thus such a technique may be counter-productive. The question may be easily resolved before induction commences, by simply asking, for example, 'what sort of holiday do you prefer?' Then proceed:

I would like you to imagine a situation in which you are on holiday. You are staying in a beautiful resort where the sun always shines and the temperature is just as you would like it. You spend part of the day relaxing and part, if you wish, exploring or in more active occupations. This is the relaxing part. Just wander down to the gardens, and look around at the peaceful scene before you. Note the mass of exotic plants and the vivid colour of the flowers. Take a deep breath...and as you breathe out relax deeper and deeper. Wander slowly towards them and as you approach them the scent is more fragrant than any you have experienced. Take a deep breath again and inhale the soft, warm and perfumed air...and as you breathe out, relax deeper and deeper. Now continue on your way, to that pretty winding pathway which takes you down to the beach. Wander along, relaxing deeper and deeper with every step. There is that beautiful beach with miles of golden sand. There, a sunshade, especially for you and beneath it a most inviting deck chair. Stroll across the sand to the chair, sit down, slip off your shoes and just lie back. Adjust the sunshade so that it is just right for you...Take a deep breath once more and relax deeper and deeper as you breathe out. Look out at the calm blue sea, the waves are lapping lazily on the beach and a fishing boat, with its colourful sail, is gently bobbing up and down. The sun is shining, the sky is blue and not a cloud in sight...Take a deep breath, and as you breathe out relax deeper and deeper than ever before...and as you relax deeper and deeper...*Go to sleep...sleep...deep, deep, sleep...deeper and deeper than ever before.*

Using another setting the age-old technique of counting sheep may be employed. After setting the appropriate scene, proceed in this way...

Look across at those beautiful green fields, the lush long grass
waving gently in the breeze. Watch those sheep grazing in the
distance, some black and some white. Take a deep breath, and as
you breathe out, relax deeper and deeper. As that first sheep
moves, the others follow, nudging his head away so as to graze on
his patch. He moves towards the fence and they follow...Take a
deep breath again and relax deeper and deeper...
That first sheep grows tired of being pushed around and jumps
over the fence—but the others follow...count them as they
jump...one...two...three...(The therapist should speak in time to
the subject's breathing.)
Relax deeper and deeper.
Four...five...six...
deeper and deeper.
Seven...eight...nine...ten...
Relax very very deeply indeed.
Tell me...what colour was that last sheep?
The subject will tell you.
Good...now take a deep breath in once more and as you breathe out
relax deeper than ever before.

There may be no end to the peaceful and relaxing situations
which can occur to the therapist. New ideas for deepening may be
invented as experience increases but these should always reinforce feelings of peace and calm and never suggest any threat to
the patient.

6. Deepening by Vogt's Fractionation Method

This is reputed to be one of the most effective methods of inducing very deep trance states, and it is claimed that it will often succeed when all others have failed. It is certainly an excellent way
of handling difficult subjects who, having entered a light hypnotic
state, upon awakening express doubts as to whether they have
actually been hypnotized at all.

The essential feature of this method is the repeated hypnotizing and awakening of the subject in rapid succession, several
times in the course of each of the first few sessions. The theory is
that each hypnotization renders the subject more suggestible, and
thus favours the induction of a deeper state at each successive attempt. One of the most effective ways of using it is that described

by Weitzenhoffer[1], which forms the basis of the following routine:

> I am now going to wake you up by counting up to *seven*.
> After I have done so...although your eyes will be open...whilst I
> am talking to you...you will begin to feel very, very drowsy and
> sleepy again.
> You will find it harder and harder to keep your eyes open...and
> to stay awake.
> Your eyes will feel very, very heavy...the eyelids will feel heavier
> and heavier...and will begin to blink.
> You will not be able to stop them blinking.
> And as they blink...you will find it more and more difficult to
> keep them open.
> They will want to close...you will not be able to stop them from
> closing.
> Every moment...as I go on talking...you will feel drowsier and
> drowsier...sleepier and sleepier.
> Your eyes will close...and you will fall into a deep, deep sleep.
> You will be in a much deeper sleep than you are now!
> I am going to count slowly up to *seven*.
> As I do so...you will open your eyes and wake up.
> But you will feel very, very drowsy...very, very sleepy.
> Your eyes will feel so heavy...so very, very tired...that you will
> not be able to keep them open for long.
> They will start to blink...you will be unable to stop them from
> blinking.
> And as they do so...your eyes will feel so very, very tired that they
> will close...and you will fall into a much, much deeper sleep!

After being awakened, the subject's eyes will either start to
blink, or he may seem to remain sleepy with his eyes half-closed.
He should be asked what is the matter with his eyes, and may
even say that he feels sleepy. Sometimes, however, he will seem
to be puzzled and say that he doesn't know, or that the light is
troubling his eyes. A simple comment at this point, to the effect
that he is feeling sleepy and that it is difficult for him to keep his
eyes open, will often suffice to start him blinking or even closing
his eyes. This must be followed up immediately:

> You see! Your eyes *are* feeling heavier and heavier!
> You *are* feeling very, very drowsy...and sleepy.
> Your eyes are closing...and you are falling into a deeper, deeper
> sleep.

Go to sleep!

Sometimes, this will be unnecessary since the eyes will not only start to blink but will also close entirely on their own. In this case, the above suggestions should be modified accordingly.

> You see! Your eyes *have* closed on their own.
> Sleep very, very deeply...very, very deeply.
> Deeper and deeper asleep...deeper and deeper asleep!

Alternatively, just as his eyes seem about to close, you can say to him authoritatively:

> *Sleep!*
> *Sleep...very, very deeply...very, very deeply!*
> *Deeper and deeper asleep...deeper and deeper asleep!*
> *Go to sleep...very, very deeply!*

Although the trance may now be further deepened by any of the usual procedures, this is not often done since the method in itself is designed to effect further deepening. Nevertheless, it is useful to deepen it further by using the counting and breathing technique before waking the subject and repeating the procedure. This should be carried out on several occasions during each of the first few sessions.

Subsequent procedures. Before being awakened, the subject can be told that whenever you either suggest sleep or even mention the word sleep, his eyes will close and he will fall into a deep sleep from which he will not awaken until told to do so.

Tell him that when you count up to seven, he will open his eyes and wake up. But as soon as you begin to talk to him, no matter what you are saying, his eyelids will begin to feel heavier and heavier...he will feel drowsier and sleepier...and that the moment he hears you mention the word sleep, or anything to do with sleep, he will be quite unable to resist the urge to close his eyes and fall into a deep, deep sleep.

When successful, and the trance has been deepened by a few more suggestions, Weitzenhoffer[1,2] advises the use of the lid catalepsy and the limb rigidity techniques, but avoiding the use of challenges in the following manner:

> Your eyes are now so tightly closed...that they feel as if the eyelids

are firmly glued together.
So tightly glued together...that it will be impossible for you to
open your eyes.
Even if you tried...you would find it quite impossible to open
them.
But you will have no wish to try!
You are just relaxing...more and more completely...and sinking
into a deeper, deeper sleep.

Alternatively, after you have stiffened the subject's arm, and
made it rigid, you can say:

You cannot bend your arm now!
It is so stiff and rigid...it is quite impossible for you to bend it.
Even if you tried...you would find it impossible to bend it.
But you will have no wish to try!
The moment I count *three*...your arm muscles will relax...the
stiffness will pass off again...and your arm will bend quite easily.
And as it does so...you will fall into a deeper, deeper sleep.

This technique is continued until the subject goes to sleep both
quickly and easily. The time it takes to achieve this will vary with
the type of subject with whom you are dealing, and how long you
are prepared to spend with him at each session. But once he has
reached this stage, you can proceed as follows:

From now on...whenever you hear me say *'Go to sleep'*...your
eyes will close immediately...and you will fall into a sleep...just
as deep as this one.

You should repeat this instruction twice, firmly, and with conviction. Then awaken the subject, and in a few seconds' time, in
an authoritative tone of voice tell him to go to sleep:

Go to sleep! Sleep deeply! Very, very deeply!

If his eyes fail to close immediately, these suggestions should be
repeated with even greater emphasis. Should they still remain
open, you should extend your first and second fingers and bring
them slowly towards his eyes, thus causing them to close instinc-
tively. As they do so, repeat the above suggestions even more emphatically. This procedure should be rehearsed over and over
again until the subject's eyes close immediately, whenever he is
instructed to go to sleep.

Some hypnotists prefer to employ a shortened version of this technique. They simply tell the subject that each time he falls asleep, his sleep will become deeper and deeper. They then proceed to hypnotize him and awaken him several times in rapid succession, until he enters the hypnotic state as soon as the induction is started.

The feedback technique. This is a variation of Vogt's method which can sometimes be extremely effective. It often succeeds with subjects who experience difficulty in achieving depth. The subject is asked to describe the exact sensations that he felt as he went into the light hypnotic state. Such sensations will be found to vary greatly in different subjects. The hypnotist takes careful note of each successive sensation, and the exact order in which they were actually experienced. During the next induction, suggestions are then made that the subject is going to feel each sensation that he did on the previous occasion, in the exact order in which they originally occurred.

This feedback technique has certain definite advantages. It avoids the suggestion of experiences that the subject may never have felt, or those to which he may have either an unconscious or even conscious resistance. Since the events suggested to him are those which have actually happened already, they are much more likely to happen again.

7. Deepening by the Dissociation Method

This depends upon the production of a fantasy in the subject's mind that he is actually watching someone else being induced into a deep hypnotic sleep. Since he begins by thus 'dissociating' himself from what is taking place, his own resistances are not aroused. The description of what is occurring, however, gradually induces him to identify himself with the supposed subject, and he begins to feel that the phenomena are actually happening to himself. He is able to allow this to happen because his resistances never become activated.

> I want you to imagine that you are standing outside the consulting-room door.
> You are beginning to feel quite interested...and as you grasp the

handle of the door...and slowly open it...this feeling of interest is increasing.
As you walk into the room...note how interested you are in what is going on.
There is a doctor in the room, who is dealing with a patient.
The doctor is wearing...

(Here you describe roughly what you, yourself, are wearing.)

The patient is wearing...

(Here you describe what your subject is actually wearing.)

Now, watch the doctor...and notice what is happening to the patient with him.
He is talking to the patient...and as he does so...something very curious is happening.
See how the patient's right hand and arm are starting to float up into the air.
His right hand is floating up...and up...and up.
Now, his whole arm is floating up...and up...and up.
And as it does so...you can see that he is falling into a deeper, deeper sleep.

(During this description, your subject's own arm usually starts to rise, as he identifies himself with the patient.)

This is an extremely powerful method of producing a deep trance state, since it depends upon what is called dissociation or temporary splitting of the subject's mind. It could be very dangerous in any undiagnosed pyschotic patient, in whom even under normal conditions the mind possesses a strong tendency to dissociate. You might consequently find it difficult if not impossible to achieve re-integration when you awaken him.

This is not a technique for the beginner nor for any therapist without psychiatric training and experience.

REFERENCES

1. Weitzenhoffer A.M., 1953. *Hypnotism: An Objective Study in Suggestibility*. Chapman and Hall, London.
2. Weitzenhoffer A.M., 1957. *General Techniques of Hypnosis*. Grune and Stratton, New York.

CHAPTER 7

Trance Resistance, Difficulties and a Test for Trance

Although in the average case when the subject is willing and co-operative the induction of hypnosis is comparatively easy to achieve, from time to time cases will be encountered in which varying degrees of difficulty will be experienced. Whenever this occurs, it is most important to try to discover the nature of the problem. For instance, if a subject fails to enter a trance state at all during the first hypnotic session, there is always some reason for this, and until this has been discovered and dealt with adequately, further attempts at induction will probably prove equally unsuccessful. It may be that the technique adopted will have to be modified to suit the needs of this particular subject, but even this cannot properly be decided until the nature of the difficulty is known.

Resistance to trance induction may be conscious or unconscious. The possibility of either or both occurring must be recognized. Undoubtedly extensive and discerning history taking should reveal the patient who is unable or unwilling to allow himself or herself to relax and alternative means of therapy must always be considered. However, if hypnotherapy is the treatment of choice for the condition diagnosed, then an attempt should certainly be made to uncover the reason for the resistance. Conscious problems must be fully discussed, doubts explained, fears allayed and misunderstandings resolved. Unconscious resistance should be fully explored. Fear of the unknown, fear of revealing past indiscretions, the skeleton in the cupboard, or of losing control. The patient has often learned to live with his problem, although he may not like it and because of that has built up a defence system which may well be impenetrable. He has learned to adapt to the threatening environment so that when his well-guarded barrier has been penetrated how would he cope with the world outside?

Perhaps the problem is not quite so concealed. Is your diagnosis correct? Hypomanic or psychotic patients are not easily hypnotizable and indeed no attempt should ever be made to treat these conditions with hypnosis. The patient may be too young to appreciate what you are saying or may be elderly with some cerebrovascular impairment. Be certain of your diagnosis before searching for other problems.

The best way of approaching this difficulty is to question the subject closely as to any difficulties that he may have felt during the induction. It is surprising how much valuable information can often be obtained from this simple measure alone. Even when the subject is unconscious of the real reason for his failure, talking it over with him will often reveal the necessary clue. Nevertheless it is also possible that he is rationalizing. However, the reason of greatest importance is what the patient *thinks* it is, and this reason cannot be lightly dismissed. Sometimes the method of induction may not suit the personality of the patient, in which case some other approach must be adopted. This is not as difficult a task as it might seem, provided that one is well acquainted with various kinds of difficulty that most commonly arise.

These can be summarized as follows:

1. Over-anxiety and fear of failure.
2. Fear of the hypnotic state itself.
3. Inadequate preparation before induction.
4. Defiance of authority and failure to establish rapport.
5. Fluctuating attention.
6. Need to prove superiority.
7. Physical discomfort.
8. Dislike of the method of induction employed.
9. Uncertainty on the part of the therapist.
10. Poor motivation and expectancy.

1. Over-anxiety and Fear of Failure

This is a very common source of difficulty. Indeed, over-anxiety to succeed with hypnosis is almost bound to interfere with successful induction. It is nearly always present to some extent in the patient who seeks psychological help and advice. Such patients have usually undergone many other kinds of treatment, none of which have succeeded in affording them the relief that they seek. Finally, as a last resort, they will even try hypnosis but with the conviction that nothing is really capable of solving their problems. They consequently attach little importance to their need to enter the trance successfully and this attitude is quite sufficient in itself to prevent them from achieving even the light trance state.

You will also meet the patient who, because of strong feelings of inferiority regards hypnosis as yet another test of his ability to perform. Since such a person is always convinced of his own inadequacy, failure is almost inevitable.

The only way of dealing with this situation is to give the patient the strongest possible reassurance and encouragement before proceeding with any further attempts at induction.

Tell him that it is not in the least important that he should succeed at the first attempt. Remind him of what happened when he first learned to ride a bicycle. During his first lesson it was impossible for him to balance on his own without somebody supporting him by holding the saddle. On the next occasion, he found himself able to remain seated and unsupported, for a few yards at a time and to proceed in a rather unsteady manner. Then, with each subsequent lesson, his control over his balance improved until he was able to manage on his own, without the need of any support at all. Tell him that he can be taught to enter the hypnotic state in easy stages in exactly the same way, so that there is actually nothing for him to worry about. Explain that deep hypnosis is neither necessary nor even desirable for most treatment purposes. Such relatively simple measures as these will often enable him to relax sufficiently to respond to future attempts at induction.

2. Fear of the Hypnotic State Itself

It sometimes happens that whilst the subject may be 'consciously' anxious and willing to be hypnotized, he may also be 'unconsciously' afraid of succumbing to the trance. When this is so, his 'unconscious' fear is usually that of 'losing control', and the mental conflict that consequently arises in his mind is quite sufficient to prevent him from entering the hypnotic state at all.

Now, this fear of losing control is much more common than might be imagined, and can manifest itself in two ways.

1. *If the subject's anxiety on this score is great* he will be quite unable to enter even the lightest hypnotic state.

2. *If he is only moderately worried* he may be able to achieve the light trance, but further deepening will usually prove impossible.

Obviously, the more you can allay his anxiety and his fears, the deeper the trance you will be likely to obtain. This particular difficulty, however, arises much less frequently when the subject's mind has been properly prepared before induction. He must be reassured that you have no intention of taking over control or of imposing *your* will upon him. That the main object of the exercise is to show him how he can regain control over himself and over his feelings and so to rid himself of the problem for which he is seeking treatment.

Not only should you give the subject the reassurance he requires regarding his fears, but you should also promise him that *nothing will be done without his prior knowledge and consent*. It is also useful to stress the fact that *it will be impossible to obtain any effect that he, himself, is unwilling to produce*.

Another excellent way of overcoming this fear of losing control is to prove to the patient that he can awaken himself from the trance at any moment he chooses. Tell him that once he has entered the trance state and you are giving him suggestions, he is to select any moment he likes, and deliberately awaken himself and should he so desire, his eyes will open and he will be wide awake again. Once he has put this to the test, you assure him that he will always be able to awaken himself immediately at any moment he wishes even before his treatment is completed. This simple procedure usually affords him all the reassurance he needs.

3. Inadequate Preparation before Induction

Most of the difficulties encountered in trance induction will be greatly lessened, if not entirely removed, if the subject's mind has been fully prepared before any attempt is made. Many of the difficulties that arise in the induction of hypnosis are due to far too little importance being given to the preparatory talk.

Just occasionally, a subject will say to you when he has been awakened:

> As you told me — I could hear everything that you said.
> At one stage, however, I thought I might have gone to sleep — but something seemed to stop me.

Now this is very important and should not be overlooked, for it shows that he could have gone deeper. He didn't — simply because at the last minute he became afraid of losing control. In such a case, full discussion may not only shed a great deal of light upon his difficulties, but he may even be able to suggest possible ways of overcoming them.

4. Defiance of Authority and Failure to Establish Rapport

Sometimes a subject will admit the fact that, during the induction of hypnosis, he experiences an irresistible impulse to oppose everything that is being suggested. Questioning will often reveal that this is a lifelong trait in his character and that even as a schoolboy he strongly resented authority. Curiously enough, ventilation and discussion of these feelings will often succeed in increasing his susceptibility. Point out to him that hypnosis is essentially a matter of teamwork, that without his full co-operation nothing can be achieved, and that you seek to exercise no more authority over him than he is willing to grant in order to treat his condition successfully.

5. Fluctuating Attention

This is a difficulty that is encountered from time to time during the induction of hypnosis. It usually occurs in the subject who has, what is aptly called, a 'grasshopper' mind. His power of concentration is poor, and his mind cannot remain fixed upon one idea, or his attention held for long enough to permit the induction to become successful. It flits incessantly from one subject to another.

The best way of dealing with this, by far, is to use a modified counting technique. This probably explains why this particular difficulty is much less frequently encountered when the eye fixation–distraction method of induction is used.

The following modification is the one which will be found most satisfactory:

> I want you to start counting slowly, to yourself...and to go on
> counting until you hear me tell you to stop.
> When you say...*one*...Close your eyes!
> When you say...*two*...Open your eyes!
> When you say...*three*...Close your eyes!
> When you say...*four*...Open your eyes.

The subject counts to himself, he opens and shuts his eyes deliberately with each alternate count. Whilst he is doing this he is quietly told how sleepy he is becoming, that his eyes are becoming more and more tired and his eyelids heavier and heavier, that presently they will want to remain closed and he will fall into a deep, deep sleep.

6. Need to Prove Superiority

From time to time, you will come across a subject to whom the mere induction of hypnosis seems to represent a challenge to his ability to perform. This particular resistance is often linked with one that we have already considered, namely defiance of authority, for once again a few simple questions will often reveal the fact that all his life the subject has resented taking orders from anyone. This is most important for if there is the slightest hint of dominance in the course of induction failure will be inevitable.

In dealing with such subjects it is necessary to emphasize, even to overemphasize, the importance of the part that they themselves play in the actual induction of hypnosis. At the same time every possible step should be taken to increase their motivation and pride of achievement. Tell them that it is only very intelligent people who make good hypnotic subjects, since a considerable degree of concentration and co-operation is required. Since, under most circumstances, the subject unconsciously tends to feel that he is the better man, this puts him upon his mettle and offers him the chance to prove it. For this reason alone, it is necessary to frame your suggestions in such a way as to challenge his ability to perform well. They should also succeed in conveying to him the impression that every effect that is produced has actually been achieved by his own efforts.

> Hold your arm out...stiff and straight...palm facing the ceiling.
> *Now, I want you to tell yourself*...that your arm is becoming stiffer and straighter...just like a steel poker.
> This needs a great deal of concentration...but you can do it quite easily...if you want to.
> Just concentrate upon letting your arm go stiff and straight.
> You want it to become so stiff...so straight...so rigid...that it will be quite impossible for *me* to bend it at the elbow.
> If you concentrate enough upon wanting this to happen...it *will* happen...it *will* become stiff and straight...so rigid...that I shall be quite unable to bend it at the elbow...until I ask you to count *three.*
> But...the moment you count *three*...your arm will bend quite easily again...and your sleep will become much, much deeper.

7. Physical Discomfort

Physical discomfort can greatly hinder the successful induction of hypnosis, therefore the subject should always be made as comfortable as possible. He should visit the toilet before settling down on the couch or chair. Draughts should be avoided, and he should be kept warm and, if necessary, given a rug. Loud and unexpected noises should be avoided if possible. Care should be taken to see that he is not holding his head and neck in a position of undue strain when he is asked to look upwards and backwards. Sometimes the subject himself when awakened will remark that he was not comfortable and that this prevented him from going into hypnosis, or that he felt quite shivery and cold or that his beck felt strained.

It must be borne in mind, however, that these simple explana-

tions are not always founded upon fact. They are often pure rationalizations of the real reason for failure, which is to be found in unconscious anxiety.

Be that as it may, always take prompt steps to correct anything that seems to be worrying the subject — real or imaginary. At the next induction he should be seated in a chair, provided with a travelling-rug or given a pillow for his head, for any measures taken to rectify his complaints will afford him considerable reassurance. He is bound to feel that he himself is helping in the induction and is thereby retaining some measure of control over the situation.

8. Dislike of the Method of Induction Employed

Sometimes a subject dislikes the method of induction or he may dislike something in the actual phrasing of your suggestions. For instance, some subjects occasionally object to the word *sleepy*. If so, you should discard it completely and substitute the word relaxed only, during the next induction. Similarly, words such as *sinking* or *falling* (i.e. into a sleep) should be avoided and *drifting* or *relaxing,* used instead. Even the word 'sleep' may be misunderstood so that the subject will say on awakening, 'I wasn't asleep, I heard every word you said.' Emphasize repeatedly that the 'sleep' to which you refer is 'hypnotic sleep' and that he should hear everything that is said to him. Indeed that he will hear everything that is going on around him but will ignore everything but the sound of your voice and of what you are saying to him. In addition always reassure the subject that nothing will be forced upon him. Whenever it is the actual induction method that the subject dislikes, always adopt an alternative procedure at the next attempt at induction.

Just occasionally a subject may say: 'I could see you sitting there all the time and it distracted my attention. I found that the light was worrying me as well.' Although this may seem both unimportant and irrelevant, don't forget to turn his chair slightly away from you or from the light at subsequent sessions. Such simple precautions always help in the induction and deepening of the hypnotic trance.

9. Uncertainty on the Part of the Therapist

There is nothing more likely to cause doubt in the mind of the patient than uncertainty on the part of the doctor. Uncertainty of diagnosis, aetiology or treatment. An unsatisfactory or dubious assessment, insufficient knowledge of his subject or an unacceptable explanation of the cause of the trouble are certainly not ingredients for success. Finally, the 'let's see if hypnosis works' attitude is doomed to failure. By using hypnosis under such conditions the doctor will only succeed in reinforcing the problem of the patient. When a diagnosis is made, then it must be made with knowledge and conviction and when treatment is suggested it must be suggested with equal knowledge and conviction. If there is uncertainty about the diagnosis, the patient should be referred on to the appropriate expert but if it is not considered that hypnotherapy is the treatment of choice, this fact must be unequivocally stated to the patient. If it is intended to treat with hypnosis, this must also be stated clearly, an explanation given as to what can be achieved in that particular state and an outline of the course to be adopted indicated to the patient. In this way he will gain confidence in the doctor and in the technique and a major hurdle on the way to a successful induction will be overcome.

10. Poor Motivation and Expectancy

Rarely does the patient who expects nothing from his treatment achieve anything. If the patient is unconvinced that hypnotherapy will help his problem, unless the doctor can show him how it could help and unless the patient then wants to recover, there will be no rapport, no confidence and no mutual understanding established, all of which are so important for a successful outcome of therapy. Transference and counter-transference play an important role in the induction process as well as in treatment and the doctor must be ever aware of this factor.

Why has the patient come for treatment in the first place? Was he (or she) dragged along by mother or spouse? Did he (or she) attend because 'you helped my friend'. Anticipating success can induce good positive motivation unless if the 'I'm much worse than she is' attitude prevails, then the management of this patient will inevitably be difficult.

Does the symptom fulfil a need or serve a purpose? One immediately thinks of the agoraphobic lady, the housebound housewife who manipulates husband and children, parents and friends because of her 'illness'. If she is unable to go out alone she is unable to do the shopping or collect the children from school. Husbands are kept from work, cinema and supermarket alike are 'no-go' areas and the entire household revolves around her incapacity. Is there a meaning to this condition or is it purely an irrational fear which will respond to the appropriate chemotherapy or desensitization technique?

Apart from the obvious anxiety surrounding any problem is the patient additionally depressed? A very considerable number of patients met with in general practice and in specialist psychiatric practice are depressed and this symptom will certainly influence any attempt at induction and treatment. *It is essential to exclude an underlying depression* when intending to treat any patient with hypnosis whatever the presenting symptom may be.

Is the problem a conversion symptom? Does the problem 'protect' the patient from some unconscious fear or emotional response too threatening to look at? Poor motivation may equally be an unconscious response in any well-guarded patient. Remember also that one reason why Freud abandoned the use of hypnosis was that he was unable to 'penetrate' sufficiently the defences of many of his patients. It is useless to induce hypnosis and then to find that the patient remains so guarded that further progress is impossible. Remember too the possibility of substitution symptoms. Always a likelihood if the patient does not really wish to recover.

Finally we are all acquainted with the patient who expects the doctor to do it all for him. 'Here I am, now *you* get me better.' Nothing is less likely. Such a patient will resist even the initial induction. Thus cynicism and scepticism may be added to the reasons for poor motivation and expectancy.

DIFFICULTIES IN TERMINATING THE TRANCE

Once the trance state has been induced and deepened, it is most unlikely that you will experience any difficulty in awakening your subject, although this has been known to occur. Remember that whilst it is generally assumed that the trance can always be terminated by simple suggestion this is not necessarily the case. This assumption depends entirely upon the old idea that the hypnotized subject was completely passive, under the control of the hypnotist and subject only to his will. This, of course, is absolutely untrue for the trance situation in reality is nothing more or less than a relationship between two individuals, each of whom must be regarded as a person in his own right. Consequently, in the rare case of a subject who declines to awaken when instructed to do so, it should be borne in mind that he has some reason, conscious or unconscious, for not complying with the suggestion. There are six main reasons for a subject's refusal to awaken:

1. *It may be a defence.*   The subject may have experienced so much pleasure and peace that he wishes the trance to continue and is reluctant to awaken to face reality again. Or he may be so anxious that he simply will not allow himself to face reality until sufficiently reassured.

2. *It may be due to hostility or negative transference on the part of the subject.*   An unconscious means of expressing hostility or resentment toward the hypnotist could manifest itself in this way. The subject may feel that he is not being treated as he would like, or may resent certain things that have occurred during his treatment. Perhaps he is saying that he doesn't really want to get better.

3. *It may be due to a misconception as to what should occur.*   There was a patient who went into a somnambulistic trance and obstinately declined to awaken when told to do so. When questioned as to why he didn't wake up, he said that the last time he was hypnotized he had to sleep it off for an hour or so. Further questioning elicited the fact that he had not in fact been hypnotized, but had undergone a drug-induced abreaction (Thiopentone). When it was explained to him that he had no drug injected into his arm this time and that consequently there was no reason why he should not awaken immediately when told to do so, he subsequently awoke without difficulty.

4. *It may be due to a post-hypnotic suggestion he dislikes.* In this case, he will avoid the necessity of complying with it by the simple expedient of remaining in the trance. Questioning will soon reveal the cause of the trouble, and the offending suggestion can be promptly withdrawn.

If the subject's dislike is not sufficiently strong to prevent him from waking, he may still unconsciously express his resentment by feeling discomfort such as headache or dizziness once he is awake. Should this occur in a case in which a post-hypnotic suggestion has been given, re-hypnotize the subject immediately and withdraw the suggestion, avoiding any necessity for compliance.

5. *It may be a conversion symptom.* The patient may have discovered the means of opting out, of converting his unacceptable emotions into a form of sleep in which he no longer has to face his problems.

6. *The subject may have fallen asleep.* Perhaps overtired, or the effects of earlier imbibed tranquillizer drugs or alcohol. Or perhaps simply the effect of a warm room, a comfortable chair and the steady and soporific drone of the voice of the hypnotist!

If a subject fails to awaken from his trance when instructed to do so, the golden rule is to ask him why he is unable to wake up. In some patients this will provide the necessary clue as to how to proceed. In other cases it may even help to ask the subject himself what to do in order to awaken him. In most instances, this will be quite sufficient to resolve the difficulty.

Erickson met this situation with some specialized hypnotherapeutic techniques, making use of the patient's behaviour pattern in order to solve the problem. He often manipulated the time factor, projecting the patient well into the future, bringing him back to a less distant but still future time, taking him still further into the future and returning him closer to the present, eventually encouraging the patient to awaken at his correct age. In an obsessional case, he would induce in the patient a compulsive need to sleep for a stated period whilst stimultaneously implanting an obsessional doubt as to whether he would be able to accomplish this. As a result of this, the trance was usually terminated within a few minutes.

A SIMPLE TEST FOR HYPNOSIS

Having acquired the ability to hypnotize, you may well ask 'how can I be sure that my patient is in hypnosis?' If you have completed your initial induction and the patient has closed his eyes you may wonder 'perhaps he's doing this to please me or because he thinks he has to'. That may indeed be so, but if at this point you begin to lose confidence then without doubt the patient will sense this by the sound of your voice and general demeanour. Most experienced clinicians maintain that once the eyes are closed and some suggestions of deepening have been given, the patient is ready for therapy. Many experimental psychologists on the other hand, argue that this is not any state other than one of attempting to behave as would a hypnotized person, of role playing or of thinking and imagining with the suggestions[1,2]. This is an idea which seems to have been perpetuated since the pronouncements of the Royal Commission of Louis XVI.

Is it necessary to prove that the subject is in hypnosis? Perhaps it is sufficient that he will 'imagine' that he is hypnotized and behave as he considers would a hypnotized person. Perhaps it is sufficient that he will respond to suggestions and begin to get better. After all, is not this the object of the exercise? Nevertheless the sceptics may still require some confirmation.

One relatively simple test may be applied which will help the doubtful doctor as well as the patient.

Tell the patient, who is apparently relaxed and with his eyes closed, that you will get up from your chair, approach him and touch the back of his hand with the point of a pin. Proceed as follows:

'Now as you sit there with your eyes closed and in this pleasant state of hypnosis I am touching the back of your hand with this pin. Just say yes when you feel it.' The patient will say 'yes'. Move the point of the pin over the back of the hand awaiting confirmation at each touch. 'Now I am going to draw a circle around the back of your hand with the blunt end of the pin and the entire area within this circle will become numb'. Move the pin around a few times. 'Now the entire area within the circle that I have drawn has become completely numb. You can feel nothing within the limits of this circle. Do you feel this?' Prod the back of the hand well *outside* the circle. The patient will say 'yes'. Gradually approach the circle and then prod the back of the hand *within* the circumscribed areas with the point of the pin. 'Do you feel this?'

Should the patient say yes, then once again draw the circle and repeat the instruction in a somewhat more assertive manner and add 'Now, *you feel absolutely nothing within this circle.* There is no pain at all when I prod the back of your hand within the circle, with the point of the pin.' Proceed to prod, repeating the instruction 'no pain, *no feeling at all'.*

'Now I'm going to prick the outside of the circle with the point of the pin and tell me every time you feel the prick.'

Proceed to do this and the patient will respond by drawing his hand away sharply. Repeat this several times moving slowly and obviously nearer to, and then well within the circumference of the circle saying nothing. If at this stage the patient answers 'yes' then he is either not in hypnosis or may still be in a light hypnoidal state where the perception of pain is still present. If he says 'no' then the likelihood is that he is simulating. However, if he says nothing at all then he is more likely to be in hypnosis.

REFERENCES

1. White R.W., 1941. A preface to the theory of hypnotism. *J. Abnorm. Psychol.*, **36,** 477–505.
2. Spanos N.P. and Barber T.X., 1974. Towards a convergence in hypnosis research. *Am. Psychol.*, **29,** 500–511.

CHAPTER 8

A Comprehensive System of Trance Induction, Deepening and Post-hypnotic Conditioning

The description which follows, will be found to be most consistently successful in securing adequate depth for all ordinary clinical purposes; only when complete analgesia or hypnoanalytical techniques are required is greater depth likely to be necessary. Provided that the problem has been fully explored, a correct diagnosis has been made and the subject's mind has been satisfactorily prepared beforehand, it should always be possible to produce a trance. Only rarely does the subject fail to become conditioned to enter the hypnotic state in future immediately it is suggested that he should do so. In a reasonably good subject, the whole routine of induction can be completed successfully in a single period of about 20 minutes. In less responsive cases the same result can easily be obtained if the subject is trained gradually over two or three consecutive sessions.

The eye fixation–distraction method is used for the initial induction, and the trance is gradually deepened by progressive relaxation, the induction of graded responses and a counting and breathing technique. Although the following description necessarily involves a great deal of repetition, this will probably prove more convenient than otherwise, since it is a full account of the routine which may be employed in the majority of cases. But whilst one would seldom fail to teach subjects to enter the hypnotic state upon a given signal, verbal or otherwise, by the use of this method, other psychological factors are also involved, such as belief, confidence, personality, experience and certainly reputation. Nevertheless, one may be greatly encouraged by the fact that most medical and dental practitioners who have been introduced to this technique and have tested it thoroughly in their own practices have not only confirmed many of the advantages described, but have subsequently incorporated it into their own routines.

As already stated, no single method can ever be said to be the best for inducing and deepening hypnosis. Each aspiring operator must gradually evolve that which is best suited to his own personality, and this may well incorporate features characteristic of a number of different techniques.

A COMPLETE ROUTINE FOR THE INDUCTION OF HYPNOSIS, TRANCE DEEPENING AND POST-HYPNOTIC CONDITIONING

Preliminary Induction

I want you to lie back comfortably in the chair.
Look upwards and backwards at a point on the ceiling of your own choosing.
Keep your eyes fixed on that point. Good!
Don't let your eyes wander from it for a single moment.
Now start counting slowly backwards, from 300.
Mentally, to yourself...not out loud.
Keep on counting...slowly and rhythmically...and go on counting until you hear me tell you to stop.
Try not to listen to me...any more than you can help.
You'll still hear everything I say...but try not to listen.
Just stick to your counting.
Let yourself go completely...limp and slack.
Breathe quietly...in...and out.
And whilst you're breathing quietly...in...and out...you can feel that your eyes are becoming very, very tired.
They may feel a little watery...the point you are looking at may begin to look a little blurred.

Already, your eyelids are beginning to feel very, very heavy and tired.
Presently, they will want to blink.
As soon as they start to blink...just let them blink as much as they like.
You see! They're starting to blink, now.
Just let everything happen...exactly as it wants to happen.
Don't try to make it happen...don't try to stop it happening.
Just let everything please itself.
Presently, your blinks will become slower...and bigger.
And as they do so...your eyes will become more and more tired.
The eyelids...heavier...and heavier.
So heavy...that they feel they are wanting to close.
As soon as they feel they want to close...let them go...just let them close...entirely on their own.
They're wanting to close, now...let them go...closing tighter and tighter...tighter and tighter.
Go to sleep!
Sleep very, very deeply.
Relax completely...and give yourself up completely to this very pleasant...relaxed...drowsy feeling.
Stop counting, now.
Just sleep...very, very deeply indeed.

Deepening by Progressive Relaxation

Now, a feeling of complete relaxation is gradually extending over your entire body.
Let the muscles of your feet and ankles relax completely.
Let them go...limp and slack.
Now, your calf muscles.
Let them go limp and slack...allow them to relax.
Now, the muscles of your thighs.
Let them relax...let them go...limp and slack.
And as the muscles of your legs and thighs become completely limp and relaxed...you can be aware of a feeling of heaviness in your lower limbs.
As though your limbs are becoming just as heavy as lead.
Let your legs and thighs go...heavy as lead.
Let them relax completely.
And as they do so...your sleep is gradually becoming deeper and deeper.

That feeling of relaxation is now spreading upwards...over your entire body.

Let your stomach muscles relax...let them go...limp and slack.

Now, the muscles of your chest...and your back.

Let them all go...limp and slack...allow them to relax.

And, as you do so...you can experience a feeling of heaviness in your body...as though your body is becoming just as heavy as lead.

As if it is wanting to sink down...deeper and deeper...into the chair.

Just let your body go...heavy as lead.

Let it relax back comfortably...deeper and deeper...into the chair.

And as it does so...you are drifting pleasantly and slowly but surely, into a deeper, deeper sleep.

Just give yourself up completely...to this very enjoyable...relaxed...drowsy...comfortable feeling.

And now, this feeling of relaxation is spreading into the muscles of your arms...your shoulders...and your neck.

Let your arm muscles relax...

Let them relax...let them go...limp and slack.

Now, your shoulder muscles.

Let them go limp and slack...allow them to relax.

Now, the muscles of your neck...and all your facial muscles....

Quite relaxed...your eyes closed...your eyelids completely relaxed....

And the muscles of your forehead....

And right to the tip of your head....

Completely relaxed....

Let your entire body relax...let it go...limp and slack.

And as you do so...your sleep is becoming deeper...deeper...deeper.

And as this feeling of complete relaxation spreads...and deepens...over your body...you have fallen into a very, very deep sleep indeed.

You are so deeply asleep, in fact...that everything that I tell you that is going to happen...will happen...exactly as I tell you.

And every feeling that I tell you that you will experience...you will experience...exactly as I tell you.

Now, sleep...very, very deeply.

Deeper and deeper asleep...deeper and deeper asleep.

Deepening by a Counting and Breathing Technique

In a few moments...I am going to count slowly up to five...and as I do so...you will take five deep breaths.

And with each breath that you take...each time you breathe out...you will become more and more relaxed...and your sleep will become deeper and deeper.

One...Deep, deep breath...more and more deeply relaxed...deeper and deeper asleep.

Two...Very deep breath...deeper and deeper relaxed...sleep becoming deeper and deeper.

Three...Deeper and deeper breath...more and more deeply relaxed...more and more deeply asleep.

Four...Very, very deep breath...deeper and deeper relaxed...sleep becoming even deeper and deeper.

Five...Very, deep breath indeed...very, very deeply relaxed...very, very deeply asleep.

And I would now like you to take one more very deep breath...fill your chest...and hold it until I say... 'Let go'.

Then, let that breath out as quickly as possible...and as you do so...you will feel yourself sagging limply back into the chair...and you will become twice as deeply relaxed as you are now...twice as deeply asleep.

Now take that very deep breath...fill your chest...and *Hold it*...(five seconds pause)...*Hold it*...(five seconds pause)...*Hold it*...(five seconds pause)...*Let go*!

Sleep very, very deeply...deeper and deeper asleep...deeper and deeper asleep.

Deepening by the Induction of Arm Heaviness

I am now going to ask you to place your arm on the arm of the chair.

And, as you do so...you will begin to be aware of a feeling of heaviness in your arm.

That feeling of heaviness is increasing...with every word that I utter.

Your arm is feeling heavier...and heavier...just as heavy as lead. *You can feel it pressing down more firmly upon the arm of the chair.*

With every breath that you take,...with every word that I utter, your arm feels heavier and heavier...heavier and heavier... (The word 'heavier' is spoken to coincide with the movement of the

patient's chest as he exhales.)
And in a few moments...your arm will feel so very, very
heavy...that, when you try to lift it...it will dropback on to your
chair, so heavy that you can't be bothered to lift it if I ask you to
do so...just like a lead weight.
And as it drops limply back...on to your chair...you will fall into
a deeper, deeper sleep, your arm, heavy aslead, so you just can't
be bothered to lift it...
Sleep...deeply asleep.

This response is now tested, following which the arm is restored
to normal.

You have now fallen into a much deeper sleep.
And, as I speak and you relax even deeper...you will notice that
all feelings of heaviness are now leaving your arm.
It is coming back to normal...and now feels just the same as
your other arm.
All that feeling of heaviness has passed away completely...and
your sleep has become even deeper...and deeper.

Deepening by the Induction of Arm Catalepsy

(This is not an essential step, and often omitted.)

As your arm rests upon the arm of the chair...I want you to
concentrate on it again.
This time...instead of feeling heavier...it will begin to feel lighter
and lighter.
Just as light as a feather...as if there is no weight in it at all.
Lighter and lighter...lighter and lighter.
So light, in fact...that as you concentrate on it, it will want to
float up in the air, just like a balloon. Just imagine a bright and
attractive balloon. It's blown up and tied with a piece of string.
The loose end of the string is attached to the index finger of your
hand resting on the arm of the chair. As the balloon floats up
into the air, the string gives a slight tug on your finger. Just
watch that balloon.
What colour is it?

The patient is surprised by the sudden question and if he is visualizing well, will think for a moment and then answer 'red' or
'blue' or whatever colour he sees it to be. Then you know he is with
you in what you are suggesting so continue...

As the balloon floats gently up into the air, the string gives a little tug at your index finger...let it happen.

Watch for the slight movement and then proceed.

The finger is rising as the string pulls gently at it. As the balloon floats upwards so the finger and the hand and the arm gently float up into the air...let it happen.

Watch for every slight movement and exploit it, gradually coaxing the arm to move upwards.

Now your arm will want to remain just where it is...suspended by the balloon...*your arm will remain just where it is suspended in mid-air...without your having to make the slightest effort to keep it there.*

When the response is positive, the gradual restoration of the arm to normal may be used as an additional deepening technique.

Now slowly the air begins to leak out of the balloon...the balloon descends...and the string around your finger falls to the ground as your arm drops heavily on to the arm of the chair. And as your arm touches the chair, sleep...deeper and deeper...deeper and deeper...deeply asleep...and your arm feels perfectly normal again. And now your arm...has returned to normal.
All that feeling of lightness and weightlessness has left it...and it is now feeling just the same as your other arm.
And your sleep has become deeper...and deeper.

Deepening by the Induction of Limb Rigidity

Now, I want you to hold your arm out...level with your shoulder...stiff and straight...with the palm facing the ceiling. And as you concentrate on your arm...you will feel that it is becoming much stiffer and straighter.
That stiffness is increasing...with every word that I say.
You can feel all the muscles tightening up...pulling your arm out...stiffer and straighter...with every word that I say...until it is beginning to feel just as stiff and rigid as a steel poker...from the shoulder to the wrist.
Now, I want you to concentrate on a steel poker.
Picture a steel poker in your mind.
And as you do so...you will feel that your arm has become just as stiff and rigid as the steel poker.

As if the elbow joint is firmly locked.
As if there is no elbow joint there at all.
So that it will be impossible for you to bend your arm at the elbow...until I count up to 'three'.
The harder you try to bend it...the stiffer and straighter...and more rigid it will become.
But, the moment I count 'three'...all the stiffness will pass away immediately...your arm will bend quite easily...and as it does so, you will fall immediately into a deeper, deeper sleep.
Stiff and straight! Just like that steel poker!
One...two...three!
Arm back to normal, absolutely normal now and sleep...deeper...deeper...deeper sleep.

Deepening by the Induction of Automatic Movements

Now place your elbow on the arm of the chair...and hold your arm upwards with the fingers pointing to the ceiling...
Now I want you to imagine that the centre of a piece of cord is tied around your wrist...and the cord is being gently pulled at each end...pulling your arm back and forth...back and forth...back and forth...
Just let it happen...
And now the cord is released...and the arm continues to swing...back and forth...until I tell you to stop...
You won't try to make it move!
You won't try to stop it moving! You will just let it please itself...and it will go on moving on its own...quite automatically...back and forth...back and forth...until I tell you to stop.

When the arm is moving freely, tell the subject that his sleep is becoming deeper and deeper, timing this so that you repeat the word deeper on each alternate forward movement of his arm.

Now, stop!
Let your arm fall back...on to the arm of the chair...and as you do so...you are falling into an even deeper, deeper sleep.
Sleep! Very, very deeply!

By now, the subject is usually in a sufficiently deep sleep to permit post-hypnotic conditioning to be attempted with a considerable chance of success.

The Induction of Post-hypnotic Conditioning

> You are now so deeply asleep...that everything that I tell you
> that is going to happen...*will* happen...*exactly* as I tell you.
> Every feeling...that I tell you that you *will* experience...you will
> experience...*exactly* as I tell you.
> And every instruction that I give you...you will carry out
> faithfully.
> Now...in a few moments...I shall waken you by counting up to
> 'seven'.
> You will wake up...feeling wonderfully better for this long sleep.
> And after you have awakened...I shall talk to you for a minute
> or two.
> Then, I shall ask you to lie back in the chair...and look straight
> into my eyes.
> Whilst you are looking at me...I shall say:
> *Go to sleep!*
> And the moment you hear me say...'Go to sleep'...your eyes will
> close immediately...and you will fall immediately into a sleep, just
> as deep as this one.

This instruction should be repeated at least once, quietly and
firmly.

> In a few moments...I am going to wake you by counting up to
> 'seven'.
> And after you have awakened...I shall talk to you for a minute
> or two.
> Then I shall ask you to lie back in the chair...and look straight
> into my eyes.
> Whilst you are looking at me...I shall say:
> *Go to sleep!*
> And the moment you hear me say...'Go to sleep'...your eyes will
> close immediately...and you will fall into a sleep, just as deep as
> this present sleep.

The subject is then awakened.

> In a few moments...when I count up to 'seven'...you will open your
> eyes...and be wide awake again.
> You will awaken feeling wonderfully better for this long sleep.
> You will awaken feeling completely relaxed...mentally and
> physically...feeling quite calm and composed.
> *One...two...three...four...five...six...seven!*

As soon as he is awake, ask him a few questions about his own feelings during the hypnosis, and briefly discuss his reactions. Then, ask him to lie back in the chair...and look straight into your eyes.

Whilst he is doing this, say to him firmly:

Go to sleep!

Usually his eyes close immediately, and he sinks into a deep hypnotic sleep.

If there is some delay and the subject's eyes do not close immediately, repeat the suggestion firmly and authoritatively, once or twice if necessary, with the result that the eyes generally close without more ado.

After waking him again, explain that the only reason that his eyes failed to close immediately lay in the fact that he just could not believe that such a thing could possibly happen. Point out to him that, despite his doubts, it did actually happen, and that when told to go to sleep again, in a few moments' time — on this occasion he will find that his eyes will close without delay. This usually proves to be the case, but if the reactions are still inclined to be sluggish, a few more rapid rehearsals will generally produce the desired result. Then proceed to consolidate this conditioning for all future occasions

From now on...*whenever you want me to give you treatment*...all I shall have to do is ask you to lie back comfortably in the chair...and look straight at me.
Whilst you are looking at me...I shall say:
'*Go to sleep!*'
And from now on...whenever you hear me say...'*Go to sleep*'...your eyes will always close immediately...and you will always fall immediately into a sleep...just as deep as this present sleep.
It doesn't matter whether it is t*omorrow...next month*...or even *next year*.
From now on...whenever you hear me say...'*Go to sleep*'...your eyes will alwyas close immediately...and you will always fall immediately into a sleep...just as deep as this present sleep.
And that is exactly what is going to happen when you see me next.

After our preliminary chat...as soon as you are ready for treatment...I shall ask you to lie back comfortably in the chair...and look straight at me.
Whilst you are looking at me...I shall say:
'Go to sleep!'
And next time...and, indeed on every future occasion when you want me to give you treatment...the moment you hear me say...'Go to sleep'...your eyes will close immediately...and you will fall immediately into a sleep...just as deep as this present sleep.
However, if you hear the words 'go to sleep' spoken by anyone else, unless you have given them permission to put you into hypnosis, and unless you really want to go into hypnosis these words will have no effect on you.
They will only be effective if I tell you to 'go to sleep' in this hypnotic way and only whenever you want me to give you treatment.

This exclusion is repeated several times. Finally awaken the subject giving him post-hypnotic suggestions of feelings of well-being and calmness and assurances that the next time he attends, he will relax even deeper into this hypnotic sleep

In a few moments...when I count *'seven'*...you will open your eyes and be wide awake again...feeling wonderfully better for this long sleep. You will wake up...feeling really fit and well...feeling completely relaxed...mentally and physically...feeling quite calm and composed...and feeling much more confidence...both in yourself...and in the future and you know that you will relax even deeper into this pleasant hypnotic sleep.
One...two...three...four...five...six...seven!

In this routine there are one or two points that are worth noting. Although the subject certainly falls asleep immediately he is told to do so, the procedure is not as dominating as it might appear. The subject has been given some choice in the matter since the conditions under which he will respond have been precisely specified. You have also written in an 'exclusion clause'. The phrase *whenever you want me to give you treatment* allows him to select the occasions upon which he will be ready to comply with the suggestion, and this feeling of independence is furthered by the phrases *whenever you lie back comfortably in the chair* and *look straight at me*, which also define the limited conditions under which he will respond. The freedom thus allowed seems to afford a great deal of reassurance, and does a lot to ensure whole-hearted co-operation. Should the first attempt at post-hypnotic conditioning fail, no further steps should be taken until the next session. Then repeat the whole induction and deepening procedures as previously but with the addition of dream induction. Whenever a positive response is obtained to this technique, the post-hypnotic conditioning routine can be suggested with every expectation of success. The technique described is rapid, reliable and efficient. Even with a subject who has never been hypnotized before, provided that his mind has been properly prepared, it rarely takes more than 2 to 3 minutes to secure spontaneous closing of the eyes and the light hypnotic state. And as already mentioned, in a good subject the whole induction and deepening routine, including post-hypnotic conditioning, can be completed in a single session of approximately 20 minutes duration. Even more difficult subjects can still be trained to go to sleep immediately it is suggested that they should do so, if they are gradually trained over several consecutive sessions.

Tell your patients that although nearly everyone is capable of being hypnotized, the susceptibility of different individuals varies a great deal. If they happen to be good subjects, they will probably enter the deep hypnotic state during the first induction; if not, they can still be taught to achieve sufficient depth for treatment purposes in the course of two or three consultations. Never attempt to induce hypnosis during the first interview. This should be devoted entirely to history taking, explanation and establishing rapport. The order of events should be as follows:

1st Session. Get to know your patient, take the case-history, and discuss the problem with him. Make a firm diagnosis and decide whether the case is suitable for hypnotherapy or whether some alternative form of treatment is more appropriate. If considered suitable, discuss the question of hypnosis, explain it fully, correct any mistaken ideas, banish doubts and fears, and generally prepare the patient's mind to accept it.

2nd Session. Begin by asking the patient whether he has any questions to put, arising from the previous discussion. If so, answer them in order to dispel any last lingering doubts. Then explain to the patient exactly what he has to do, what you will do, and exactly what he may expect to happen. Induce light hypnosis, and deepen it by the use of progressive relaxation and limb-heaviness and, occasionally, limb catalepsy.

3rd Session. Discuss with the patient his reactions to the previous session and correct any misconceptions he may still hold. Induce and deepen hypnosis as before, following with limb rigidity and terminating with automatic movement.

4th Session. Once again, the patient's reactions are thoroughly ventilated and discussed. Then repeat the entire induction and deepening procedure with the addition of the counting and breathing technique, followed by post-hypnotic conditioning. This is usually successful and the subject subsequently enters the hypnotic state immediately, whenever he is instructed to do so. Should any difficulty arise, the whole process is repeated at the next session, any further attempt at conditioning being preceded by dream induction.

With this system of gradual training, one should rarely encounter a patient who cannot be taught to enter the hypnotic state immediately the appropriate suggestion or signal is given. The scheme just described, however, is far from being rigid. Carefully watch the manner in which the subject reacts to each phase of the induction and deepening process, and if his responses indicate a considerable degree of susceptibility, then one may proceed to the stage of automatic movement during the first hypnotic session. Indeed, whenever the subject is really susceptible, the entire conditioning routine can be completed in a single session.

The scheme described may be adopted by the beginner and should prove generally successful. Practice is essential. However anyone who wishes to succeed with hypnosis must formulate his own individual technique through painstaking trial and error, but it is hoped that the description of this routine may afford some assistance to those who are trying to develop their own particular methods.

PART TWO

SOME PHENOMENA OF HYPNOSIS AND THE USE OF ADVANCED TECHNIQUES

CHAPTER 9

The Common Phenomena of Hypnosis

Curious and unusual as many of the hypnotic phenomena may seem, most of them have their counterpart in everyday life and can be reproduced at least to a minor extent in the waking state. Moreover, they can often be seen and induced in perfectly normal individuals as a result of post-hypnotic suggestion, following which they subsequently appear after the subject has been awakened. Many of them can also be self-induced by those who have mastered the technqiue of self-hypnosis.

The phenomena of hypnosis have often been separated into two distinct categories—the physiological and the psychological—but it is difficult to draw any hard and fast division between them. As we know, alterations in bodily functions often occur solely as a result of changes in the psychical state. For instance, when a man becomes paralysed by fright his complete inability to move is due to his mental state and is certainly not the result of any injury or damage to his muscles. Similarly during the hypnotic state the muscles and sense organs often display abnormalities in function simply because the mental state of the subject has been altered. The alterations usually encountered in the course of hypnosis affect both voluntary and involuntary muscles, the sense organs, the memory, mental activity and the emotions.

Many of these phenomena are incorporated into the Harvard Group Scale of Hypnotic Susceptibility[1].

Alterations in the Voluntary Muscles

Suggestion exercises an extraordinary influence over the functions of the voluntary muscles, the activity of which can nearly always be influenced to a high degree. During hypnosis, the movements of these muscles can either be inhibited or excited.

1. *Relaxation.* Suggestions of muscular relaxation seem to induce a feeling of laziness in the subject and a pronounced disinclination to move his limbs; he may even feel unable to make up his mind whether to do so or not. He never actually loses the power to move them even though he may be told that he is unable to do so, but as hypnosis deepens so muscular tonus diminishes, sometimes to a point beyond voluntary control.

2. *Paralysis of muscle groups.* This may effect only small groups of muscles such as those of the eyelids or may be extended to larger groups such as the muscles of the limbs and body. The actual distribution of the paralysis never corresponds exactly to that of the motor nerves but follows the subject's own idea of how a paralysed person would behave. If the subject is told that he has entirely lost the use of all the muscles of his limbs and body he will be quite powerless to get up out of his chair. This occurs simply because the suggestion has aroused in the subject's mind a firm conviction that his muscles are completely useless. Such paralyses are indistinguishable from true hysterical paralyses that arise spontaneously in the absence of hypnosis.

Sometimes the subject is unable to move a paralysed limb because he can no longer voluntarily contract his muscles. In other cases every attempt at voluntary movement is actively opposed and rendered futile by contracture of the antagonistic muscles. The subject may be deprived temporarily of the power of speech, or told that he will only be able to pronounce his own name and will otherwise be quite dumb. It can be made impossible for him to write whilst still retaining his ability to shuffle a pack of cards or play the piano. The prohibited actions will only become possible again when the necessary permission is given.

These effects will vary greatly from subject to subject. In some people it will be easier to influence one particular set of muscles than any others. For instance, it may be possible to prevent one person from opening his eyes, yet be quite impossible to affect his speech. Another may be rendered quite dumb, yet all attempts to prohibit him from writing will fail completely.

3. *Rigid catalepsies.* Catalepsy is said to occur when a limb remains in any position in which it has been placed by the hypnotist. Such postures can often be maintained for long periods of time far exceeding those possible by voluntary effort, without being followed by the pain and fatigue that one would normally expect after such excessive muscular exertion.

The essential requirement for the production of catalepsy is that the subject should accept the idea of the particular attitude involved. Sometimes the arm of a hypnotized subject can be raised, supported in the air and then released. The limb will remain exactly where it was left although not a word will have been spoken. Despite this, the subject firmly believes that his arm must remain so. In another subject the arm will probably fall, yet if again raised and if he is told that it will now remain in the air, this will undoubtedly happen. Indeed there is no need to speak to him at all, for one or two upward jerks of the wrist alone will cause him to understand what is intended to take place. Erickson believed that catalepsy occurred because the subject becomes so intensely absorbed that he is unresponsive to ordinary stimuli.

Cataleptic rigidity can be induced in any limb or even in the entire body by direct suggestion, for example an arm can be stiffened so that it is impossible for a second person to bend it. The rigidity can be increased by concentrating the patient's attention upon the limb. Cataleptic rigidity can be terminated immediately by the appropriate counter-suggestion.

One of the favourite tricks of the stage hypnotist is the production of a cataleptic rigidity of the whole body. The hypnotized subject is then supported by one chair placed under his head and another under his heels (the 'human bridge' effect). Not only will his body fail to sag, but it will be capable of supporting the weight of a 14-stone man. To heighten the effect, a slimly built girl is usually selected as the subject. Dramatic as this may be, this particular phenomenon *must never be used for demonstration purposes.* It is bound to involve unwarranted strain upon muscles, joints and ligaments, all of which can be just as easily injured in the hypnotic as in the waking state, for suggested catalepsy is never accompanied by physical changes in the tissues. Consequently bones can be just as easily broken and joints just as easily strained as in the normal state.

4. *Increased muscular performance.* This is largely due to an inability to feel fatigue for long periods at a time. Thus in hypnosis we find that the subject can maintain uncomfortable attitudes and perform tasks with much less discomfort and fatigue than when wide awake.

In everyday life, we generally work well below our true capacity and have considerable reserves of power to call upon in times of stress. In the hypnotic state these can be utilized even though they lie outside voluntary effort. Under normal circumstances few of us would be capable of climbing a rope to reach a trap-door in the roof, yet if every exit were blocked by fire and this represented our only means of escape, most of us would be able to manage it. The fact that such reserves can be tapped under hypnosis has been used advantageously in the field of sport but account must be taken of other existing problems. Many athletes have been enabled to attain their maximum effort instead of putting up merely an average performance. It should be remembered, however, that nobody can be caused to exceed their own individual capacity although this is often much greater than would appear from their normal achievements.

5. *Automatic movements.* Not only can muscular action be inhibited by suggestion but it can also be excited and made automatic. If a subject is told that his left arm will gradually rise into the air, it will do so even though he may make no voluntary effort whatever. It will seldom occur to him to resist unless his motivation has been misjudged.

Voluntary movements are not difficult to distinguish from involuntary ones since they are usually smooth and executed with steady ease. On the other hand, even when the subject is passive, involuntary movements are characterized by a certain amount of slowness and jerkiness. This is sometimes greatly exaggerated, and involuntary movements that are executed without the subject's will are often accompanied by strong muscular contractions and trembling. This shows the presence of two antagonistic forces—the suggestion of the hypnotist, and the will of the subject. The latter is resisting the suggestion that his arm will rise, and this displays itself in the trembling.

A useful test of automatic movement is to rotate the subject's hands around each other in a circular fashion, in front of the body. When his hands are released, the tendency to continue the movement will persist, particularly if he believes that he has to go on turning. If he is then told that he cannot stop, no matter how hard he tries, he will find that although his hands may bump into each other, he will be quite unable to discontinue the movement. When this phenomenon is elicited, it usually signifies that a medium if not deeper stage of hypnosis has been reached.

Before considering the phenomena affecting the involuntary muscles, there are two specific muscular reactions occurring during the induction of hypnosis which are worthy of attention.

1. *Passive hypnosis.* Occasionally the subject becomes so passive that even the strongest suggestions are insufficient to overcome the muscular relaxation that has occurred. In such cases the arms will drop after having been raised despite all suggestions to the contrary. It may even be difficult to persuade the subject to answer questions.

In most inductions hypnosis will be passive in the early stages. Very often, once the eyes have closed, the head will drop forwards, backwards or sideways because the supporting muscles have become so relaxed. Indeed, there are many transitional stages between active and passive hypnosis, and the one can easily pass into the other.

2. *Oculomotor disturbances.* Although in the majority of cases hypnosis is characterized by closure of the eyes, this is by no means essential; but in most cases the eyes do close and, except in somnambulism, cannot be opened again without terminating the hypnosis. Even when the subject remains in a deep trance with his eyes open, he usually feels heaviness in his eyelids and a desire to close them.

The initial closing of the eyes is sometimes gentle, sometimes spasmodic, and is not always complete, but this does not interfere with hypnosis. Once the eyes are closed, the lids frequently quiver, but this is not important. It is a sure indication that the patient is on the threshold of hypnosis and in some instances is a sign of increasing rather than decreasing depth. The eyeballs often roll upwards as the eyes are closing and may remain in this position; in other cases they return to their natural position as soon as the eyes are closed. If they do not only the white sclerotics will be visible if the eyelids are gently raised.

Alterations in the Involuntary Muscles, Organs and Glands

Many functions and activities of the body are quite outside voluntary control. They are controlled and regulated by the unconscious mind, by action through the thalamus and the autonomic nervous system. The circulatory, respiratory, alimentary and excretory systems and the endocrine glands are all largely controlled in this manner.

The effects that hypnosis can produce that transcend all voluntary control are important to our understanding of the use of this method in the treatment of psychosomatic conditions, for the activity of both organs and glands can often be influenced by the emotions. Fear, for instance, causes an increase in the secretion of adrenaline and a more rapid heart beat.

Suggestion, particularly in the hypnotic state, can exercise the same effect, which will be greatly heightened if the appropriate emotion is simultaneously evoked. The control by suggestion, of the mind and body, thus becomes more understandable. The unconscious mind has the power to inhibit or excite the autonomic nervous system, and since in the hypnotic state the unconscious mind becomes more accessible to suggestion, much of the influence exerted under hypnosis becomes explicable. Unfortunately, however, we do not yet know exactly how this comes about.

1. *The heart.* The heart rate can be both accelerated and retarded by suggestion during hypnosis. Such changes can be conditioned to verbal cues, once they have resulted from emotional stimulation in the first place.

2. *The blood vessels.* Lloyd Tuckey[2] found that the smaller arteries and capillaries were almost invariably contracted in hypnosis, so that even deep wounds tended to produce little or no haemorrhage. This is confirmed by many dental surgeons who report a definite decrease in bleeding following the extraction of teeth under deep hypnosis. Subsequent investigations have verified the fact that suggestion can exercise a certain amount of influence on the blood vessels. Forel[3] also found that local flushing could be induced by suggestion, and this is not surprising when one considers how easily the vasomotor system is influenced by mental processes. Embarrassment will cause blushing, fear will cause pallor. In the treatment of certain dermatological conditions, hyperaemia of the skin may be produced by direct verbal suggestion. Additionally one indicator of anxiety is excessive palmar perspiration. This is due to capillary dilatation and is followed by a drop in temperature. The induction of hypnosis results in a decrease in anxiety, constriction of the capillaries, dry palms and a rise in local temperature. This can easily be recorded.

The blood pressure can also be influenced. Suggestions of relaxation and calmness will lower the blood pressure and pulse rate, whereas suggestions of excitement and agitation will certainly raise them. Indeed, it is the fact that disturbed emotional states play such an important part in essential hypertension that enables hypnosis to be of great value in the treatment of this condition particularly if self-hypnosis is routinely used.

3. *The respiratory system.* When the eyes close in response to suggestion during the induction of hypnosis, the respiration rate becomes diminished as the subject experiences a feeling of restful calm. As hypnosis proceeds the breathing becomes slower and more superficial, although it deepens both at the commencement and the termination of the hypnotic state.

Suggestion can also produce considerable variations of both respiration rate and respiratory excursion. Increases in pulmonary ventilation up to 50 per cent have been obtained in a resting hypnotized subject to whom it had been suggested that heavy work was being performed. But though these facts are of some significance in contributing to the success of hypnosis in the treatment of bronchial asthma and bronchospasm, they are not as important as its ability to control the emotional factors underlying the attacks.

4. *The alimentary system.* It has been shown that when a deeply hypnotized subject was told that he was eating an imaginary meal of beef and protein, this suggestion produced an increased secretion of gastric juice. Similarly, when imaginary fats were substituted for the protein, contraction of the gall bladder followed, accompanied by an increased flow of lipase and bile. These facts are hardly surprising since the mere suggestion of an appetizing meal can cause our mouths to water. It has also been reported that increased and decreased gastric acidity could be produced by suggestions of enjoyment or disgust.

Peristalsis can certainly be influenced very strongly and efficiently by suggestion, and because of this the bowel actions can often be regulated under hypnosis. If a very deeply hypnotized subject is told that his bowels will act as a specified time, the suggestion is quite likely to succeed. Indeed, when the hypnosis is accompanied by an amnesia, it will seldom fail. It is even possible to arrest the action of aperient drugs by suggestion, although this is less frequent. Water has been given to the hypnotic subject and represented either as a strong purgative or emetic. The appropriate reaction followed.

5. *The secretions.* Secretion of both saliva and perspiration have been reported to have been induced by suggestion. Under hypnosis the eyes can be caused to water if it is suggested to the patient that he is smelling an onion. Similarly, the secretion of tears can be induced by the suggestion of a strong emotion.

Lactation can also be facilitated by hypnotic suggestion and the secretion of milk increased to a considerable extent. However it seems to be doubtful whether the secretion of urine can be affected by suggestion, since in many of the cases reported it is the act of micturition and not that of secretion that has been modified.

6. *Changes in metabolism.* When it is suggested to a deeply hypnotized subject that he has not eaten anything for several days, a fall in blood sugar results. If it is then suggested that he is enjoying an imaginary meal of pastry, cream cakes and sugar, a rise

in blood sugar will occur, although he has actually eaten nothing. The blood sugar level is always increased by adrenaline, so whenever strong emotions such as terror or anger are aroused, more adrenaline is released into the blood stream and the blood sugar rises to mobilize the body for action and provide a sufficient fuel supply for anticipated increased muscular demands. Since emotional states such as these can easily be produced by hypnotic suggestion with the consequent release of adrenaline, its effect upon the blood sugar becomes quite understandable.

7. *Anatomical and biochemical changes.* It would be foolish to deny the possibility of effecting physical change by means of hypnosis, but gullibility should be avoided since the hypnotic subject, knowing that certain things are expected of him, may try to comply with the hypnotist's demands and later develop an amnesia for his actions. There is no doubt, however, that organic changes can be brought about by mental processes.

Menstruation can often be induced or arrested by hypnotic suggestion. This is hardly surprising when one realizes how often psychical influences in everyday life can change the pattern. For instance periods not infrequently become irregular in women who are anxious and apprehensive, as when awaiting a surgical operation.

Bleeding of the nose and skin resulting from suggestion, even when the most elaborate precautions have been taken to prevent the subject from causing a wound, have been reported by many of the older hypnotists. Such phenomena bear a strong resemblance to the stigmata recognized by the Roman Catholic Church when bleeding of the skin is said to occur in sites corresponding to the wounds of Christ. Such reports as these should always be accepted with caution in view of the ever-existing possibility of unconscious deception.

Blistering, or marks resembling blisters, have been reported by many observers. In a typical experiment, a pencil was pressed upon the skin in the morning and the subject was told that it was red-hot and that his skin was being burned. He was then awakened, and after the interval of several hours a blister appeared on the skin in the exact shape of the pencil. This phenomenon is extensively described, together with a comprehensive commentary on the literature on the subject by Chertok[4]. He unhesitatingly confirms that somatic effects can be produced by psychic processes.

Weals have also been produced by hypnotic suggestion, but it should not be forgotten that some people have been known to develop them under conditions of mental excitement without any hypnosis. It has also been reported in recent years that they have occurred spontaneously in the course of profound emotional drug-induced abreactions. Obviously, reports of these kinds of hypnotic experiment should be received with a certain amount of reserve. Moll[5] stated that whilst it is not denied that anatomical changes can be produced by suggestion, *the evidence of such changes having taken place must be unimpeachable before it can be accepted.* Such results, if and when they occur, can only be interpreted as an autonomic response to an emotional stimulus.

Modification of allergic skin responses. It has been known for many years that the symptoms of both asthma and hay fever could be relieved by direct suggestion under hypnosis. In 1958 A. A. Mason and S. Black[6] described how allergic skin responses were abolished during the treatment of a case of asthma and hay fever by hypnosis. In addition to the relief of the patient's symptoms, the skin reactions to injected pollens also disappeared. A Prausnitz–Kustner reaction was performed and when the patient's serum was injected into the arm of a non-sensitive volunteer, his skin produced allergic reactions to the allergens to which the patient was now apparently insensitive, proving that although the patient's allergic symptoms had been abolished by hypnotic suggestion, her blood remained unchanged.

In 1963 Black *et al.*[7] reported four cases in which the Mantoux reaction was inhibited by direct suggestion under hypnosis. Although histologically there was no observable change in the degree of cellular infiltration, there was evidence that the exudation of fluid had been inhibited. They thus concluded that the Mantoux-positive reaction could be inhibited by direct suggestion under hypnosis to give a Mantoux-negative result, and that a vascular constituent of the reaction is probably involved in the mechanism of inhibition.

Alterations in the Sense Organs

In deep hypnosis the five special senses, sight, hearing, smell, taste and touch, can all be influenced by suggestion, and the subject's perception through any one of them may be either increased or diminished.

1. *Sight.* The power of vision can often be increased far beyond the subject's normal voluntary effort. In a typical experiment, it is first established that a very short-sighted person, without his glasses, cannot read a printed page at a greater distance than 12 inches. With his glasses he can read the same size of print at the distance of 1 to 2 yards. Under deep hypnosis, he is then told that his sight without glasses will become much keener than normal and that he will be able to read at a much greater distance, but when the hypnotist raps upon the table his sight will immediately revert to normal again. He then opens his eyes whilst still remaining in the trance state, and it will be found that he is able to read a different page of the same print at a distance of over 2 yards *without glasses*. As he continues to read the hypnotist unexpectedly raps upon the table and the subject will immediately break off in the middle of a sentence and will be quite unable to continue until the page is brought to within a distance of 12 inches, which respresents his normal performance.

Similarly, the power of vision can be decreased and even abolished if suggestions of partial or total blindness are made. Electroencephalograph tracings reveal the fact that whenever it was suggested that the subject could not see brain-waves appeared which were identical with those found in the case of a totally blind person, or in one whose eyes were shut. Erickson[8] has also succeeded in inducing colour-blindness through the use of hypnotic suggestion.

2. *Hearing.* This can be rendered much more acute in the hypnotic state. A deeply hypnotized subject can sometimes hear a clock ticking in an adjoining room which is quite inaudible to him in the waking state, and which nobody else can hear. In fact, it can be stopped and started and the subject will be able to tell exactly when this occurs. Such a case has been described by Mason[9], who considered that it is probably due to the fact that,

in the hypnotized subject, all external sensory stimuli are minimized so that he is able to bring the whole of his concentration to bear upon whatever task he is called upon to perform. In other words, he hears better because he has nothing to distract him.

Partial or even total deafness can also be induced by hypnotic suggestion. In the case of total deafness, a gun can be fired unexpectedly behind the subject, and not only will he show no sign of having heard anything but he will display no rise of blood pressure whatever. It should be remembered, however, that in such a case he will also be unable to hear the hypnotist's voice and will lose contact completely unless suitable precautions have been taken. Therefore an exclusion may be introduced by saying to the subject that he will hear nothing but your voice. In addition, before any such experiments are made, the subject should always be told that his hearing will become normal again upon a given signal, such as a tap upon his shoulder, in which case he will awaken with his function fully restored.

For practical purposes this phenomenon is most useful in treating tinnitus. Patients suffering from this apparently intractable condition are often referred for hypnotherapy. The reduction of anxiety through the use of hetero-hypnosis and self-hypnosis, discussion of anxiety-producing situations and the suggestion of the abolition of those unpleasant sounds in the ear will prove of considerable benefit. It is essential of course, to ensure that no pathological condition exists in the ear before attempting treatment.

Both blindness and deafness induced by suggestion are purely mental phenomena. A simple command will suffice to restore the functions of both sight and hearing. The corresponding organ of sense still performs its usual functions, but the impressions and stimuli fail to reach consciousness.

3. *Smell.* The older hypnotists claimed that the sense of smell could be greatly increased by hypnotic suggestion. An acute sense of smell is known to be normal in many animals for a dog will easily recognize his master by the scent. It was held that under certain circumstances this keenness of scent could be attained by human beings as the result of strong suggestion.

Experiments have been described in which gloves and handkerchiefs have been restored to their rightful owners who were guided only by a sense of smell. Braid successfully conducted such experiments but found that when the subject's nasal passages were blocked all attempts failed. Conversely, the sense of smell can also be diminished or even abolished by suggestion in the deep trance state, so that irritating vapours can be inhaled without the slightest discomfort.

4. *Taste.*   This can be both increased and diminished in hypnosis. Complete absence of taste may be suggested or specific taste sensations temporarily obliterated. Equally, variations of taste may be obtained, for example a favourite trick of stage hypnotists is to give the unfortunate 'volunteer' an onion to eat and to tell him that it is a deliciously sweet and juicy orange. The subject will respond accordingly much to the amusement of the audience. In aversion therapy using hypnosis, a cigarette or an alcoholic drink may be suggested to taste foul and disgusting and so on.

5. *Touch.*   Both Bramwell[10] and Moll[5] earlier claimed that tactile sense can be intensified in hypnosis. In fact it is not difficult to achieve some variation in the sensation of touch in the average hypnotic subject. Alterations in the sensation of touch are frequently used as a test for hypnosis and pain can be diminished or abolished by hypnotic suggestion. Numbness produced in the hand may be transferred to the gums and is used for this purpose in dentistry. Chronic pain may be transferred to other more manageable parts of the body in a similar way. These uses are discussed in the appropriate chapter.

Paraesthesias

Numbness, tingling, itching, sensations of coldness and increased sensitivity to pain, pressure, temperature and touch may be relatively easy to induce under hypnosis. Paraesthesias of vision, taste and smell may also be produced.

REFERENCES

1. Hilgard E.R., 1965. *Hypnotic Susceptibility.* Harcourt, Brace, Jovanovich, New York.
2. Tuckey C.L., 1921. *Treatment by Hypnotism and Suggestion.* Bailliere, Tindall and Cox, London.

3. Forel A., 1949. *Hypnotism.* Allied, New York.
4. Chertok L., 1981. *Sense and Nonsense in Psychotherapy: The Challenge of Hypnosis.* Pergamon, Oxford.
5. Moll A., 1890. *Hypnotism.* Walter Scott, London.
6. Mason A.A. and Black S., 1960. Allergic skin responses abolished under treatment of asthma and hay fever by hypnosis. *Lancet,* **ii,** 877.
7. Black S., Humphrey J.H. and Niven J.S.F., 1963. Inhibition of Mantoux reaction by direct suggestion under hypnosis. *Br. Med. J.,* **1,** 1649–1652.
8. Erickson M.H., 1939. The induction of colour blindness by a technique of hypnotic suggestion. *J. Gen. Psychol.,* **20,** 61.
9. Mason, A.A., 1960. *Hypnotism for Medical and Dental Practitioners.* Secker and Warburg, London.
10. Bramwell J.M., 1903. *Hypnotism, its History, Practice and Theory.* Grant Richards, London.

CHAPTER 10

Somnambulism and Other Phenomena

All kinds of sensory delusions can be produced in deep hypnotic states, many of which are so remarkable that anyone seeing them for the first time may well be excused for doubting the reality of the phenomena. In everyday life, we all depend so completely upon our sense organs that it seems incredible that a few words or phrases can succeed in placing the hypnotic subject in entirely different surroundings. But before many phenomena such as these can be elicited, a very deep or even somnambulistic trance is usually essential.

SOMNAMBULISM

The discovery of this condition is attributed to a follower of Mesmer, the Marquis Chastenet de Puységur (see Chapter 1).

It is generally considered to be one of the deepest stages of hypnosis, and one of the most reliable tests of this condition is to cause the subject to open his eyes without waking from his trance. He will be able to see quite clearly, to talk and to walk about whilst still remaining deeply hypnotized, and will continue to carry out all the suggestions made to him by the hypnotist. Occasionally, but not very often, the subject may appear drowsy in the somnambulistic state; this can easily be remedied if suggestions of alertness are given to him when he will become just as wide awake as in his normal state. Indeed, it can sometimes be very difficult to tell whether a good somnambule is actually in a hypnotic state or not and the only criterion by which this may be judged is the extent to which the subject will respond to suggestion. Other tests of somnambulism are found in the subject's ability to produce hallucinations, to carry out bizarre and complicated post-hypnotic suggestions, to establish major anaesthesia to pain and to produce complete amnesia for the events of the trance state. Some of these phenomena have already been discussed, but others, such as illusions and hallucinations, must now be considered in some detail.

Unfortunately, under ordinary circumstances only some 5 per cent of the hypnotizable population are capable of achieving the somnambulistic state and in medical work the average will probably prove to be even fewer. Generally speaking, it can be said that children are more readily induced into somnambulism than adults, and people who are natural sleep-walkers or automatic writers will often prove to be potential somnambules. With careful training, however, these figures can be considerably improved upon. Erickson has succeeded in inducing somnambulism in difficult subjects only after several hours of continuous sleep suggestions, but very few hypnotists possess either the patience or the necessary skill to induce these deep states in average individuals.

Illusions and Hallucinations

Delusions of the senses are usually classified as '*illusions*' or '*hallucinations*', and before considering them, it is well to define exactly what is meant by these terms: *a delusion* is a false belief, *an illusion* is a false interpretation of an existing object, and *a hallucination* is the perception of an object or person where nothing really exists.

For instance, if a cushion is taken for a cat, we speak of an illusion. But if a cat is perceived when there is actually nothing there, we call it a hallucination. On the whole, it is easier to induce an illusion than a hallucination, for in the absence of an external object the suggestion will frequently fail. Both illusions and hallucinations can be produced in connection with any of the five senses, and may be either positive or negative. If a subject is told

that he can see something that is not really there, the resulting
hallucination is a positive one, but when he is told that he cannot
see something that is actually present, a negative hallucination
is produced. However, it should be noted that in order not to see
something that is really there, the object must first be perceived
before it can be abolished, although this is an unconscious perception of which the subject is unaware.

Moll[1] described a convincing experiment which tends to prove
that the subject recognizes the object of a negative hallucination,
even though there is no conscious perception of it. He took a match
and marked it with a spot of ink, and suggested to a somnambulistic subject that this match would become invisible. He then took
29 other matches and put the whole 30 on the table in such a manner that the subject could still see the ink spot.

When asked how many matches were on the table, the subject
replied, '29'. Whilst his back was turned, the marked match was
moved in such a way that the ink spot could no longer be seen.

The subject once again counted the matches and said there were
now 30 of them on the table. This shows clearly that the marked
match could only remain invisible as long as the subject could distinguish it from the others. It seems certain that in negative hallucinations the subject always retains a dim consciousness of the
true situation.

It is generally considered that the negative hallucination is
probably the deepest of all hypnotic phenomena, and as such is
the most difficult to obtain.

1. *Positive hallucinations.* Hallucinations of sight are usually
more readily induced when the subject's eyes remain closed. He
will then see objects or persons with his eyes shut exactly as he
does in dreams. It will even seem to him that his eyes are open
since we are all unaware in our dreams that our eyes are shut. It
should be noted, however, that hallucinations of sight and hearing are only likely to succeed when very deep trance states have
been achieved. Generally speaking, it is found that the senses of
taste and touch are more easily influenced than others. All the
organs of sense can be deceived in this way. A sudden blow upon
a desk may be interpreted as a gun shot. A subject can be induced
to hear music in the absence of any external stimulus. Water may

be represented as neat whisky, and its consumption will be followed by the usual manifestations of insobriety. Told that a raw potato is an apple, the subject will eat it with every appearance of enjoyment, and strong ammonia will be smelt with pleasure if it has been presented as eau-de-cologne. If given a rubber ball for an onion, when the subject smells it his eyes will fill with tears.

The expression on the subject's face as he complies with such suggestions corresponds exactly with what one would expect had the real article been employed and the thoroughness of the deception is clearly reflected in his reactions. No epicure could show more delight than does the hypnotic who sits down to a hallucinated meal of his favourite dishes.

The stage hypnotist depends upon the production of hallucinations such as these for the entertainment value of his performance, but it cannot be too strongly emphasized that hallucinations of this kind which violate the dignity of the subject should never be indulged in by the medical profession. Even when demonstrating hallucinations for scientific purposes the approval of the subject should be sought before any experiments are made and he should always be treated with the same consideration and respect that he would receive if he were awake. Although mild hallucinations are sometimes possible in medium-depth hypnosis, one can be sure that the more bizarre and complex they become, the deeper the trance that has been achieved.

When a deep somnambulistic stage has been reached, the subject will be able to open his eyes without waking from his trance. In order to test this, he may be instructed in the following manner:

> In a few moments...when I count up to *five*...you will open your eyes...but you will *not* wake up from this deep sleep.
> You will be able to see quite clearly...but you will still remain very, very deeply asleep,
> It may be that things will seem a little hazy or blurred at first...but in a few moments...everything will become quite clear...although you will still remain in this very, very deep sleep.
> You will be able to see clearly...everything that I point out to you!

In this state positive visual hallucinations can be produced which will evoke exactly the same emotional reactions and behaviour that would be expected were the stimulus a real one. The subject will shrink with terror when told that he is confronted with a tiger, or will pick up and fondle a cat.

Hallucinations can also be produced as a result of post-hypnotic suggestion. A subject can be told during hypnosis that at 12 o'clock tomorrow morning his forehead will begin to itch and will continue to do so until he relieves it by rubbing. This will actually occur at the stated time.

2. *Negative hallucinations.* These are possible only in the deepest somnambulistic states, and even then the instructions given to the subject have to be very carefully and precisely worded. When successful, he will be unable to recognize the presence of either an object or a person with which he is confronted. The importance of framing suggestions explicitly with the utmost care is shown in the two following examples, which produce widely different results.

1. If the subject is told: 'From now on you will only be able to see me. You will not be able to see Mr Blank although he is still here', he will be able to talk to Mr Blank, to answer his questions and even be able to feel him. But he will *not* be able to see him.

2. If, on the other hand, the subject is told: 'After you wake up Mr Blank will have disappeared completely. You will not be able to see Mr Blank, to hear Mr Blank or to feel Mr Blank', he will stare straight at the chair in which Mr Blank is sitting and ask where he has gone. If spoken to by Mr Blank he will be unable to hear him, and if he is asked to examine the chair still occupied by Mr Blank he will feel something there but will be unable to interpret it correctly and will probably suggest that Mr Blank has left his overcoat on the chair.

When a fountain-pen is held in front of the subject's eyes, he will recognize it, but if it is then relinquished to Mr Blank, one of two things will happen according to the interpretation he puts upon it. If he then considers that when Mr Blank is holding it, it has become his property and consequently a part of him, the pen will vanish completely. But if he still interprets the pen as belonging to someone else, it will appear to him to be floating unsupported in the air. In this particular experiment the senses of vision, hearing and touch are all simultaneously affected.

This phenomenon is useful in order to demonstrate the depth of hypnosis in a given subject during, for example, an instructional course. A negative hallucination produced in one subject and a positive hallucination in another is a very convincing argument for other phenomena which may be used in treatment.

Hallucinations are not solely of academic interest and frequently have therapeutic applications. Crystal and mirror gazing under hypnosis are both forms of visual hallucination. When instructed to gaze into the crystal or mirror, the subject may both see and describe scenes that arise from his own unconscious conflicts and emotional disturbances. This technique is frequently used in hypnoanalysis.

As in the case of hypnotic analgesia, hallucinations that have been induced must always be removed before the subject is awakened and allowed to leave.

Methods of producing hallucinations. Although in somnambulism it is not difficult to enable the subject to remain in his trance with his eyes open, it is not always easy to get him to hallucinate objects or persons under these conditions. Wolberg[2] has described two excellent techniques for achieving these results.

1. The hypnotist tells the subject that he is going to pick up a small bottle, and to picture him doing so. He will feel curious as to what is in the bottle and will notice a flower on the label. He will realize that the bottle contains perfume and he will picture a flower. As he does so, he will smell the perfume. The hypnotist then places the bottle under the subject's nose whilst simultaneously removing a cork from an actual bottle to convey the necessary sound. The subject is then told that as soon as he smells the perfume, he is to raise his hand. This experiment is carried out with the subject's eyes closed, and when successful produces a positive hallucination of smell.

2. The hypnotist then teaches the subject how to open his eyes without waking, by giving him the following suggestions.

> I want you to imagine that I am holding a bottle of water in front of your eyes.
> You will notice that it is colourless...but as you watch it...it is

gradually becoming pinker and pinker...and changing to a
reddish colour.
As soon as you see the colour changing...let your right (or left)
index finger rise.

The subject responds accordingly (this is known as the ideomotor signal) and the suggestions are continued.

Although you are still deeply asleep...you are going to be able to
open your eyes without waking.
Your eyes will open slowly...but you will *not* wake up from this
deep, deep sleep.
Things may seem a little hazy at first...but they will gradually
become quite clear...and you will remain very, very deeply
asleep...even though your eyes are wide open.
You will stay asleep with your eyes open...until I tell you to
close them again.
You will be able to stand up...or walk about...just as a person
walks in his sleep.
You will see everything that I point out to you.
When you open your eyes...you will notice that I am holding a
bottle of clear fluid in front of your eyes.
As you watch it...you will see the colour of the fluid slowly
becoming pinker and pinker...until it becomes quite red...just as
it did when your eyes were shut.
As soon as you see the colour changing...please lift up your
index finger.
Now open your eyes, slowly...very slowly...open your eyes.
Never mind if things look a little blurred at first...as you look at
the bottle...they will gradually become clear...and you will see
the colour changing...first to pink...then to red.
Open your eyes slowly...wider and wider.

As the subject does so, a bottle of water is held in front of his
eyes, which he gazes at until he notices the colour change, and
raises his index finger. Once this has occurred, he can be told that
as he looks at the table, he will see a candlestick with a burning
candle. He is told to go over to the table and blow out the candle.
This suggestion is repeated several times.

Many subjects are able to hallucinate well with their eyes closed,
but have difficulty in doing so with their eyes open. In such cases
a very simple object may be suggested. When the subject signifies

that he can see this clearly, tell him that when he opens his eyes he will remain deeply hypnotized but will still be able to see that particular object.

Three Effective Demonstrations

For each of the following demonstrations a deeply hypnotized somnambule, capable of opening his or her eyes without waking from the trance, is required.

1. The hypnotized subject reclines in a chair with eyes closed. A volunteer sits close by, and is instructed to close his eyes and to try to simulate the hypnotic state. The hypnotist then produces a small bottle containing fluid which he represents to be a very delightful perfume. He tells them that they will each smell it in turn and derive the greatest pleasure and enjoyment from doing so. The bottle is then placed under the nose of the hypnotized subject, who smells it repeatedly with enthusiasm. When asked what it smells like, the subject invariably names a favourite scent. The bottle is then presented to the non-hypnotized volunteer, who takes one deep sniff only and turns his head away in disgust. It actually contains ammonia.

2. The deeply hypnotized subject is told that presently he will open his eyes and will be able to see quite clearly, without waking from his trance. One minute after his eyes open, he will hear a noise like a cat mewing, and will look around to see where it is coming from. He will then see a kitten walk round the side of his chair, and will bend down, pick it up and stroke it. He is then told to open his eyes without waking and within the prescribed time limit he will comply with these suggestions in a most convincing manner.

This experiment demonstrates hallucinations of hearing, sight and touch. Before embarking upon it, however, it is always advisable to make sure that the subject neither dislikes, nor is allergic to cats. If fond of dogs, the suggestion of a puppy barking can be substituted.

3. Once again, the hypnotic subject is told that he will presently be able to open his eyes without waking. He is also told that, when his eyes are open, an object standing on the table will have completely disappeared and that he will not be able to see it. After

he has opened his eyes, he is asked to pass this object which is on the table, in full view. He will carefully scrutinize the table and fail to discover it there. A pen or notepad can then be placed on top of the object and, to the utter astonishment of the subject, will appear to be floating unsupported in the air just above the table.

This experiment demonstrates a negative hallucination of sight. With a good somnambule, both this demonstration and the one previously described can be even more effectively performed in the waking state, as the result of post-hypnotic suggestion.

SOME PSYCHOLOGICAL PHENOMENA OF HYPNOSIS

The psychological phenomena characteristic of the hypnotic state can be most conveniently discussed under the headings of memory, mental activity and emotions.

Memory

This determines every other psychical activity for all the higher mental functions are dependent upon memory, which consists essentially of four important factors so far as hypnosis is concerned. These are:

1. The power of assimilating ideas.
2. The power of retaining ideas.
3. The power of recalling ideas.
4. The power of recognizing ideas and locating them accurately in the past.

The part these play is clearly shown in the following example. Let us take some event we can remember from the past, such as a severe reprimanding from a teacher. In such a case, the memory acts in four ways:

1. What was said at the time was assimilated by it.
2. What was said at the time was retained in it.
3. The memory can recall and reproduce exactly what was said.
4. It can be placed in its exact position in time by recalling its relation to other events, such as being in the school.

There are also three other factors upon which the powers of retention and recall ultimately depend: firstly, the more forcibly or dramatically an event or idea strikes us at the time, the more likely it is to be remembered; secondly, the more frequently an experience is repeated, the more easily it will be remembered; thirdly, the more distant such an experience is in time, the more difficult it will be to remember.

It was originally thought that the subject always had amnesia upon waking for everything that had happened during the trance, but this is certainly not correct. In the lighter hypnotic stages, the memory is usually unaffected. During the trance, the subject will remember everything of which he was conscious in everyday life, and when it is terminated he will recollect accurately everything that has occurred during the hypnosis. In the deeper hypnotic states, however, it is a very different matter. There is frequently a complete amnesia upon waking, and the subject is astonished to hear what he has actually been doing during the trance. But it must not be assumed that this is necessarily the case, since certain individuals who readily achieve a deep trance can still recall spontaneously everything that has occurred during the trance. And in other cases, the mere association of ideas will be sufficient to restore the missing memory. Moll[1] quoted the following example.

'I suggest to a hypnotic that he is at a concert. He hears various pieces of music amongst which is the overture to *Martha*. He goes into the bar, drinks his beer, and talks to imaginary people. On awakening, he can remember nothing of all this. I then ask him if he knows the opera *Martha*. This one word will suffice to recall nearly all the events of the hypnosis.'

Bernheim went so far as to state that the memory could be recovered in all cases by means of strong, persistent suggestion in the subsequent waking state. Indeed, it was one of his experiments to illustrate this that influenced Freud in his development of the technique of psychoanalysis.

It is a well-known fact that some memories which are thought to have been entirely forgotten, and consequently inaccessible in the waking state, can be recalled during hypnosis. This remarkable phenomenon is termed hypermnesia, and is the opposite to amnesia. Certainly not all of life's events and experiences are recorded in the mind. Many however, may be so, even if quite trivial. Since it would be impossible to retain everything, they may be discarded and become no longer available for recall. On the other hand, more significant events that are charged with emotion, pleasant or unpleasant, can usually be recalled at will, or through an association of ideas. Even so, if these memories are associated with such humiliating and painful experiences that their restoration to consciousness would arouse considerable anxiety, it will be impossible to revive them. Such memories have been repressed below the level of conscious awareness, but may be recalled in hypnosis in some subjects. This object is often achieved in a deep trance state by employing the technique known as age-regression, in itself a most fascinating phenomenon. Nevertheless it must be clearly understood that a hypnotized subject may still confabulate or lie wilfully even when under hypnosis (Orne[3]).

Age-regression

In deep hypnosis, an adult can be told that he is going back in time, in place and in memory, perhaps even to childhood, and that he will be able to relive experiences that he underwent at that particular age. As a result, if he is regressed to the age of 5 years, he will begin to talk and act exactly as if he were a small boy again, and will be able to recount experiences and events of that period which he could not possibly remember in the waking state. Indeed, if he is taken back successively through several different ages and is asked to write his name at each age, his handwriting will change progressively until it becomes quite childish both in character and performance.

Many authorities today consider that hypnotic regression is an artefact and that the subject is merely playing a role, but another view is that the regressed subject frequently does reproduce early patterns of behaviour far too accurately to permit the possibility of simulation alone. Erickson and Kubie[4] recognized two distinct types of age-regression:

1. In the first type, the subject does actually return to an earlier stage of development, with a total amnesia for all events subsequent to that period. When regressed to 5 years of age he will readily remember things that happened to him at this period of his life but will have completely forgotten everything that fol-

lowed. He may even fail to recognize the hypnotist himself, whom naturally enough he has not yet met, and who may consequently have to identify himself with someone with whom the subject was familiar at this particular age.

2. In the second type the subject never succeeds in actually returning to an earlier stage of development but behaves exactly as he imagines a child of that age would behave. Despite this, the hypnotic subject will always be able to simulate earlier patterns of behaviour far more accurately than a subject in the waking state, and he will still be able to remember at the regressed level things that are beyond conscious recall in his adult life. All this can happen without any subsequent amnesia for the trance.

In true regression of the first type (which is sometimes referred to as *revivification*) the changed immature handwriting will often be found to correspond closely to that in old school books of that particular period. Moreover, the way in which it is performed will sometimes carry further conviction.

Some experimental psychologists have offered even more evidence in an attempt to prove that the subject is merely simulating the sort of response that he considers a hypnotized person would produce if being age-regressed.

However, the purpose of the exercise should not be overlooked. Whether to produce an abreaction or to help in the psychoanalytic phase of treatment, it is an attempt to revive memories of past experiences which might have played some part in the origin of the patient's problem. From the clinical point of view, what is important is what the patient says, what he believes to be true, what may be true or perhaps even what he wants you to believe is true. It is up to the therapist to use this information for the benefit of his client.

It should be understood however, as is elsewhere also stated, this recall is not regression. It is simply remembering. Regression is reliving an event with all its physical and psychological experiences simultaneously expressed.

Sometimes the revived memories of the regressed subject can be checked. It has been reported that when an adult subject, regressed to her seventh birthday, was asked what day of the week it was, she replied 'Friday' without the slightest hesitation, and subsequent investigation proved this to be true. This is a feat of memory that few of us could accomplish in the waking state.

Methods of producing age-regression.   There are several different methods of producing age-regression. The simplest of these is just to tell the deeply hypnotized subject that, upon a given signal, he will once again feel that he is at a particular age—say 10 years old. It is always wise to specify some special day such as a birthday or Christmas day. The subject is told that he will feel exactly as if he were 10 years old again, and will experience everything that he formerly did upon that occasion. A little time should be allowed for these suggestions to take effect, and then the signal should be given. It is helpful to ask the subject to give an ideomotor signal (raising a finger) as soon as he feels that he is 10 years old. He can than be questioned as to who he is, where he is, how old he is, what he is doing and what presents he has received.

No matter what technique is used, it is necessary that the hypnotist should be fitted into the regressive pattern. It is obvious that if the subject is taken back to a period of his life prior to meeting the hypnotist, as far as he is concerned the latter does not even exist. It is true that such a situation seems to arise but rarely, for in most cases the subject either continues to accept the hypnotist as such, or spontaneously fits him into the regressive situation. There would, however, be a real danger of losing contact if he failed to do so. It is consequently wise for the hypnotist to include in his instructions to the subject the suggestion that he will become identified as an observer of the events that occurred at that particular time of his life.

Once any specific phase of regression is ended, the subject should be told to sleep deeply again before any further regression is attempted, or before he is returned to his normal age. In attempting regression for the first time, a relatively simple and uncomplicated technique may be employed:

> Whilst you are in this deep sleep...time no longer matters...you will presently be able to go back quite easily to any earlier period of your life.
> You are gradually going back to the time when you were 6 years old...you will feel that you are gradually getting smaller...smaller and smaller...that your arms and legs are

getting smaller...that your body is getting smaller...
In a few moments now...you will feel that you are 6 years old
again...and that it is your birthday.
You are exactly 6 years old.
As soon as you feel that you are exactly 6 years old...please raise
your right (or left) index finger.

Wolberg[2] precedes this by first taking the subject back to yesterday, and questioning him about what he did and what meals
he ate. He then takes him back to the very first consultation. He
is asked to describe it, how he was feeling and what clothes he
wore. He is told that he will actually see himself talking to the
doctor once again. This is a modification of the most powerful of
all methods which was originally described by Erickson. It consists of a combination of disorientation and reorientation. The
subject is slowly but completely disorientated both for time and
place. A general state of confusion is first produced by suggesting
to the subject that he finds it more and more difficult to remember what day of the week it is, what the date is , what the month
is and what year it is. As these suggestions are given, the patient
becomes more confounded and as this occurs he is slowly reorien-
tated to the particular age required.

It must be emphasized that this technique is not for amateurs.
The patient may even become dissociated if the situation is not
properly controlled and if the hypnotist is unable to handle the
regression. Considerable experience is essential also in dealing
with any possible emotional response.

Additionally although it is necessary that age-regression should
be both fully described and demonstrated when teaching hypnosis, it should never be used for idle experimentation. There is
always the risk of unwittingly regressing a subject to an age at
which some traumatic emotional experience had occurred, in
which case the reactions might be both severe and difficult to deal
with. For this reason alone, the technique of age-regression is ordinarily best restricted to those with psychiatric or clinical psychological experience, and that even for treatment purposes it is
best avoided by general medical and dental practitioners.

Mental Activity

Just as in the normal state, the mental activity in hypnosis depends upon the attention paid by the subject. In deep hypnosis, the subject's attention is primarily directed towards the hypnotist, so that other objects or persons hardly seem to exist so far as he is concerned.

Rapport. This can best be defined as a state of affinity existing between subject and hypnotist and should be present at the very onset of hypnosis. It is of such a nature that it tends to prevent the subject from responding to any stimuli other than those arising from the hypnotist himself unless he instructs the subject otherwise. Even when it is not as strong as this, it will still cause the subject to respond more effectively to suggestions from the hypnotist himself, than those from other people.

In the early days of hypnosis, it was believed that a subject would only respond to the suggestions of his original hypnotist, and would ignore those from anyone else unless instructed otherwise. This rapport could easily be transferred to another person, in which case the hypnotist himself would lose contact with the subject. It was also thought that the subject could only be awakened by the individual with whom he was in rapport.

Although such complete rapport does sometimes occur, it is more frequently present to a lesser degree. It is, however, mistaken to consider rapport as being merely the product of suggestion. It is very much more than that. Erickson claimed that one can never be sure what it actually includes, that it expresses the attitude of the subject towards his surroundings and is very definitely a phenomenon of hypnosis. Essentially, rapport seems to be a kind of mental sympathy which gradually develops through repetition into a state of exaggerated belief and trust on the part of the subject which often leads to a form of emotional attachment and a positive transference between subject and hypnotist.

We have already seen that these conditions begin to exist before trance induction is even attempted. Indeed, induction will only be likely to succeed when the hypnotist has first convinced the subject that he is to be trusted implicitly and that whatever he says is to be believed and relied upon. Only in this way can anxieties relating to the trance be reduced to a bare minimum. But one must not think that rapport consists of nothing more than this initial approach, strengthened by various deepening techniques which result in increasing the subject's trust and belief. The work of Freud and the psychoanalytical school has demonstrated that something much more fundamental exists. They consider rapport between subject and hypnotist to resemble a child–parent relationship. This is a phenomenon that regularly occurs in psychoanalysis, and is a state in which the subject unconsciously regresses and adopts the attitude of a child towards his parent, with all its exaggerated trust, belief, affection and acceptance of authority. In this respect, it can be said to resemble the transference situation that exists in most good doctor–patient relationships, the difference being merely one of degree. In hypnosis this regression is much more complete and results in a diminution of the subject's ability to evaluate critically the situation that has developed.

The fact that rapport can either be transferred to, or shared with another person should the hypnotist so desire, can often be important in the therapeutic field. This applies particularly to obstetrics, for should the hypnotist be unable to attend the confinement, the patient can be placed in rapport with the obstetrician or midwife, and will then follow their instructions just as faithfully as if they had been given by the hypnotist.

The sense and judgement of time. The evidence as to whether in the hypnotic state a subject is able to judge the passage of time more accurately than in the waking state is conflicting in nature.

It is certainly true that if the hypnotized subject is asked to perform a task after a specified number of minutes, he will usually do so with a fair degree of accuracy. Similarly, he will perform an act as the result of a post-hypnotic suggestion, after a prescribed interval of time. The most comprehensive account of this phenomenon was given by Bramwell[5], whose hypnotic subjects were unbelievably accurate in their judgement of time. Unfortunately, however, no subsequent investigator has succeeded in duplicating his results. Indeed, controlled experiments tend to show that the ability to estimate time is no greater in the hypnotic than in the waking state, provided that sufficient concentration is devoted to the task.

Calculations carried out in the unconscious mind are not invariably exact. Sometimes suggestions are not executed punctually when an abstract period of time has been given. Even so, they will usually approximate fairly closely to the specified moment. This unconscious estimation of time is not unknown in everyday life. Some people can judge time in the waking state with remarkable accuracy, whilst others can do the same during sleep. They are able to waken themselves at a predetermined hour without hearing a clock strike or an alarm bell ring.

Personality changes. Under deep hypnosis, the subject can be made to believe that he is a totally different personality, and will act the role of the suggested character in a most convincing manner. Moll[1] pointed out that in such cases not only do many memories connected with the subject's own personality disappear, but he tries to connect the remaining ones with his suggested personality and will sometimes create new ones appropriate to it. For instance, when a subject was told that he was Frederick the Great, he promptly walked with a crutch in the well-known gait, *but he knew nothing of railways.*

If during hypnosis several different personalities are suggested, each successive change is usually accompanied by a loss of memory of that which preceded it. One hypnotized subject was unable to remember as Napoleon what he had done as Frederick the Great. These changes of personality in hypnotic subjects have often been compared with the performances of actors, yet few actors seem to identify themselves so completely with a character as does the hypnotic subject. This is because the latter is not distracted in any way by sense perceptions, whereas the actor cannot avoid being affected to some extent by them.

Because of the ability to produce personality change under hypnosis, the problem of multiple personality has been extensively investigated through the use of hypnosis. The classical example is that of a female patient of Thigben and Cleckley, clearly described in the book 'The Three Faces of Eve'[6].

The Emotions

The emotional changes that arise spontaneously as feelings towards the hypnotic state and the hypnotist have already been discussed. But quite apart from these, the general feelings of the subject can be readily influenced by hypnotic suggestion. Desire and dislike can easily be suggested, particularly in deep hypnotic states. Sadness or cheerfulness can readily be induced in deep hypnosis and may alternate very quickly. Similarly, emotions such as love, hate, fear, anger and anxiety are easy to evoke by means of suggestion. Indeed, many moods can be artificially induced under hypnosis if a specific situation is suggested which tends to arouse that mood. For instance, if after being told to hallucinate some person he dislikes intensely, he is told that he is being insulted by him, the hypnotic subject will appear very angry. Under such circumstances, the facial expression, attitude and behaviour of the subject show quite convincingly what he is actually feeling.

Post-hypnotic Amnesia

After somnambulism, the subject usually experiences a loss of memory on waking, the extent of which varies with the depth of the trance. This may or may not occur following medium or even deep trances, and when it does, the resulting amnesia is only partial. Indeed, it can be said that complete post-hypnotic amnesia is only likely to be found in the deepest of hypnotic states.

Although no amnesia may be observed following the first few hypnotic sessions, it can still appear upon some subsequent occasion. It is sometimes spontaneous and occurs in the absence of any suggestions from the hypnotist. At other times, it can be induced by direct suggestions to this effect. When it appears, it always means that some degree of dissociation has actually occurred. The events of the trance state are forgotten, and the amnesia seems to resemble that for dreams which follows normal sleep. Even a good subject will be unlikely to develop an amnesia if he is instructed to remember what has occurred during his trance.

Amnesia will only arise if the subject has no objection to it, conscious or unconscious. The more important the memory is to a subject in his occupation, the more difficulty there is likely to be in successfully inducing an amnesia.

Another unconscious obstacle that is difficult to overcome arises when the personality of the subject is such that he feels that at all costs he must retain some degree of control. Although he may enter the deep trance state, he will either remember everything that has occurred, or at least sufficient to satisfy his needs. This can sometimes be countered by telling him that he will remember one or two of the more trivial incidents, but will forget all the rest. On the whole, it is true to say that if the subject does wish to remember something, he will almost certainly do so.

Amnesia is most complete immediately the trance state is terminated but sometimes begins to break down, hours, days or weeks later. In this case, it is probable that fresh associations enter the subject's mind which tend to restore his memory. When complete amnesia can be induced in a somnambulistic subject, he may often be caused to forget certain aspects of his waking life. He can even be told that he will not remember being hypnotized, and will subsequently deny that anything has happened.

Complete amnesia is an invaluable asset when it can be secured. It convinces the subject in no uncertain manner that he has really been hypnotized, and ensures deep trance production on future occasions. Amnesia always seems to strengthen the effect of post-hypnotic suggestion and is most useful from the therapeutic point of view, for since the patient will have no recollection of what has been said, he will be unable to criticize the suggestions he has been given during the trance. They will consequently take effect much more rapidly and powerfully. Although the events of the trance are forgotten when complete amnesia occurs, they can usually be remembered in subsequent trance states, unless instructions to the contrary have been given.

One patient was given a post-hypnotic suggestion that he would not remember the recall of a certain event which he had abreacted during hypnoanalytic treatment by one of us (D.W.). He subsequently consented to the discussion of his case history at a lecture given to a medical audience and when questioned about his memory of his experiences during regression he replied 'I don't remember, because the doctor told me to forget.'

Methods of producing post-hypnotic amnesia. At each hypnotic session, before waking the subject it is wise to suggest that every time he enters a trance, he will remember less and less of what has occurred, until eventually he will be able to remember nothing at all concerning his hypnosis. If this occurs, it will obviously be the result of continued post-hypnotic suggestion.

1. Amnesia can sometimes be produced in the deep trance state by direct suggestion alone. When applied forcefully, it can be very powerful indeed and, provided that the trance is deep enough, will often prove successful.

> You are now in a very, very deep sleep indeed...so deep, in fact...that, after you wake up...*you will not be able to remember anything that has happened during this deep sleep.*
> After you wake up...*if you try to remember what has occurred during your sleep...your mind will go completely blank...and you will not be able to remember anything that has taken place.*
> After you wake up...*you will not be able to remember anything that has been said...or done...during this deep sleep.*

2. Sometimes it is wiser to adopt a much milder, more persuasive approach, which will be much less likely to prejudice further attempts.

> You are now in so deep a sleep...that, after you wake up...*you will have no desire whatever to remember what has occurred during your sleep.*
> You won't feel that you want to remember anything that has happened during this deep sleep.
> Your sleep is becoming so deep...that you will tend to forget everything that has happened since you went to sleep.

In therapeutic work the following suggestions may be added to provide increased motivation.

> *The less you remember of what I say to you, during this sleep...the more quickly and powerfully this treatment will act...so that you will not want to remember anything...after you wake up.*

Amnesias produced by this method are seldom complete at first, but can sometimes be rendered total by constant repetition over a number of sessions.

We have already noted the fact that both hypnosis itself and loss of memory seem to offer a threat to the peace of mind of certain subjects. In such cases, Wolberg[2] would suggest to the subject that he will remember some trivial event of the trance, but will develop amnesia for the rest of it. This allays the subject's fear of losing control completely. Should this fail and the subject remembers everything, he would proceed in the following manner during the next trance session:

3. The subject is told that he is to imagine that he is at home, asleep. He will then have a short dream, after which his eyes will open and he will wake up with a start. He will feel that he has just awakened from a sound sleep. He will remember the dream vividly, but immediately after describing it, he will only have a vague recollection of other events of the trance and may even forget some of them when questioned.

4. If a partial amnesia is secured as a result of these suggestions, they are followed up in the next trance, and the subject is told:

> Forgetting is a perfectly normal process…it is easy to forget if you divert your attention to other things.
> Last time, you forgot certain things that happened whilst you were asleep.
> Today you will probably forget many more…possibly everything that happens during the trance.

Before waking the subject, the above dream sequence is repeated. These two techniques can be constantly repeated over a number of sessions to train the subject gradually to achieve amnesia.

Weitzenhoffer[7] has found it effective to use a modified 'fractionation' method. He repeatedly awakens and rehypnotizes his subjects, each time suggesting that they will forget more and more of the happenings in the trance. He pointed out that since amnesia and depth of hypnosis are intimately related, this is a very convenient way of dealing with the two problems simultaneously.

5. A method which is sometimes used with success is the so-called blackboard technique.

I want you to imagine that you can see a blackboard...and that I am standing in front of it with a piece of chalk in my hand.
Just picture that blackboard...and as soon as you can see it quite clearly...please signal with your index finger.

(The subject's finger rises.)

Now, as you watch that blackboard...you can see me writing on it with the chalk.
You can see what I am writing...I am writing the word MEMORY.
You can see that word quite clearly.
As soon as you can see that word...please raise your index finger.

(Once again, the subject's finger rises.)

As you go on watching the blackboard...you can see that I have taken a wet duster...and am cleaning the writing off the board.
And as the word...MEMORY...disappears from the blackboard...so will everything that has happened during your sleep also disappear from your mind...just as if your mind were being cleaned like the blackboard.
As soon as you can see that the word has disappeared...and the blackboard is clear and blank...please raise your index finger.

(The subject's finger rises.)

In a few moments...when I wake you...you will not remember anything that has happened whilst you were asleep.
If you try to remember what has happened...your mind will remain quite blank...just like that blackboard, after it had been cleaned.
After you wake up...you will not be able to remember anything that has happened during your deep sleep.

Amnesia is a complicated and sometimes unpredictable phenomenon. As we have seen, it can vary from the simple forgetting that is found in hypnosis, to the much more significant and severe loss of memory caused by the repression of traumatic experiences, the recollection of which could arouse a severe emotional response.

PARAMNESIAS

These can be readily induced in hypnosis, particularly in the deeper stages. They differ from the amnesias in that the subject is told that he will only forget specific things, such as his name, his birthday or even the meanings of words. Aphasias can thus be produced. The subject may be deprived of the power to speak at all, or simply rendered unable to pronounce a particular word or consonant. Moreover, false memories can also be induced. If the subject is told in deep hypnosis that a number of entirely imaginary events have occurred, when he awakens he will remember them as actual facts. This is one of the major problems which may arise in the use of hypnosis in criminology. If the investigator is unwary or inexperienced, he may easily cue his subject and produce false 'memories' or pseudomemories.

REFERENCES

1. Moll A., 1890. *Hypnotism.* Walter Scott, London
2. Wolberg L.R., 1948. *Medical Hypnosis,* Vol. 1. Grune and Stratton, New York.
3. Orne M.T., 1979. The use and misuse of hypnosis in court. *Int. J. Clin. Exp Hypnosis* **XXVII** 311–341.
4. Erickson M.H. and Kubie L.S., 1941. The successful treatment of a case of acute hysterical depression by a return under hypnosis to a critical phase of childhood. *Psychoanal. Q.,* **10,** 583.
5. Bramwell J.M., 1903. *Hypnotism, its History, Practice and Theory.* Grant Richards, London.
6. Thigben C.H. and Cleckley H.M., 1957. *The Three Faces of Eve.* Secker and Warburg, London.
7. Weitzenhoffer A.M., 1957. *General Techniques of Hypnosis.* Grune and Stratton, New York.

CHAPTER 11

Post-hypnotic Suggestion and Other Techniques

POST-HYPNOTIC SUGGESTION

This is the phenomenon in which suggestions that are given during the trance state are caused to take effect after the subject has been awakened. But for this, the therapeutic value of hypnosis would be almost negligible. Most patients, having entered the hypnotic state, will comply with any reasonable suggestions given and will respond, whilst in hypnosis, for example to deepening techniques. Others will respond to suggestions given whilst *in* hypnosis, that some act be carried out *after* the hypnosis has been terminated. No satisfactory evidence has been produced to explain this occurrence. Wolberg[1] described a post-hypnotic suggestion as 'any phenomenon induced during hypnosis which may be executed post-hypnotically on suggestion'. Although it is generally believed that such responses will only be effective in the somnambule, Wolberg also found, as have most experienced therapists, that in some cases a relatively light trance is sufficient for the suggestion to be effective. It was also considered essential that amnesia must follow the suggestions given, but this, as has already been said, is certainly not the case. Amnesia will occur however if the instruction is given 'to forget' in very deep trance subjects. Generally speaking however, most post-hypnotic suggestions will be more effective when a deep trance state, followed by amnesia, has been produced. There is no doubt that amnesia greatly increases the force of post-hypnotic suggestion.

One of the most characteristic features of the post-hypnotic response is its compulsive nature. That is, that the suggestion cannot be resisted. This resistance may sometimes be overcome but it can take a tremendous effort and be extremely disturbing to do so. If the effort to resist is persisted in, anxiety may build up and eventually will only be relieved by compliance with the post-hypnotic instructions. In addition, Wolberg confirmed that post-hypnotic suggestions that are reasonable and in keeping with the personality of the individual are usually carried out. Unreasonable or ridiculous suggestions may be rejected even if the subject is a somnambule.

Moll[2] considered that the phenomenon of post-hypnotic suggestion is hardly as curious as it may seem, since it can be compared to a similar kind of behaviour that occurs in everyday life. He quoted the following example:

I give a letter to Mr X who has called on me, and ask him to post it on his way home if he passes a letter-box. He puts the letter in his pocket and subsequently meets a friend and walks home with him, passing a letter-box on the way. Whilst engaged in conversation, Mr X apparently did not notice the box, but threw the letter into it without interrupting the conversation. Later on, it occurred to him that he had a letter to post. He had only a dim recollection of having done so, and only by feeling in his pocket and finding no letter there could he convince himself that he had indeed executed the commission.

The particular feature to be noticed here is that Mr X has performed a specified act *without the intervention of his will,* and one of the most striking features of post-hypnotic suggestion is the fact that it is carried out under precisely the same conditions. Moll also called attention to the fact that it is not the post-hypnotic command itself—not what was actually said to the subject at the time—*but the idea of carrying out the instruction* that becomes conscious at the appointed time. For instance, if it is suggested to the hypnotic subject that he will ask for an apple, half an hour after he wakes up, he will certainly do so. But it is not the fact that he has been told to ask for an apple that will occur to him at the appropriate moment. It will be the idea that he would like an apple and had better ask for one that will rise into his conscious mind. Even in normal life, ordinary occurrences can sometimes produce similar ideas through suggestion. A healthy patient has frequently become convinced that he is suffering from heart disease as a result of overhearing some casual conversation about a severe cardiac condition.

It is remarkable to what extent post-hypnotic suggestions are carried out at the right moment. This can be appointed in two ways: (1) *By an external signal* such as a sign given by the hypnotist, or the striking of a clock. (2) *By fixing an abstract period—* after so many minutes, hours or days. In the latter case, the accuracy is often less precise than in the former, although a very close approximation will usually occur.

The first of these methods involves no new mental phenomenon at all, for in normal life the striking of a clock often calls to mind something that we wished to do at a particular time, and we promptly proceed to do it. How often have you wanted to write a letter tomorrow, and have tied a knot in your handkerchief to remind you of the fact. The knot and the letter have become so closely associated in your consciousness that, although you may have completely forgotten what you intended to do, when you see the knot the next day the idea of writing the letter arises from your unconscious mind into consciousness again.

The following examples illustrate the various kinds of predetermined signals used in post-hypnotic suggestion:

1. 'When you hear me rap on the table twice...you will lie back in your chair and fall into a deep sleep.'

This is an audible external signal.

2. 'When you see me straighten my tie...you will get up from your chair and then sit down again.'

This is a predetermined visual signal, suggested by the hypnotist.

3. 'Ten minutes after you wake up...you will bend down and take off your right shoe.'

In this case a period of time—10 minutes—has been fixed. Specifying the time in this way, however, may not always be successful, for some subjects' perception of time may be poorer than others, or they may even become so interested in what is taking place that they tend to lose track of time. But even after the specified interval has elapsed and the subject has shown no sign of complying with the instruction, it does not necessarily mean that the suggestion has failed. Indeed, it is more than likely that if in general conversation some casual remark is made about the subject's shoes, he will probably become restless, look down at his feet, and eventually take off his shoe.

There are several ways in which the patient can avoid complying with such suggestions. He may wake spontaneously, his hypnotic sleep may change into ordinary sleep, he may become restless and obviously concerned or he may develop such severe signs of increasing anxiety and nervous agitation that the hypnotist will have no choice but to awaken him, after cancelling the offending instruction. Under these circumstances, however, the hypnotist is present and able to take prompt steps to counter the suggestion, or replace it with one that is more acceptable. *It is not always the actual suggestion that is made, but the way the subject interprets it that determines the way he responds, and whether he finds it acceptable or not.*

This question of interpretation is of the greatest possible importance. Suggestions to be acted upon post-hypnotically must always be carefully and precisely worded, not only to ensure that their meaning is fully understood by the subject, but also to avoid the slightest risk of ambiguity or possibility of misinterpretation. It is not always easy to foresee the latter occurrence, for our intentions often seem so clear to us that we are only too prone to assume that they are equally clear to the subject. This is not invariably the case, as the following example from the experience of one of us (J.H.) will show:

During the second world war, I had a patient who was a member of a British Red Cross Detachment. He was a man in his late thirties, strictly brought up, very religious, and who never in his life had been known to use bad language. He was sadly lacking in self-confidence and dreaded one of his tests for promotion, in which he had to command a squad in stretcher drill. He was an excellent somnambule with complete amnesia, and I gave him the post-hypnotic suggestions that the moment he stood up in front of his squad, all traces of nervousness would disappear and he would be able to give his commands and drill the men *just like an army sergeant-major.* During the actual tests, much to my discomfiture he proceeded to address his squad in the following terms: Squad 'shun! As you were! Jump to it, you blankety-blank, pot-bellied lot of so-and-so's!

It is obvious that his own literal interpretation of my instruction varied widely from my own innocent intention that he should drill his squad with the confidence of an army sergeant-major. Careless wording was entirely responsible for this unfortunate and embarrassing incident which took place in the presence of a large number of onlookers. This need for formulating one's instructions clearly and unambiguously is equally important at every stage of hypnosis, for it should never be forgotten that the hypnotic subject tends to take everything literally, sometimes with unexpected and surprising results.

Sometimes a post-hypnotic suggestion will only be carried out if the subject has been provided with a logical reason for the suggested act.

If a subject is told to take a glass of water and throw it over the desk, he may well refrain from doing so, but if it is first suggested to him that the desk is on fire, he will comply without the slightest hesitation. Similarly, if he is told to steal Dr Blank's fountain-pen when his back is turned, he will certainly not do so. But if it is represented to him that it is really your fountain-pen, which Dr Blank has pocketed, and that the only chance of regaining the property is for him to take it back, he will probably oblige.

In certain cases, seemingly harmless suggestions can arouse sufficient anxiety to prevent their fulfilment because of an association with the subject's own unconscious mental conflicts. For this reason, always watch the subject's reactions carefully, so that any such suggestion can either be rephrased or withdrawn if it appears to arouse uneasiness or anxiety. This can be important, for if such suggestions are post-hypnotic and the subject fails to realize their full implications at the time, some psychological disturbance could quite easily result.

The phrasing of post-hypnotic suggestions may also determine whether they are executed or not. If either the wording or manner of delivery of such suggestions betrays the slightest lack of confidence on the part of the hypnotist that they will be carried out, the subject will detect this immediately and will be better able to resist. When, however, the suggestion conveys to him the belief and conviction that he is expected to comply, he will be much more likely to do so. When in doubt about the success of a post-hypnotic suggestion, it should never be given. There is no situation using hypnosis, in which failure is more likely to occur, than when the therapist fears that he will fail.

The effect and duration of post-hypnotic suggestions can be very prolonged. Many authentic instances have been reported in which they have been carried out months or even years after they have been given.

A young married woman aged 26 years, sought hypnotic treatment for her psoriasis. In the course of her interview she asked the therapist (J.H.) if he remembered her. When he apologized she reminded him that he had treated her previously for insomnia when she was only 11 years old. Once again she was simply told to go to sleep and she lapsed into complete somnambulism after an interval of 15 years.

There is no doubt that the effects of post-hypnotic suggestion can be greatly enhanced if the suggestion is repeated frequently. Indeed, if repeated often enough, such suggestions tend to become permanent since it is probable that a conditioned response is established. This may partly explain why patients who have improved under hypnotherapy do not generally tend to relapse.

Another method of increasing the strength of a post-hypnotic suggestion is to couple it with some normal experience, so that a reasonable explanation becomes possible in the subject's mind. Under hypnosis, a subject can be told:

After you wake up...you will drink a glass of water.

Better still, a much clearer indication can be given by saying:

Five minutes after you wake up...you will drink a glass of water.

The best way of putting it, however, would be to say:

As soon as you wake up...you will begin to feel thirsty.
Your mouth will become dry and parched...and in a few

minutes...you will drink a glass of water.

Each of these suggestions would need to be repeated, but the last would require less frequent repetition than either of the others. It would none the less influence the subject far more powerfully for, once again, he has been given a logical reason for the suggested act.

Rationalization

Baudouin[3] remarked that the subject of a post-hypnotic suggestion usually thinks that he is activated by his own will and often justifies or rationalizes by finding an excellent reason for what he does.

For example when post-hypnotic amnesia is present, and the subject upon waking is unable to remember the particular instruction that has been given once the action has been performed and if he is asked why he had done it, he will often produce the most ingenious rationalizations for his conduct. Suppose he has been told that, two minutes after he wakes up, he will take off his right shoe. Provided that he has developed a deep trance followed by amnesia, he will faithfully carry out this instruction. Since he is quite unable to remember having been told to do this, when he is asked why he has removed his shoe, he will generally give some plausible yet entirely false explanation of his action which completely satisfies himself. He will probably say, 'My foot was itching', or 'My sock had become creased and uncomfortable'. Indeed, the more bizarre or incongruous the post-hypnotic suggestion is, the more astonishing such rationalizations are likely to be. Several instances have been recorded in which post-hypnotic suggestions have been chosen for which it would be difficult to find logical explanations:

1. A subject was told that five minutes after he woke up, he would leave the lecture room and return with an umbrella from the hall. He would then unfurl the umbrella and walk round the room with it open. When asked why he had done this, he calmly remarked, 'I thought I would like to find out if anybody present was superstitious.'

Moll[2] gave an account of some really incongruous post-hypnotic suggestions which were none the less explained by the subject to his own complete satisfaction.

2. A subject was told that when he woke up, he would take a flower-pot from the window-sill, wrap it in a cloth, put it on the couch and bow to it three times. When asked for his reasons for performing this remarkable series of actions, he replied, 'When I woke up and saw the flower-pot there, I thought that since it happens to be a cold day, the flower-pot ought to be warmed a little or else the plant might die. So I wrapped it in a cloth, and as the couch is nearer to the fire I thought I had better put the flower-pot on it. I then bowed because I was so pleased with myself for having such a bright idea.'

Although most amnesic subjects do rationalize, this is not always the case. Sometimes a subject will say, 'The idea just occurred to me to do so', or 'Something made me feel that I should do it'. However, it is not unknown for the subject simply to say 'I did it because you told me to'. He has no amnesia for the instruction and this answer is the safest of all. Generally speaking, no matter how silly or absurd the suggested action may be, it has to be performed, and thus the subject feels it necessary to provide himself with a logical reason for doing it. Such explanations are needed because, being wide awake, the subject is fully aware of what he has just done.

To the stage hypnotist, the post-hypnotic suggestion is the mainstay of his performance, and the more amusing he can make such suggestions, the better the audience is pleased. One well-known performer used to return several subjects to their places in the audience with the post-hypnotic suggestion that whenever he snapped his fingers, they would stand upon their seats and cry 'peanuts'. Such exhibitions may be undesirable and degrading and there is always the risk that when a number of subjects are being used in this way, the hypnotist may lose track of some of the suggestions he has given and the subject return home without the instruction having been removed.

An instance is reported in which a secretary had been told by a stage hypnotist that, whenever she heard the tune *I'm so tired,* she would immediately fall into a deep hypnotic sleep. During his performance, he secretly signalled to the orchestra from time to time, and on each occasion the tune was played, the subject promptly fell asleep. Unfortunately, the performer omitted to cancel this instruction with the result that two days later when she heard an office-boy whistling this tune she promptly fell asleep at her work. Unfortunately, stage performances of hypnotism do not all end as harmlessly as these cases illustrated. Considerable embarrassment and much distress may be caused to innumerable subjects who in their ignorance or curiosity, or for a variety of unknown reasons, offer themselves as willing subjects for the benefit of the entertainer. These problems are discussed in Chapter 26.

A great deal of discussion has taken place as to whether the post-hypnotic performance of a suggested act occurs in the normal waking state, or whether at the moment of its execution the subject re-enters a spontaneous self-limiting trance. Quite often a good subject will seem rather dazed and develop a rather glassy far-away look in his eyes as he carries out the suggested action, as if he were behaving quite automatically. It has also been noticed that, the more incongruous or ridiculous the post-hypnotic suggestion may be, the more likely the subject is to develop a complete amnesia, possibly in order to avoid embarrassment or anxiety.

Erickson and Erickson[4] conducted a systematic investigation of post-hypnotic behaviour and concluded that when the hypnotized subject is instructed to execute some act post-hypnotically, he invariably develops spontaneously a hypnotic trance. This trance is of brief duration, occurs in direct relation to the performance of the post-hypnotic act, and apparently constitutes an essential part of the process of response to, and execution of the post-hypnotic command. They further pointed out that the development of this trance state as part of the post-hypnotic performance requires for its appearance neither suggestion nor instruction. It develops at the moment of initiation of the post-hypnotic act, and usually persists for only a moment or two, so that it is easily overlooked. If there is no amnesia for the original trance and the post-hypnotic suggestion that has been given, or if the amnesia is weakened so that the subject remembers it before he carries it out, this spontaneous trance many not develop. In this case, the suggestion is complied with either voluntarily or through a feeling of compulsion.

Post-hypnotic Conditioning in Hypnosis

Bernheim[5] said 'There is no hypnotism, there is only suggestion' and 'suggestion is not everything but in everything there is an element of suggestion'. Post-hypnotic suggestion, in one form or another is involved with almost every therapeutic modality in which hypnosis is used, be it deliberately covert, discretely subtle or overtly authoritarian. All suggestion, however implanted, is intended to be acted upon either during or after the hypnotic session has terminated.

Post-hypnotic suggestion is not only invaluable in the therapeutic application of hypnosis, but is also extremely useful in facilitating future trance induction and protecting the subject against accidental hypnosis. In the latter case, an easily hypnotized person may even be prevented from being hypnotized by some unqualified individual.

The first induction of a hypnotic trance can be a laborious and time-consuming process. Indeed, it may take anything from 15 minutes up to many hours to secure satisfactory depth, and if it were necessary to repeat this procedure in full on every subsequent occasion, the practical uses of hypnosis would be extremely limited. So much time and energy would have to be spent upon induction alone that there would be little left for therapeutic purposes. Should this in fact occur, the therapist should question his assessment and diagnosis of the case as well as his own technique. As already described, conditioning the subject by post-hypnotic suggestion to enter the trance state upon a given signal, verbal or otherwise, is easily accomplished. This can always be done for deep trance subjects, and for many who achieve medium-depth hypnosis only.

The somnambulistic subject is so highly suggestible, even in the waking state, that it is wise to protect him against unexpected hypnosis. This can easily be effected by telling him, in the deep hypnotic state, that under normal circumstances nobody except yourself will be able to hypnotize him in future. Should, however, the necessity for hypnosis ever arise, he will then be able to respond to any other doctor or dental surgeon who posseses special knowledge and experience of hypnosis. Various authorities have doubted whether this does afford complete protection. Moll[2] considered that the chief danger does not arise from susceptibility to hypnosis as such, but from susceptibility to accidental hypnosis, or hypnosis against the subject's will. As an example of the efficiency of such protective suggestions, one case which occurred to one of us (J.H.) may be quoted in which, entirely without knowledge or intention, it was actually put to the test.

A schoolgirl, aged 14 years, was a somnambule and it was judged wise to protect her in this manner. About 12 months later, whilst on holiday she went to see a stage exhibition of hypnosis together with her parents. In the course of this, the performer rashly claimed that he would guarantee to hypnotize anyone in the theatre. This so annoyed the father that, knowing the protection that had been given, he promptly challenged the hypnotist to hypnotize his daughter. Despite his efforts, the performer was quite unable to induce even the lightest hypnotic state, and excused himself to the audience on the grounds that this was one of the very rare cases in which a person was completely unhypnotizable. The father then announced that this was very curious, since the child was accustomed to enter the deep hypnotic state whenever her doctor simply told her to go to sleep!

Dangers of the Post-hypnotic Suggestion

Many of these have already been discussed, the most common situation for problems to arise being when hypnosis is used for purposes of entertainment.

However hypnotherapy even if used by an expert is not without its problems. The failure to take an adequate history and, for example, to diagnose anxiety alone and miss a background of depressive illness, may end in disaster. Reduction of a secondary anxiety or of other symptoms such as phobic illness where the patient is additionally depressed may allow that patient to view his depression in the cold light of day without the overlay of anxiety which prevented him from taking further action. It is of paramount importance fully to understand the problem being treated. Any psychotic illness in remission may result in an acute exacerbation if suggestions are made which could cause conflict in the patient's mind and a post-hypnotic suggestion of loss of symptoms when the latter is a conversion symptom may well result in symptom substitution.

Failure to remove a post-hypnotic suggestion after it has fulfilled its purpose may bring additional problems. Worst of all perhaps, is the failure of the patient to respond to the suggestion when that suggestion is an essential adjunct to successful treatment. This will not only result in a further reinforcement of the patient's problems but will do little to enhance the reputation of the therapist.

No matter how profound, scientific or advanced may be the discussions on the effects of suggestion and suggestibility, or of susceptibility or hypnotizability, there is as yet no valid explanation of the reason for the effectiveness of the post-hypnotic suggestion. It is a sad reflection of our knowledge of the hypnotic *state* that whilst psychological explanations are plentiful the neurophysiology of the positive response remains an enigma—why it should work and be therapeutic in some subjects. Why it may not work in others may be more obvious. Although the term 'post-hypnotic' suggestion implies a response in the waking state to a suggestion given whilst the patient is in hypnosis, that suggestion is inherent in any form of re-learning whether dynamically or behaviourally acquired. It must be emphasized that the intention of all suggestion, however given, *must* be that it is for the ultimate benefit of the patient.

SELF-HYPNOSIS OR AUTO-HYPNOSIS

This involves the production of a self-induced hypnotic trance without the intervention of another person. The subject either learns or is taught how to enter the hypnotic state on his own, whenever he needs to make use of it. Although the technique is more easily learned by subjects who have previously entered medium or deep trance states, it is not difficult to acquire without any former subjective experience of hypnosis. Many persons who practise hypnosis have also taught themselves self-hypnosis at some time or other. Some therapists consider that all hypnosis is self-hypnosis and this idea should be conveyed to the patient. Nevertheless, most clinicians teach self-hypnosis through hetero-hypnosis and some of the methods which may be used are later described. According to Sacerdote[6], self-hypnosis, taught through hetero-hypnotic experiences, is effective as a method for physical and emotional tranquillization in nearly all subjects. Fromm *et al.*[7] made the important observation that 'expansive, free-floating attention and ego receptivity to stimuli coming from within are state specific for self-hypnosis, while concentrative attention and receptivity to stimuli coming from one outside source—the hypnotist on whom the subject concentrates his attention—are state specific for laboratory-defined hetero-hypnosis'. (Laboratory-defined hypnosis is that in which the wording and practices of standardized hypnotic susceptibility scales are accepted).

Some Uses of Self-hypnosis

Whatever the experimental findings, there is no doubt of the clinical benefits of self-hypnosis. These may be listed as follows:

1. As an aid to relaxation and to reduce the patient's general level of anxiety.

2. To repeat and thus to reinforce the preceding therapeutic session.

3. To help deal with anticipated future events which would otherwise produce unacceptable symptoms.

4. To encourage the independence of the patient and at a carefully selected point in the psychotherapeutic relationship to help disengage from the transference.

More specific advantages are found in the use of self-hypnosis to induce feelings of calmness and relaxation during pregnancy and to assist with labour, in abating attacks of asthma and migraine, in reducing the discomfort of pruritis and for use in pain relief and in dentistry.

An excellent practical use of self-hypnosis was described by Olson[8] at the 9th International Congress of Hypnosis and Psychosomatic Medicine, in his programme of training lower, middle and upper levels of executives, in self-hypnosis for general relaxation, anger control, self-confidence, sleep difficulties and various tension symptoms. At the same Congress, Davidson *et al.*[9] reported on a controlled study of 50 primigravidae using self-hypnosis training cassettes. The results supported the hypothesis that the hypnotically prepared women report less pain and have a more positive attitude to their labours and having further children. They found that audiotaped self-hypnosis training is an effective low cost, non-invasive adjunct in the practical support of producing a normal healthy baby in a normal healthy mother. A useful and fascinating study was reported by Swirsky-Sacchetti and Margolis[10]. In this, a comprehensive self-hypnosis training programme to decrease stress and to assess the amount of clotting factor used for bleeding in haemophiliacs was compared with a control group. It was found that the treatment group significantly reduced the amount of factor concentrate used to control bleeding in comparison with the controls. General distress level was also significantly reduced and the training was extremely cost effective. These results emphasized the value of self-hypnosis if used to complement the medical management of this unpleasant and potentially dangerous condition. Without doubt, a similar technique could be applied as an adjunct to the treatment of many other medical conditions.

Whilst eye closure and light or even medium-depth hypnosis are relatively easy to obtain, deep hypnosis is a much more difficult matter. Part of this difficulty lies in the fact that since the subject has to be his own hypnotist, he is faced with the problem of having to play both an active and a passive role at one and the same time. Because of this, although the state of mind that is self-induced is very similar to that produced by a hypnotist, it is usually on a lighter plane. The subject has to retain a certain degree of conscious control and activity in order to direct operations, and thus cannot allow himself to go too deeply. On the other hand, when he enters a trance state induced by a hypnotist, he can let himself go completely and doesn't need to worry about anything that is likely to happen or anything that is being done. He can consequently allow himself to go so deeply that his conscious mind becomes inactive and needs to play no part in what is taking place. In self-hypnosis, a part of the conscious mind must necessarily remain active in order to control the hypnosis and direct what is to happen in the self-induced trance. Roughly speaking, it is as though the conscious mind assumes the role of the hypnotist in making the suggestions which enter the unconscious part of the mind, where they are first accepted and then acted upon.

Before teaching a subject self-hypnosis, always discuss the matter with him in the waking state:

> I am going to teach you how to put yourself into the hypnotic state whenever you need to make use of it. You will not run the slightest risk because you will always be able to waken yourself whenever you wish to do so. If you go to sleep whenever I tell you to, you are equally bound to wake up when I tell you to do so. This is because you are allowing me to control what is taking place.
> Similarly, if you go to sleep on your own when you tell yourself that this will happen, then you are equally bound to wake up when you tell yourself to do so. This time, you see, *you* are in complete control of what is happening. So there is no risk whatever of putting yourself to sleep and being unable to wake yourself up whenever you wish to do so.
> During your hypnotic sleep, you will be able to relax completely…you will be able to think clearly…and you will be able to give yourself whatever *reasonable* suggestions you wish…and they will act just as if I had given them to you, myself.
> Whenever you hypnotize yourself…you will be able to remember the kind of suggestions I have been giving you…and you will be able to administer them to yourself.

Also tell the patient that if he uses and practises self-hypnosis morning and evening he will achieve a more rapid improvement. Explain it to him that through the use of self-hypnosis twice daily, he will really be receiving the equivalent of treatment fourteen times weekly instead of just once each week when he attends your clinic. Inevitably therefore, treatment time will be reduced. There is no doubt that the motivation of any patient may be judged by the application with which he will pursue this advice.

Self-hypnosis by Suggestion in the Hypnotic State

This is probably the most reliable method of instruction in the use of self-hypnosis.

After an explanation of the relevant uses of self-hypnosis, the patient is asked where he would most likely carry out the exercises. He is told that the regime would require twice daily sessions—once in the morning to prepare himself for the day ahead and once in the evening, to produce feelings of calmness and to neutralize any stress which may have been experienced in difficult or unexpected situations during the previous hours. Additionally to prepare him for the evening and for a peaceful and restful night. Before commencing, he is asked to deal with any immediate problems that require attention so that he will not have to be bothered with thoughts of needing to hurry through the exercises and also to ask anyone else in the house not to disturb him unless it happens to be a matter of urgency. The patient must be reassured that if he is called he will immediately open his eyes and be ready to deal with whatever is required of him.

The patient is then put into hypnosis by one of the methods previously described. Of these, the writer (D.W.) prefers the method of eye fixation with progressive relaxation. After the usual suggestions of feelings of calmness and composure the patient is aroused. Without further discussion he is then told to imagine himself at home, or wherever the self-hypnosis is to be used, and having made the initial preparations indicated above he is told to go and sit in the chair he has chosen, to look straight ahead at a fixed point, to imagine that he is in *your* consulting room and to talk *with* you, but silently, whilst you once again repeat the induction process, but this time—in the first person. He is then once again aroused with suggestions given to himself, of feelings of well being etc.

The patient then repeats the entire process once more. This time, by himself but closely observed by the therapist. He is asked to give a signal (raising the right index finger) when the end of each stage is reached so that the process may be monitored and the patient helped gently into the next stage.

Self-hypnosis Through Post-hypnotic Suggestion

Another method of teaching a subject to induce self-hypnosis is through the use of post-hypnotic suggestion. It seems doubtful, however, as to whether this procedure is really entitled to be called self-hypnosis since it has certainly not been initiated by the subject's unaided efforts. It is a power that has been delegated to him by the hypnotist which is indistinguishable in its mode of operation from any other form of post-hypnotic suggestion. As might be expected, the subject who is taught in this way will be able to enter the trance state much more rapidly, often in response to a self-administered signal, and will probably be able to achieve greater depth. This can be very useful therapeutically when it is necessary for the patient to induce the trance state rapidly, in order to avert a threatened attack, for example of asthma or migraine.

When teaching self-hypnosis using this method, put the subject into as deep a trance as possible and proceed to give him the following instructions:

> You are now in so deep a sleep...*that everything that I tell you that is going to happen...will happen...exactly as I tell you.*
> And every feeling...that I tell you that you will experience...you will experience...exactly as I tell you.
> And these same things will continue to happen to you...and you will continue to experience these same feelings...just as strongly...just as surely...just as powerfully...when you are back home...as when you are with me, in this room.
> I am now going to teach you how to go into this deep sleep, whenever you wish to do so...even though you are no longer with me.
> All you will have to do is to lie back in a chair...fix your eyes upon a spot on the ceiling...and count slowly up to *five.*
> As you do so...your eyes will rapidly become more and more tired...your eyelids heavier and heavier...*and the moment you have reached the count of five...your eyes will close immediately...and you will fall immediately into a sleep...just as deep as this one.*
> Whilst you are in this deep sleep...stage by stage, you will be able to suggest complete relaxation of all the muscles of your body...exactly as I do...and all other suggestions that you give yourself for your own good...will act...just as effectively as if I had given them to you, myself. Should any unexpected emergency arise during your deep sleep...you will automatically wake up immediately...fully prepared to take any necessary action.
> After you have given yourself treatment...as soon as you are ready to wake yourself...you will count slowly down from *five* to one...*and the moment you reach the count of one...your eyes will*

open...and you will be wide awake again...feeling much better than before you went to sleep.

Then awaken the subject and talk to him for a few minutes, after which tell him to lie back in the chair and put himself straight off to sleep again. Whilst asleep, he is to relax all his muscles, and once he feels this relaxation he is to wake himself up. Rehearse him in this procedure several times until it occurs quite automatically. Finally conclude by putting him back into a deep trance, and adding these further instructions:

Whenever you are with me...and you put yourself into this deep sleep...you will always be able to hear everything that I say to you...and you will always carry out any instructions that I give you. *Even when you are alone...you will always be able to put yourself into this deep sleep...whenever you wish to do so...by lying back in a chair...staring at a spot on the ceiling...and counting slowly up to five.*
Whilst you are in this deep sleep...you will neither listen to...nor accept suggestions from anyone other than myself.
But your own reasonable suggestions will always take effect...more and more powerfully as you become more proficient. You will only use this self-hypnosis for your own benefit...*you will never use if for the purpose of demonstrations or entertainment.*

Self-hypnosis by Suggestion in the Waking State

When teaching self-hypnosis in the waking state without the use of post-hypnotic suggestion, after having given the preliminary explanations and assurances, proceed in the following manner:

Now, I want you to listen carefully to the instructions I am going to give you...and after I have finished...I shall ask you to lie back in the chair and put yourself right off to sleep...by doing exactly what I've told you. When I tell you to put yourself to sleep...you will lie back in the chair...and fix your eyes upon a spot on the ceiling. Don't let your eyes wander from this spot...and while you are staring at it...you will repeat to yourself...over and over again...that your eyes are becoming very, very tired...that your eyelids are feeling heavier and heavier...that they will want to blink...and that as they blink...they will feel that they want to

close...that they are wanting to close...that you want them to close...and that you will let them close as soon as they want to. You'll find that if you keep on saying these things over and over again to yourself...your eyes will very soon close of their own accord...and you will have no desire to open them...until you tell yourself to do so. Once your eyes have closed...and you have fallen into a light hypnotic sleep...I want you to tell yourself...that all the muscles of your legs and thighs are becoming completely relaxed...all the muscles of your chest, body and stomach are becoming limp and slack...and that all the muscles of your neck, your shoulders and your arms are becoming completely and utterly relaxed.
Keep on repeating these suggestions...over and over again...until you do feel relaxed...then, tell yourself that you will open your eyes and be wide awake again, the moment you count *from five to one* ...feeling very much better than when you went to sleep.

Repeat these instructions once, to make sure that the subject knows exactly what he has to do. Then tell him to put himself to sleep, and that you will not utter another word until he has done so and awakened himself again. This procedure rarely fails. Indeed, it often succeeds in people who have never previously been hypnotized, provided that the preliminary talk and explanations have carried conviction. As one would expect, the previous subjective experience of hetero-hypnosis facilitates it greatly, even though no post-hypnotic suggestion is used.

The subject is told to practise this twice daily until his next attendance. On the next occasion, tell him that after he has put himself to sleep and produced relaxation, he is to hold his arm out stiff and straight, level with his shoulder and with the palm upwards facing the ceiling. He is then to tell himself, over and over again, that his arm is becoming stiff and straight from the shoulder to the wrist, just like a steel poker, and that it will feel so stiff and straight that he will be quite unable to bend it until he counts up to three. In fact, the harder he tries to bend it, the stiffer and straighter it will become. As soon as he feels this stiffness, he is to try to bend it and when he finds that he cannot, he is to relax it again by counting up to three. Then he is to waken himself.

This often succeeds at the first attempt. If it doesn't, it is important to tell him that as he practises and becomes more proficient, he will eventually succeed. Follow it up by teaching him how to induce automatic movement, by resting his elbow on the arm of the chair and imagining the cord tied round his wrist as already described in the orthodox deepening techniques.

Finally, prove to him that other reasonable suggestions that he gives himself will also work. Tell him for example, to see himself doing what he intends to be doing for the rest of the day, going where he thinks he will go and seeing who he intends to see etc., whilst remaining completely calm and relaxed. Finally, telling himself that he will feel fit and well and much better than before the self-hypnosis. When this is concluded he is to awaken himself by using the method of counting backwards from five to one.

No matter what method of instruction has been adopted, once the subject has mastered the technique of the self-induced trance, he will be able to apply suggestion to himself exactly as the hypnotist does. He will normally remember the therapeutic suggestions he has been given and will make use of these, rewording and rephrasing them to suit himself. Normally, he will not go beyond this, but since in deep-trance subjects it is sometimes possible to enlarge the field of self-hypnotic phenomena to include self-induced analgesias, it is necessary for the hypnotist to take the protective measure of imposing strict limitations upon such capabilities. It could be extremely dangerous if the subject were left with the ability to remove pain or other symptoms at will, in the absence of medical supervision. In the case of such complaints as dysmenorrhoea or migraine, the ability to remove pain self-hypnotically can be restricted by the hypnotist to this particular pain alone, as and when it occurs. Similarly, a subject can be told that he will only be able to produce dental analgesia for himself when he is actually sitting in his dentist's chair.

Brief Hypnosis (An Instant Method of Self-hypnosis)

This is a simple, easily acquired and useful technique taught by one of us (D.W.) for inducing immediate feelings of calmness.

One of the stages of the induction of hypnosis commonly used is that in which the action of exhalation is paired with feelings of calmness and this is utilized each time the patient attends for treatment. Thus he gets to know this and to recognize its value very early on. It is practised in this way.

Hypnosis is induced to eye closure and the patient's attention is drawn to his quiet and regular breathing. An explanation of what is happening is given in simple terms:

> When you breathe in you fill your lungs, when you breathe out you empty them. When you breathe in you stretch the muscles of your chest, when you breathe out you let go of tension in those muscles. Now as you breathe out and let go of tension in the muscles of your chest—at that point let go of tension from every part of your body, just flop into the chair and see the word calm in your thoughts. Calm...calm...calm...

(The words are paired with the patient's rate of exhalation.)

> As you breathe out and see the word calm in your thoughts—additionally say the word calm—silently in your mind and every trace of tension in your body and in your mind will disappear.

This is repeated and practised several times.

He is told, whilst in hypnosis, that if ever he anticipates or experiences some stressful situation whilst in the waking state all that he need do is to take a deeper breath and as he allows the air to leave his lungs, to see the word calm in his thoughts, say it silently in his mind and all tension and anxiety will immediately disappear.

He is then asked to imagine some situation of stress which could possible occur in his everyday life and to *experience this situation actually occurring.* That when he is actually *in* that situation to give an ideomotor signal (raising the right index finger)...

> Now—take a deep breath—hold for a second and...let go and the word is calm...see it, say it, think it, experience it...and all the tension goes.
> Give me a signal when the tension has gone...

(The right index finger moves again.)

This exercise is practised repeatedly and the patient is told that he can use it at any time and anywhere should he feel the need. He will at all times use it with his eyes open and whilst he is wide awake in the normal course of any day. Nobody will be aware of what he is doing since as far as any close observer will notice, he will simply be taking a deep breath.

Your patient will soon report that this exercise is one of the most useful and effective in the entire area of hypnotherapeutic techniques. It may be used to reduce a wide range of nervous symptoms from simple anxiety to psychosomatic and phobic responses.

Doubts and Difficulties in the Use of Self-hypnosis

A very important phase of treatment has been described but equally important are the difficulties which may arise.

Patients will often complain of lack of time—'twenty minutes twice a day doctor—I've barely got twenty seconds', lack of concentration, lack of facilities or other unconvincing reasons. The truth will more likely be lack of motivation and the therapist should seriously consider the advisability of continuing treatment. The patient should have understood from the outset that the doctor can only show the way—it is up to the patient to follow—that is something that nobody else can do for him.

On the other hand, patients may not yet be ready to use self-hypnosis. Patients lean heavily on the advice of the doctor and may still need that support. The doctor must judge correctly when they are ready for independence. Immature persons and those with personality or other emotional difficulties may not be ready to let go. There is also the powerful influence of the transference which must be recognized and dealt with in a way so that no harm will befall the patient.

Sacerdote[6] summarized some of the difficulties encountered by subjects during self-hypnosis as follows:

1. Incomplete dissociative experiences.
2. Anxieties about self-control.
3. Doubts about the reality of the self-hypnotic state.
4. The possibility that negative attitude, habits and expectation may act counter-therapeutically as post-hypnotic suggestions.

Nevertheless, the acceptance of the use of self-hypnosis as a necessary stage in treatment and assiduous application to the exercises will bring considerable benefit to the majority of patients. In addition to the specific treatment for which it is being applied, self-hypnosis will help to bring down the level of anxiety at which the patient has hitherto been functioning, his mind will become clearer, his concentration will improve, he will feel more stable and self-reliant and there must inevitably result an overall improvement in feelings of general well-being and physical health.

The Use of Tape Recordings

There will be found a hard core of patients who, although hypnotizable and responding well to therapy are just unable to use self-hypnosis. They may be extremely good subjects in the consulting room. In the privacy of their own homes however, they find themselves unable to settle or to relax, to cut off from the external environment or from those internal thoughts and ideas, or to concentrate sufficiently to allow themselves to go into hypnosis. Or perhaps they claim to fall asleep in the midst of it all. Again, some immature or dependent patients lean heavily on the personality of the therapist, or the transference may be too powerful to allow acceptance of anything but actual one-to-one therapy, so that self-hypnosis in any form is unacceptable.

The first author preferred the direct command 'go to sleep' recorded on the tape but few of us have the authority with which he was gifted, to achieve a positive response to this command when given by remote control as it were. Additionally there are situations in which a deliberately slow, soothing and permissive technique is preferable, such as when using a tape on an aeroplane. Since the most important use of self-hypnosis is to reduce the level of anxiety then it is recommended that the latter technique be generally employed. However, the final arbiter must be the personality and response of the patient to hetero-hypnosis and so the decision as to which method of induction to use must be left to the therapist.

Preparation of the Tape Recording

The patient should be asked where he will be using the tape, will he be sitting on a chair or propped up on a couch or on the bed?

Additionally, a pair of earphones may be useful to block out any external sounds especially if the tape is to be used elsewhere than in the home. He is warned not to loan the tape to any member of the family or friends since it is tailored especially to suit him and may result in adverse effects should it be used by anybody else. When the subject is ready to commence, open the recording as follows:

> This tape is made especially for the use of Mr John Smith and will not be effective if used by any other person.

The machine is switched off and normal induction is commenced to eye closure and a generalized feeling of relaxation. When his eyes are closed and he is in light hypnosis, the patient is told to imagine himself at home or wherever he will be when he uses the tape. If there is anybody else around he is instructed to tell them not to disturb him unless it is vitally important. If he is called, you must say that he will immediately open his eyes, switch off the tape and be awake and alert and ready to deal with any problems. If he is alone and is suddenly alerted, for example by the telephone, once again he will be awake and fully in control of all his senses. He is additionally advised to attend to all the things that have to be done, or in the case of the housewife for example, to make sure that she has not left the kettle on the stove or the dinner in the oven—so that relaxation can continue without other preoccupations. Following these essential preparations the machine is switched on again and the recording is continued. A normal induction is commenced and the entire procedure is recorded on the tape. All special instructions are included and any particular items of desensitization are added. The tape is concluded with suggestions of ego-strengthening and feelings of calmness and well-being. Finally and more assertively, the usual instruction by counting, to eyes open is given 'awake, alert, feeling really fine and ready to get on with the day'.

When the patient is awake, the recording is concluded with the repeated admonition that it will be ineffective if used by any other person. Whether the latter suggestion will be accepted by anyone else listening to the tape depends upon the personality and the problems of that individual but nevertheless, it is a wise precaution to include that particular exclusion.

The main disadvantage to the use of tape recordings is that the patient never really uses self-hypnosis. That is, he continues to depend upon the tape and therefore upon hetero-hypnosis, instead of becoming self-reliant. However, it is wise to prepare such a tape in the event of the patient being otherwise unable to use self-hypnosis. It is of course a safe procedure provided that the instructions are given correctly.

The Dangers of Tape Recordings

The wholesale manufacture of tapes for sale across the counter in chemist stores and supermarkets is fraught with danger and all patients should be strongly warned against their purchase. They are advertised as the panacea for almost all ills. For the treatment of anxiety, depression, concentration and sleep difficulties, weight problems, stammering, nail biting and so on.

The problems are considerable. In the first instance, every tape *must be tailored to suit the particular patient for whom it is prepared.* The subject *must* be known to the therapist and his problem fully explored. The dangers of treating depression by hypnosis alone are fully discussed in another chapter. Lack of concentration, certain sleep difficulties and excessive drinking for example, may again be symptoms of depression, unrecognized by the patient. Hypnosis as such may relieve any anxiety component of a depressive illness just as some tranquillizer drugs do. The listener could then take a cold, hard look at his depressed mood and life as he sees it—possibly with disastrous results.

Then again, the problems of weight control could be much too serious to be treated simply by suggestion made on a tape recording. The patient may be suffering from bulimia and the condition could easily swing over to anorexia and even more difficulties would then arise.

Subjects may go into light or deep hypnosis when listening to a tape or they may be somnambules. No-one is available to monitor that person's response. A mass-produced tape recording can take no account of the type of person who will be listening to it. Conditions are being treated, the causes of which are entirely un-

known, in subjects who have never been seen or questioned by
the so-called therapist. Additionally, such tapes may be acquired
by children or very elderly people, when the dangers could be even
greater or may be used for improper purposes once acquired.
Legislation is urgently required to eliminate this possible abuse.

THE EGO-STRENGTHENING TECHNIQUE

Psychotherapy of this kind need be neither difficult nor complicated, provided that certain fundamental requirements of the patient are borne in mind. For this purpose his psychological
responses to his illness can be conveniently divided into two
groups:

1. Those arising as a consequence of the illness itself, such as
anxiety, fear, tension and agitation.

2. Those arising from defects in his own personality, such as
nervousness, lack of confidence, dependence and maladjustment.
General psychotherapeutic suggestions now known as 'ego-
strengthening' (J.H.) to combat these, may be planned and many
can be adopted as standard ones which remain unchanged from
case to case. Others will naturally have to be added or varied to
suit each individual and tailored to his particular complaint and
personality. If once the habit is developed of using such a technique in every case that is treated under hypnosis before proceeding with the main direction of therapy it will be found to pay
handsome dividends. Not only will the patient obtain more rapid
relief from his symptoms, but he will display obvious improvement in other ways. He will become more self-reliant, more confident and more able to adjust to his environment, and thus much
less prone to relapse. In fact, *this combination of* ego-strengthening *suggestions and symptom-relief may often enable the therapist
to deal successfully with many cases without having to resort to
alternative procedures.* Naturally, he will still encounter some
problems in which a relatively simple investigation and superficial analysis of the patient's current environmental difficulties
and his reactions to them will render his treatment both speedier
and more effective. Even under these circumstances, the same
basic scheme in framing therapeutic suggestions may be adopted

incorporating any others that may seem desirable as a result of investigation. Additionally dental surgeons and specialists in many fields are successfully using a specially constructed and shortened version of the standard technique in their everyday work.

The basis of the technique has of course its origin in Coué's idea of autosuggestion[11] and his classic formula 'every day, in every way, I am getting better and better'.

In the construction of an ego-strengthening technique, quite apart from the actual suggestions themselves, it is essential that particular attention should be paid to such significant factors as *'rhythm', 'repetition', the interpolation of appropriate 'pauses'*, and the *'stressing of certain important words and phrases'*. Repetition is often achieved by expressing the same fundamental idea in two or three different ways. This tends to avoid excessive monotony. Some words and phrases are stressed because of their importance and significance to the patient himself. Other words are stressed and suitable pauses included with the sole purpose of emphasizing the rhythm of the delivery which will contribute to its success. The manipulation of these factors should become self-evident as the routine is described.

First, let us refer briefly to the question of trance depth. One of the advantages of this technique is the fact that a deep trance is certainly not essential. Nevertheless, as in most hypnotherapeutic methods, the deeper the trance, the more rapidly improvement will occur and the shorter the duration of a course of treatment will be. The patient who has been conditioned to enter the hypnotic state upon a given signal, verbal or otherwise, can usually be regarded as having attained sufficient depth for treatment to be effective. Yet even this is not absolutely necessary since a satisfactory response can often be obtained in light trance states only. Under these circumstances, however, one would naturally expect treatment to be continued over a longer period and the results to manifest themselves more slowly. Methods of trance induction and deepening are of little significance and can be safely left to individual preference, although it is important that the patient should be rendered as fully relaxed, mentally and physically, as possible, and it is well worthwhile spending a little extra time to attain this objective.

In the following detailed account and analysis, the first author describes in full the routine used in dealing with such cases as anxiety states, tension states, phobias, etc. Most of it is equally applicable as a prelude to the treatment of asthma, migraine and various psychosomatic conditions. It lends itself admirably to shortening, adaptation and the addition of specialized suggestions in accordance with individual needs, both of the patient and of the therapist.

A Typical Ego-strengthening Routine

Once the patient is in a trance state and is as fully relaxed as possible, proceed as follows:

> You have now become *so* deeply relaxed...*so* deeply asleep...that your mind has become *so* sensitive...*so* receptive to what I say...that *everything* that I put into your mind...will sink *so* deeply into the unconscious part of your mind...and will cause so deep and lasting an impression there...that *nothing* will eradicate it.

This tends to prepare the patient's mind to receive the suggestions that follow. Notice the stressing and repetition of the word 'so' which not only adds force to the ideas presented, but also strongly emphasizes the rhythmic quality of the delivery.

> Consequently...these things that I put into your unconscious mind...will begin to exercise a greater and greater influence over the way you think...over the way you feel...over the way you behave.

This is the first indication to the patient that he will begin to feel a gradual change in his thoughts, feelings and actions, as a result of the suggestions he is about to receive.

> And...because these things *will* remain...firmly imbedded in the unconscious part of your mind...after you have left here...when you are no longer with me...they will continue to exercise the same great influence...over your *thoughts*...your *feelings*...and your *actions*...*just* as strongly...*just* as surely...*just* as powerfully...when you are back home...or at work...as when you are with me in this room.

Here you will notice the introduction of the first unobtrusive post-hypnotic suggestion to the effect that the patient can expect the same changes to continue in his everyday life, after the trance state has been terminated. Note also that so far, all the suggestions have been directed towards the modification of the three fundamental psychological processes—*'thinking'*, *'feeling'*, and *'acting'*. These words have been stressed because of their importance to the patient, and the word *'just'*, in order to add to the rhythmic quality of the delivery. Repetition has been ensured by the use of three different words—*'strongly'*, *'surely'*, *'powerfully'*—all of which convey the same essential idea. Those familiar with the original descriptions of this technique will realize that these groups of suggestions are entirely new. Clinical results confirm that their addition gives increased force to the effectiveness of the basic routine.

> You are now so *very deeply asleep*...that *everything* that I tell you that is going to happen to you...*for your own good*...*will* happen...*exactly* as I tell you.
> And *every feeling*...that I tell you that you will experience...you *will* experience...*exactly* as I tell you.
> And these same things *will continue to happen* to you...*every day*...and you *will continue to experience* these same feelings...*every day*...*just* as strongly...*just* as surely...*just* as powerfully...when you are back home...or at work...as when you are with me in this room.

Here we have repetition, not only of single words or phrases, but of the same group of expectations and ideas already expressed—'driving them home'—as it were. The patient begins to expect that he will not only experience something in the course of the trance, but that he will continue to benefit from this even when he is no longer receiving active treatment. This post-hypnotic effect is of great importance, for the success of treatment under hypnosis depends upon the simple fact that the suggestions last longer than the trance itself. The words *'will'* and *'exactly'*, together with other phrases of significance to the patient, are pronounced with increased emphasis to add force and authority to the suggestions, and although the continued interpolation of *'pauses'* will be noted, particular attention is not drawn to them. Let us repeat one phrase in a slightly different manner:

Just as strongly...(pause)...*just* as surely...(pause)...*just* as powerfully...(pause).

and observe how the stressing of the word '*just*' helps to drive the idea home, almost like the blows of a hammer, and this, taken in conjunction with the pauses, establishes a rhythmical quality to the delivery similar to the beat of a metronome. In this connection, most of us tend to pay far too little attention to the importance of pauses in our work with hypnosis. Although this may be partly due to the limitations on our time, this is not invariably the case. After all, when we give the patient a drug we are quite content to allow sufficient time for it to take effect, and if only we adopted the same attitude of mind when working with a patient in a hypnotic trance there is no doubt that our results would become greatly enhanced.

As a result of this brief analysis of the mode of construction and delivery of these suggestive routines, one should now be able to detect these devices whenever they are used. Throughout the rest of this technique, the same cardinal principles are strictly observed, of 'repetition', 'stressing' and the use of 'synonymous words and phrases' intermingled with 'pauses' to secure a smooth rhythmic delivery.

During this deep sleep...*you* are going to feel physically *stronger* and *fitter* in every way.
You will feel *more* alert...*more* wide awake...*more* energetic.
You will become *much* less easily tired...*much* less easily fatigued...*much* less easily discouraged...*much* less easily depressed.
Every day...you will become *so deeply interested* in whatever you are doing...in whatever is going on around you...that your mind will become *completely distracted away from yourself.*
You will no longer *think nearly so much about yourself*...you will no longer *dwell nearly so much upon yourself and your difficulties*...and you will become *much less conscious of yourself*...*much less pre-occupied with yourself*...*and with your own feelings.*
Every day...your nerves will become *stronger and steadier*...your mind *calmer and clearer*...*more composed*...*more placid*...*more tranquil.* You will become *much less easily worried*...*much less easily agitated*...*much less easily fearful and apprehensive*...*much*

less easily upset.

Here are the first group of actual *'ego-strengthening'* suggestions, intended to improve the patient's general condition, to
strengthen his weaknesses, to increase his confidence and to allay
his anxieties. It will be noted as we proceed how they have been
designed, not only to alleviate most of the complaints made by the
average neurotic patient, but also to improve and mitigate those
defects which have contributed largely to his illness.

> You will be able to *think more clearly*...you will be able to
> *concentrate more easily.*
> You will be able to *give up your whole undivided attention to*
> *whatever you are doing...to the complete exclusion of everything*
> *else.*
> Consequently...*your memory will rapidly improve*...and you will
> be able to *see things in their true perspective...without*
> *magnifying your difficulties...without ever allowing them to get*
> *out of proportion.*
> Every day...you will become *emotionally much calmer...much*
> *more settled...much less easily disturbed.*
> Every day...you will become...and *you* will remain...*more and*
> *more completely relaxed...*and *less tense* each day...*both mentally*
> *and physically*...even when you are no longer attending here.
> And *as* you become...and *as* you remain...*more relaxed...and less*
> *tense* each day...*so*...you will develop *much more confidence in*
> *yourself*...more confidence in your ability to *do*...not only what
> you *have*...to do each day...but more confidence in your ability to
> do whatever you *ought* to be able to do...*without fear of*
> *failure...without fear of consequences...without unnecessary*
> *anxiety...without uneasiness.*
> Because of this...*every day*...you will feel *more and more*
> *independent...more able to 'stick up for yourself'...to stand upon*
> *your own feet...to hold your own*...no matter how difficult or trying
> things may be.

You have probably noticed how much more positive and defini-
tive the suggestions have become as the treatment proceeds.

> Every day...you will feel a *greater feeling of personal well-being...A*
> *greater feeling of personal safety...and security*...than you have felt
> for a long, long time.
> And because all these things *will* begin to happen...*exactly* as I

tell you they will happen...*more and more
rapidly...powerfully...and completely*...with every treatment I
give you...you will feel *much happier...much more
contented...much more optimistic* in every way.
You will consequently become much more able to *rely upon...to
depend upon...yourself...your own efforts...your own
judgement...your own opinions.* You will feel *much less need*...to
have to *rely upon*...or to *depend upon...other people.*

This routine, the full version of which has been described, will
be equally valuable if preceding suggestions of symptom relief or
other more involved techniques. Constant repetition at the beginning of each treatment session strengthens the 'ego-defences' to
such an extent that it not only renders the symptoms more vulnerable to direct suggestion and lessens the likelihood of relapse,
but will often enable a patient to co-operate eventually in an analytical investigation he was formerly ill-equipped to face.

No matter what particular branch of therapeutic activity in
which one may be engaged, patients will respond more rapidly
and effectively to treatment if a rational explanation is given in
advance of exactly what it is proposed to do, why it is being done,
and what they can reasonably expect to happen. Consequently, it
may be helpful to explain to the patient, in the waking state, why
and how he can expect this method to work.

When you first went to school, I'm sure you can remember
sometimes being given a short piece of poetry to learn off by heart
so that you could recite it next morning without the book.
And how did you set about this task?
I expect that you read the poem over and over again at home,
possibly aloud, and each time you did so, a little bit more of it
became stuck in your mind until eventually you could recite the
whole of it from memory, without referring to the book.
Now this treatment acts in exactly the same way because it is
also a *'learning process'*, only instead of having to do it all
yourself, every time I repeat these suggestions to you, more and
more of them will stick in your unconscious mind so that you
will gradually notice yourself improving in your everyday life,
even when you are no longer with me.
This will happen more quickly and easily than when you are wide
awake because, whenever you enter a trance state, your memory
becomes greatly improved, and your powers of concentration

greatly increased.

Begin every treatment session of ego-strengthening with this particular sequence of suggestions as soon as the induction and deepening of hypnosis has been completed. The suggestions are given slowly and deliberately, and those specifically directed towards lessening of symptoms should be left to the end, since this seems to render them more effective. Indeed, in certain psychosomatic cases in which the loss of symptoms is the principal objective, a somewhat abbreviated version may be used before proceeding with the main suggestions to that effect. In neurotic anxiety, tension and phobic states, however, it should always be employed in full, coupled at times with a relatively superficial analysis of the patient's current problems and difficulties. Used regularly in this way, its efficacy can be surprising. Often, many patients recover as a result of this technique alone, usually within Wolberg's suggested limit of 20 sessions of short-term psychotherapy.

It is certainly not intended that this verbatim account should be adopted in the precise form that has been described. It is the principle that is worthy of attention, and the sequence outlined should be regarded simply as a guide to the individual therapist in framing his own suggestions to conform with his own personality, method of approach and style of delivery. It is impossible to suggest here the varying inflections of the voice, but the same cardinal rules of construction, stresses and pauses etc. should be used in order to maintain a rhythmical quality from start to finish.

The following case history, with a somewhat unexpected result, seems to illustrate the effectiveness of this technique.

The patient was a young man, a salesman aged 28, and happily married. He had been suffering from 'claustrophobia' for about 7 years and was quite incapable of remaining in confined spaces without developing acute attacks of panic and anxiety. Curiously enough, he had never previously sought treatment for this condition. Recently, he had been moved to the top floor of an eight-storey block of flats. Since he found it impossible to use the lift (or elevator) he was compelled to climb the stairs several times a day, and this was making his life intolerable. Obviously motivation was strong. He was a highly-strung, anxious individual, lacking in confidence, but otherwise fairly well integrated, with no gross personality defects. No significant factors emerged from routine investigation of his childhood, his family history, or his prevailing environmental circumstances.

It was concluded that only an analytical approach would be likely to solve this problem. Unfortunately, however, whilst he was easily taught to enter the hypnotic state upon a given signal, the simpler methods of analytical investigation failed to produce any clues whatsoever, and it proved impossible to deepen his hypnosis sufficiently to use the more involved hypnoanalytical techniques.

He attended for treatment once a week, and since mentioning his incapacity seemed to distress him greatly, no further reference was made either to 'claustrophobia' or to the difficulty he was experiencing with the lift. The 'ego-strengthening' technique alone was continued, with no attempt whatever at direct symptom removal. It was hoped that he would eventually improve sufficiently to permit this, or that it would become possible to obtain the greater depth necessary for further analysis. Certainly after a few weeks he became much calmer and less tense, and seemed to be gaining more confidence in himself. Nevertheless, when he attended for his eleventh session, it was noted that he was looking extremely pleased with himself. Apparently, several days before, he was carrying home a load of timber with which he intended to make book cases, and whilst passing the lift and faced with eight flights of stairs to climb, he suddenly felt that he might be able to overcome his fears sufficiently to try to use it. This he did, on the spur of the moment, and subsequently experienced no further difficulty whatever.

Ego-assertive Retraining

In the concept of ego-strengthening as originally described, the ego is intended to include all those psychological processes concerned with the issue of personal identity—the self. Ego-strength implies that the stronger the ego—the more likely will the individual be able to withstand all those difficult and threatening situations of which life appears to be composed.

Treatment is addressed mainly to self-image, in other words, what we think of ourselves and how we see ourselves in the world and as a consequence, how we respond. Ego-strengthening is the technique by means of which these feelings can be altered, by suggestion under hypnosis, without recourse to complicated psychological or psychoanalytical interventions. Simultaneous with treatment along these lines, additional enhancement of the patient's self-confidence in certain specific situations may be required.

This may be achieved by a modification of the technique described by Wolpe and Lazarus[12] and known as 'assertive training' which lends itself ideally for use with hypnosis. It is the obvious corollary to ego-strengthening and the combination of these methods has been called ego-assertive retraining (Waxman[13]). Positive suggestions of feelings of self-assertion are paired with feelings of calmness and composure, control and confidence, in particular situations formerly interpreted as threatening and in which some of the more common manifestations of fear would otherwise occur. This technique thus additionally utilizes Wolpe's method for the reciprocal inhibition or anxiety[14].

Those behavioural responses which may result from anxiety themselves will compound that anxiety. As a result, a variety of somatic effects may manifest themselves, stammering, blushing, tachycardia or gastrointestinal symptoms being amongst the most common. Consequently, any thought or anticipation perhaps, of some social engagement or of a one-to-one interview may invoke a similar response and the actual experience of that feared situation could be a disaster. Life becomes a continuous battle for survival. Assertive training implies promoting such change in a patient's response in his interpersonal relationships so that he is no longer anxious and thus performance is improved.

In treatment, anxiety is first relieved by the induction and deepening of the hypnotic state.

The therapist then adopts the role of that particular 'important' person with whom it is anticipated, the patient may be confronted. He 'challenges' the patient accordingly. A simple 'good morning'—may initially suffice. The patient is then shown in hypnosis that he can comfortably reply 'good morning—how are you?' and remain perfectly calm and symptom-free whilst doing so. Further discussion then continues, appropriate to the status and role that the therapist has assumed and the patient is encouraged to reply positively and without anxiety. He is shown thereby that he is able to remain symptom-free in otherwise anxiety-provoking situations.

The conversation must slowly assume a more provocative line and the patient demonstrates that he can reply accordingly and with confidence yet without aggressive or otherwise unacceptable feelings. He is sent away after each session, to practice '*in vivo*' what he has already learned that he can achieve in hypnosis. It is essential to establish a hierarchy of anticipated events for the week ahead at the commencement of every session so that practical retraining may be effectively programmed.

A Typical Ego-assertive Routine

The patient is put in hypnosis and the trance state is deepened. Proceed as follows:

> You are completely calm and in a deeply relaxed state. I want you to see yourself at work and attending your weekly departmental meeting. You are sitting in the manager's office. The others are seated rather informally about the room. See that situation and confirm that you are there with the usual signal.'

The patient raises his right index finger. Now ask the patient where he is sitting.

> Patient 'On the chair by the door.'
> Therapist 'Are there any empty seats?'
> Patient 'Yes, the armchair by the desk.'
> Therapist 'You are feeling totally calm and relaxed. Go and sit in the armchair...tell me when you are sitting in the armchair and feeling totally calm and relaxed.'

After a few moments the patient will give the ideomotor signal.

> Therapist 'You will remain totally calm and relaxed...and now the manager is opening the meeting...'
> Therapist as manager (very assertively) 'Good morning gentlemen. We will have department reports first of all.'
> Therapist 'He's looking at you.'

Therapist as manager 'What have you got to tell us?'
Therapist 'You feel completely calm and relaxed and full of confidence. Completely at ease and comfortable in yourself. Speak up now. Answer him...'
Patient 'Well sir, I think...'
Therapist 'Forget about sir—speak up—you don't think— you know—speak out!'
Patient 'We have two problems, I'm sorry to say.'
Therapist 'Forget about being sorry, you have no reason to apologize! It's your department—you are in charge of it and you are in charge of yourself!'
Patient 'We have some problems regarding staff. Two of our typists are off sick and one is on holiday.'
Therapist as manager 'Can't you get replacements?'
Patient 'Unfortunately no...'
Therapist 'Stop apologizing—it's not your fault. Speak up.'
Patient 'Personnel say that all replacements are on attachment elsewhere.'
Therapist as manager (even more aggressively) 'Then what are you going to do about it?'
Therapist 'Speak up and speak out (remain quite calm and relaxed)—It's your department. You are in charge of the department, of the situation and of yourself, now speak!'
Patient 'I'll get on to them and tell them that we must have immediate replacements.'

Continue in this way simulating the manager speaking very aggressively and showing the patient that he can reply assertively but politely and remaining calm and in control throughout the interview.

A wide range of situations may be dealt with in this manner working through various aspects of the patient's life events.

It must be understood that assertive retraining involves dealing not only with the emotions of anxiety invoked by the pressure of some person or persons that the patient may consider threatening in the authoritarian sense. It may also include the difficulties which many people experience with their peers or in achieving successful interpersonal relationships or in the ability to express friendship, affection and love. The person may feel such a social misfit, that even life itself may become unacceptable. He or she may act out and even indulge in anti-social behaviour.

THE 'IDEOMOTOR FINGER-SIGNALLING' TECHNIQUE

Erickson[15] was the first to describe the use of symbolic movements of the head for 'yes' and 'no' answers when patients found it difficult to talk whilst in a trance state. Le Cron[16] employed a Chevreul pendulum for the same purpose, and subsequently added the use of unconsciously controlled finger movements to obtain 'yes', 'no' and 'I don't want to answer' responses. This has since been used extensively and its many possibilities widely explored by David Cheek[17]. In numerous instances it can be used effectively to investigate the presence and nature of unconscious material, and the principal upon which it depends can best be described as follows:

When we prepare a patient's mind for the acceptance of hypnosis, we show him how to pay attention to some part of the body, and *not* to pay attention to another. We show him how to relax his muscles—and that muscles that are contracted constantly in fear will begin to hurt because of the restricted circulation of blood through those muscles. We can then go on to teach him how muscles can react 'unconsciously', and thus establish a method of communication at an unconscious level by using the unconscious movements of the finger muscles to indicate the answers 'yes', 'no', or 'I don't want to answer' to the questions that are put to him. The following approach will be found to be most effective:

> I want you to put both hands on your lap...and I'll show you how
> you can learn to answer questions at an unconscious level.
> When you are talking to people...you have often seen them nod
> their heads when they agree with you...and shake their heads
> when they disagree with what you are saying.
> And they don't even know they are doing so.
> The movement is completely unconscious.
> Now...I'm going to teach your unconscious mind how it can
> answer questions by causing one finger to rise for the answer
> '*Yes*'—a different one for the answer '*No*', etc.
> Just let your hands lie idly upon your lap.
> I want you to think the thought...'*yes*'...'*yes*'...'*yes*'...over and over
> again.
> And as you do so...you will soon feel one of your fingers
> beginning to lift up on its own...from your lap.
> It's just like getting a swing going...you have to keep pushing it

at intervals.
You do this by keeping on thinking...'*yes*'.
And whilst you keep thinking...'*yes*'...you are not thinking of
'*no*'...or of any other answer.
Just keep on thinking...'*yes*'...'*yes*'...'*yes*'.
There...you see.
The fore-finger of your *right* hand is slowly lifting up.
Put it down again.
Now...think the thought...'*no*'...'*no*'...'*no*'...over and over again.
And...as you do so...one of your other fingers will slowly rise.
It may be on the same hand...or it may be on the other hand.
There you are.
It's the fore-finger of your *left* hand.
So...if I ask your unconscious mind a question...and the answer
is '*yes*'...after it has considered the question...it will cause your
right forefinger to rise.
If...on the other hand...the answer is '*no*'...your *left* fore-finger will
rise.

A third finger may, of course, be conditioned to signify the response '*I would prefer not to answer*', should this be considered
desirable.

Now...I'm going to ask your unconscious mind one or two questions.
Your conscious mind doesn't know the real cause of your illness.
But your 'unconscious' mind does.
And it can help us...in this way...to get to the real root of your
trouble.
Is your unconscious mind ready to help?

The *right* fore-finger slowly rises...'Yes'.

Does it object to being questioned in this way?

The *left* fore-finger slowly rises...'No'.

As an example of the usefulness of this technique, let us suppose that we have reason to believe that our patient suffered some
traumatic experience in childhood, which has been repressed and
which consequently he is quite unable to remember. The precise
age can often be pin-pointed in the following manner:

Did something unpleasant happen to you before you were 15
years old?

(Finger signals...*'Yes'*.)

Did it happen before you were 10 years old?

(Finger signals...*'Yes'*.)

Did it happen before you were 5 years old?

(Finger signals...*'No'*.)

Did it happen when you were 9?

(Finger signals...*'No'*.)

Did it happen when you were 8?

(Finger signals...*'No'*.)

Did it happen when you were 7?

(Finger signals...*'Yes'*.)

Provided that you ask the right questions, all of which must be capable of being answered by a simple *'Yes'* or *'No'*, it is surprising how much valuable information you can obtain in this way.

It is not difficult to tell whether such answers are really unconsciously determined. Watch carefully the nature of the finger movement. An answer at a conscious level will result in an *immediate* movement, whereas an unconscious answer will be much more delayed and the consequent finger movement much slower and jerkier.

It must always be remembered however, that an ideomotor response is not necessarily proof of infallibility.

Occasionally these techniques can be used successfully in general practice to uncover the nature of significant conflicts that lie just below the surface. Except in the case of war or traumatic neuroses, neither of them are likely to elicit a highly charged emotional release that might be too difficult to control. In the unlikely event of this occurring, the hypnosis should be terminated immediately and the patient referred to a psychiatrist for further treatment. Difficulties of this kind are much more likely to arise if the continued investigation of the material obtained, and its subsequent treatment, proceeds upon hypnoanalytical rather than simple psychotherapeutic lines. Because of this, it is probably wisest for the general practitioner to confine himself to the simple techniques just described, and to avoid other hypnoanalytical methods and even age-regression as means of further investigation.

REFERENCES

1. Wolberg L.R., 1948. *Medical Hypnosis*, Vol. 1. Grune and Stratton, New York.
2. Moll A., 1890. *Hypnotism.* Walter Scott, London.
3. Baudouin C., 1920. *Suggestion and Autosuggestion.* George Allen and Unwin, London.
4. Erickson M.H. and Erickson E.M., 1941. Concerning the nature and character of post-hypnotic behaviour. *J. Gen. Psychol.*, **24,** 95.
5. Bernheim H., 1900. *Suggestive Therapeutics. A Treatise on the Nature and Uses of Hypnotism* (trans Herter). Putnam, New York.
6. Sacerdote P., 1981. Teaching self-hypnosis to adults. *Int. J. Clin. Exp. Hypnosis*, **XXIX,** 3, 282–299.
7. Fromm E., Brown D.P., Hurt S.W. *et al.*, 1981. The phenomena and characteristics of self-hypnosis. *Int. J. Clin. Exp. Hypnosis*, **XXIX,** 189–246.
8. Olson H.A., 1982. Self-hypnosis in the reduction of executive stress. Paper read at the 9th International Congress of Hypnosis and Psychosomatic Medicine, Glasgow.
9. Davidson G.P., Garbett N.D. and Tozer S.G., 1985. An investigation into audiotaped self-hypnosis training in pregnancy and labour. In *Modern Trends in Hypnosis* (eds Waxman, Misra, Gibson, Basker). Plenum, New York.
10. Swirsky-Sacchetti T. and Margolis C.G., 1986. The effects of a comprehensive self-hypnosis training programme on the use of factor VIII in severe haemophilia. *Int. J. Clin. Exp. Hypnosis*, **XXXIV,** 71–83.
11. Coué E., 1923. *My Method.* Heinemann, London.
12. Wolpe J. and Lazarus A.A., 1966. *Behaviour Therapy Techniques.* Pergamon, Oxford.
13. Waxman D., 1981. *Hypnosis: A Guide for Patients and Practitioners.* George Allen and Unwin, London.
14. Wolpe J., 1958. *Psychotherapy by Reciprocal Inhibition.* Stanford, California.
15. Erickson M.H., 1952. Deep trance states and their induction. In *Experimental Hypnosis* (ed Le Cron). Macmillan, New York.

16. Le Cron L.M., 1952. *Experimental Hypnosis*. Macmillan, New York.
17. Cheek, D.P. and Le Cron L.M., 1968. *Clinical Hypnotherapy*. Grune and Stratton, New York.

CHAPTER 12

Hypnoanalysis and Analytical Psychotherapy

We know that in neurotic illness, the patient's symptoms may be maintained as a defence against unconscious mental conflicts, which are either superficial or deep. The problem, particularly in the more severe cases, is to 'uncover' these conflicts and the associated emotional difficulties underlying the illness, and to help the patient to recognize and deal with them. However, it must be understood from the outset that the recovery of memories of 'forgotten' events and experiences does not necessarily effect therapeutic change.

As has been pointed out, many of the milder neurotic illnesses, in which conflicts involved could be relatively superficial and amenable to some of the simpler forms of investigation, can be treated by the general practitioner. Others, however, arising from deeper conflicts and personality defects, will require a more penetrating form of analysis, conducted in accordance with orthodox psychoanalytical principles. The object is to purge the unconscious of repressed inner strivings and emotions often arising from inimical experiences and conditionings in the past, so that the individual is no longer threatened by anxiety and his ego is strengthened to the point where it can cope realistically with both external and internal stresses. Psychoanalytic therapy thus involves a drastic re-organization of the patient's psychic apparatus so that, freed from the need to retain relevant repressed material, he is enabled to adapt himself to reality and to fulfil his basic psychological needs. Unfortunately, psychoanalysis has to be continued over long periods of time, even years, because of the patient's resistance to abandoning his defences or relinquishing the advantages he is deriving from his neurosis.

Obviously, the scope of psychoanalysis is strictly limited by virtue of time and expense. Moreover, although the root causes of the patient's illness are to be found in the past, many of the immediate difficulties for which he is anxiously seeking relief are situated in the present. Consequently, the ideal treatment should be relatively short, a matter of months rather than years, and must attempt to afford the patient speedy relief from his symptoms through the alleviation of his current problems. It would also deal to a limited extent with some of the personality problems that have contributed to his illness.

Unfortunately such a treatment has not yet been discovered, but there is little doubt that hypnotherapy and hypnoanalysis constitute the nearest approach. Even Freud in his later years indicated that the eventual solution to the problem might well lie within the field of hypnosis.

Additionally, many psychoanalysts object to short-term psychotherapy on the grounds that it leaves the deepest personality problems untouched. Wolberg[1], however, has pointed out that psychotherapy is no mining operation that depends for its results entirely upon excavated psychic ore. He defines it as a human interaction embracing a variety of dimensions, psychological and social, verbal and non-verbal. Such complex elements as *'faith'*, *'hope'*, *'trust'*, *'acquisition of insight'*, *'restoration of confidence and self-control'*, *'self-realization'*, and the *'development of the capacity to love'* are involved. This probably explains the value of the regular use of an 'ego-strengthening' technique at each hypnotherapeutic session.

Although in short-term psychotherapy we are mainly dealing with immediate and superficial problems, we may still succeed in influencing the total personality in depth, including the unconscious. Indeed, the human warmth and feeling experienced by a patient in a single session with a sympathetic therapist may often achieve more profound alterations than years of probing by a detached therapist intent upon wearing down resistance. Nor is the unconscious being entirely neglected, for even during short-term therapy, repressed psychic material may still be uncovered and dealt with.

Nevertheless, in short-term therapy we must be prepared to accept limited goals. It requires a great deal of time to alter deep-seated personality problems, and thus we may have to content ourselves with the immediate objective of symptom relief and rehabilitation of the patient. Wolberg considered that we can reasonably expect short-term psychotherapy to succeed in achieving the following results in the average patient:

1. The relief of symptoms.

2. Restoration to the level of functioning that existed prior to the present illness.

3. An understanding of some of the forces that precipitated the illness.

4. Recognition of some of the personality defects that prevent the patient from adjusting to himself and to his environment.

5. A knowledge of how these arose from past experiences and childhood conditionings.

6. Recognition of the relationship between such defects and the present illness.

If these tasks are successfully accomplished (and they may be considerably facilitated by the employment of hypnoanalysis), we may often expect even greater developments as the patient applies himself to making the necessary adjustments he has learned during treatment.

Hypnoanalysis, like psychoanalysis, can be divided into two stages. The first is analytic and relates to the uncovering of unconscious fears, impulses and memories and the way in which they prevent the patient from adjusting to himself and his surroundings. The second stage is synthetic in the sense that through insight and re-education the patient is helped to establish new habits of thought, new patterns of behaviour, and consequently to build up his self-confidence and control in order to face life anew. We must remember, however, that hypnoanalysis differs from psychoanalysis in that *the therapist must on no account remain passive.* In any form of short-term therapy, one cannot permit the patient to become bogged down in resistance until somehow or other he muddles through. Resistances have to be dealt with gently and discretely before they paralyse progress, and it is in situations such as these that hypnosis can prove invaluable.

Regarding the selection of cases for hypnotherapy or short-term psychotherapy, Wolberg considered it best to assume that every patient is capable of benefiting from short-term treatment unless he proves refractory to it. If the therapist approaches each patient with the intention of doing as much as he can in up to 20 sessions, he will enable the patient to take advantage of short-term therapy up to the limit of his ability to profit therefrom. Should this fail to produce the necessary degree of improvement, prolonged therapy can always follow.

At this point, it must be made clear that the intention is to show how the treatment of certain selected cases can be facilitated and shortened by the use of hypnosis. Indeed, the methods employed are largely those with which psychiatrists are already well acquainted. They can, however, be rendered more rapid and effective through the simultaneous use of the hypnotic state and certain of its special techniques.

Whenever it is proposed to use hypnoanalysis, it is always advisable to induce as deep a hypnotic state as possible. With gradual training, many patients can be taught to enter a sufficiently deep trance to permit the use of some, if not all, of the techniques described. The best results will naturally be obtained when the hypnosis is deep enough to enable the patient to recover forgotten memories of his earlier life or childhood. It will be much easier for him to do this if he is able to develop a posthypnotic amnesia, which will temporarily protect him from the unpleasant necessity of having to face up to painful memories and experiences upon awakening. These can subsequently be restored to consciousness, as and when he feels strong enough to cope with them. In inducing such an amnesia, the use of direct suggestion should not be necessary. It should be more effective to employ a permissive method. During the trance tell the patient that after he awakens, *he will be able to remember just as much as he wishes, but that anything that he does not want to remember, he will be able to forget.*

Some hypnoanalytical methods—free association, dream induction and automatic writing—often need only a light or medium trance. Other procedures such as hypnotic drawing, play therapy, dramatic recall, crystal or mirror gazing, age-regression and experimental conflicts will invariably require deep or somnambulistic trances. It is always imperative, however, that the patient should be able to talk and answer questions during hypnosis without awakening from the trance.

The objective of the analysis is that through the interpretation of the patient's free associations, his dreams and his transference relationship with the analyst, an attempt is made to arrive at an understanding of how experiences and conditionings of his early life are determining his emotional reactions to the present (Wolberg[2]). The ultimate aim of psychoanalysis being the reintegration of the individual in his relationships to the world, to people and to himself.

The therapist must be warned against revealing forgotten memories and repressed emotions and being unable to deal with them. The patient must not be allowed to remain in limbo so to speak, with his raw wounds exposed.

With the concluded, although perhaps not completed analysis, many patients will be left with the thought 'well thank you for telling me why I am as I am doctor, but now how do I get better?'

Any therapist attempting analysis must at all costs avoid falling into this trap. It must be understood that repression has a reason and that reason is for the protection of the patient. No attempt must be made to 'penetrate' the unconscious and to release repressed material unless the therapist is prepared to deal with that which emerges.

Free Association

The induction of the hypnotic state itself will often remove many resistances to free association. The material tends to flow much more readily and a single session will often produce more information than several in the waking state. Medium-depth hypnosis will sometimes suffice, but the deeper the trance the more easily will resistance be overcome.

The patient is told to allow his mind to wander and to report each consecutive thought or idea that enters his mind, no matter how trivial or irrelevant it may seem. Some apparently insignificant things are often most important, so he must not withhold anything at all. Should he feel reluctant to talk, he is to mention it and describe any emotions such as fear, resentment or anger that he may be feeling at the time.

The analyst should listen passively and avoid interrupting the patient's train of thought. But he should note carefully not only what the patient says but how he says it, for his mood, facial expression and tone of voice will often betray the presence of conflicts that he has not thought fit to mention. Should this occur, his attention should be drawn to his behaviour and he should be questioned about it in order to direct his further associations into the required channel.

Not every patient will display the same ability to express thoughts freely, without restraint. It may sometimes be very difficult, for such thoughts are often distressing recollections or things that the patient feels too ashamed to mention. Only training will enable him to learn how to associate freely. Occasionally encouragement and even urgent commands from the analyst will not succeed in overcoming the block in his associations. In such cases, one may try to circumvent the resistance by an adaptation of the Freudian technique of placing a hand on the patient's forehead and telling him that at the count of five he will think of a word or get a mental picture of something connected with the material under discussion.

Dream Induction

The patient may be stimulated to dream on command during the hypnotic session, or it may be suggested to him post-hypnotically that he will dream at night during his normal sleep. The nature of the problems to be dreamed about can be suggested. Hypnotic dreams have all the characteristics of spontaneous dreams, and are dynamically just as significant. Wolberg[2] considered that the dreams that follow the first attempts at hypnosis are tremendously significant and often contain the essence of the patient's problem.

Either a medium or deep trance will usually be necessary and the patient may be gradually trained to develop this ability to dream in response to hypnotic suggestion. At first it is probably best to suggest during hypnosis that he will have a dream the same night, during his sleep, and that he will report it at his next session. If successful these instructions are repeated, but in addition the patient will be instructed to dream about a specific subject. He is then told that he will have a dream immediately before awakening from his trance. Finally, he is instructed to dream during his trance and to relate it and discuss it without waking.

Dreams that are revealed under hypnosis should not usually be interpreted in the waking state. The patient will often be able to interpret his own spontaneous or hypnotic dreams much more accurately while in a trance, since the dream symbolism is much more apparent during the hypnotic state.

Automatic Writing

The technique of automatic writing is taught by placing a pencil in the patient's hand during his trance and suggesting that his hand and arm feel as if they are completely detached and no longer belong to him. It is then suggested that his hand will begin to write and will move along quite automatically so that he will not be aware of what he is writing.

The product of such writing is usually quite different from the patient's normal writing. It is often quite undecipherable. Letters are badly formed, words run together and sentences are incomplete and fragmented. Whenever the patient is able to open his eyes without awakening from his trance, he can be instructed to write the full meaning of his communication underneath the automatic writing. If he is unable to open his eyes without awakening, he can be given the post-hypnotic suggestion that the meaning of his automatic writing will be quite clear to him after he awakens. It is always best to let the patient translate it for himself since he alone is able to supply the material that has been omitted or condensed beyond recognition.

Although the first attempts may end in failure, gradual training may often result in success. Some patients can acquire the technique in very light trances. A few may even be able to write automatically upon suggestion in the waking state. The disadvantage is that such patients may be quite unable to give the real meaning of their communications, which would only become apparent in the deep hypnotic state.

Hypnotic Drawing

The best results will only be obtained when the patient can achieve a somnambulistic trance in which he is able to open his eyes without waking. He may either be instructed to draw whatever he likes, or subjects may be suggested to him by the therapist.

In his drawings, the patient may reveal unconscious attitudes towards members of his family, his wife and children or even the physician. Sometimes he can be requested to illustrate some specific dream or experience that he has had. Even more information can often be obtained if the patient is asked to make up a story about his drawing.

The technique of hypnotic drawing may also be advantageously combined with age-regression. Under these circumstances the patient will frequently be able to express in his drawings attitudes and feelings that are deeply repressed at the adult level.

Play Therapy

Again the patient must be able to open his eyes and handle the materials without awakening from his trance. Many of the resistances that adults display towards play therapy are eliminated in the hypnotic state. Indeed, as soon as the patient realizes that he is not expected to remain passive, and need not wait for directions from the therapist, he usually plays with the materials with great enthusiasm. Play therapy is particularly useful to the patient as a means of expressing unconscious aggression or jealousy towards parents or other children.

The usual equipment consists of a series of dolls representing an adult man and woman, an old man and woman, a boy and a girl about 10 years of age, a boy and a girl of 4, and a baby. Various animals, articles of furniture (including a bed large enough to accommodate the dolls), trains, cars, guns, soldiers, together with crayons, paper and pencils are useful additions. 'Plasticine' may often afford the patient a useful outlet for displaying aggressive or destructive tendencies. The patient should be told to play or build as he likes and to talk about what he is doing. Sometimes the therapist himself will select what is to be used, and will suggest situations based upon material that has been obtained through free association. The patient projects his feelings on to the dolls because he is able, in this way, to dissociate himself from them.

When information is required about conflicts from which the patient suffered in childhood, play therapy can usefully be employed at regressed age levels. Whenever one has gained a general idea of the chief incidents in the patient's life, regression to the age at which these incidents occurred and setting the stage with appropriate materials will greatly facilitate the therapeutic process.

Dramatic Techniques

In deep hypnosis the waking resistances to dramatization are readily removed. The patient is instructed to reproduce traumatic incidents and to act out emotional situations and experiences as if he were living through them once again. He usually does this so vividly that he feels as though he were actually participating in the experience. Indeed the emotional reaction may be so intense that considerable abreaction may be achieved.

The best example of dramatization used in this way is found in the treatment of war neuroses. When the patient is told to relive the traumatic scene, he responds with intense fear and rage in a most realistic manner. He will often scream with terror or pain, and will protect himself by shooting or bayoneting his enemies. Occasionally the same reaction may be produced in re-enacting traumatic incidents that have occurred in civilian life. When it is possible to regress the patient to the age or period at which he suffered the traumatic experience, this technique will become even more effective.

Sometimes the analyst remains passive after setting the scene and encouraging the patient to re-enact the incident, at other times he may have to take a more active role and represent one of the characters in the dramatic scene. Dramatics are particularly successful in affording the patient the opportunity to express repressed aggression.

Regression

During hypnosis, two distinct types of regression may be induced. In the first type, the patient acts in accordance with his current adult conception of himself at an earlier age period. He behaves as he believes he would have done as a child of the suggested age level. This is consequently a simulated reproduction of a past period of life and is really 'remembering'.

The second type is entirely different both in character and in significance. This involves an actual return to an earlier age period, with a true revivification of the same patterns of behaviour that originally existed at that particular time. It does not depend upon current memories, recollections or reconstructions of a bygone age. It is as though the present and all life's experiences subsequent to the suggested age have been blotted out completely. This will include the hypnotist himself, who will consequently have to assume the role of some passive observer or of someone known to the patient during this earlier period, such as a teacher, a relative or a neighbour, for it will obviously be difficult for the patient to converse with someone he will not meet until years later on. This is regression in a true sense, and in this state the patient is able to recapture memories and relive events and impulses that have long been forgotten and repressed.

Regression may often be usefully combined with other hypnoanalytical techniques such as dream induction, play therapy, drawing, dramatics, automatic writing and crystal or mirror gazing. When these methods are employed at a regressed age level, material emerges that would otherwise be quite unobtainable at an adult age level.

A somnambulistic trance is usually essential and post-hypnotic amnesia can be a great asset. There are two main methods of producing regression:

1. The patient is slowly disorientated as to time and place, first as regards the day of the week, then the week itself, and finally the month and the year. When he is sufficiently confused, he is

re-orientated to any desired period of his life. When it is necessary to investigate any particular symptom, he is told to remember and to live through the time when he first developed the symptom.

2. In very good subjects, the patient may be brought directly to the required age level without this preliminary disorientation. He is told that he is going back into the past and that he will feel as if he were once again living in the periods suggested to him. As he goes back, he will feel himself getting smaller and smaller. His arms and legs are getting smaller and smaller, and he is going back to the time when he was ten years old. As soon as he feels that he is exactly ten years old, he is to raise his hand.

Before waking the patient, in this instance it is always best to tell him that he will forget everything that has occurred. The memories and material that have been recovered may be too distressing and painful for him to face right away in the waking state. He can be told that as soon as he feels able to tolerate this material, he will gradually bring it back into consciousness.

Crystal and Mirror Gazing

This technique can only be employed when the patient enters a sufficiently deep hypnotic state to permit him to open his eyes without waking. The patient is told that he will be able to open his eyes and see quite clearly, although he will still remain deeply asleep. He will look into the crystal or mirror (which is so placed as to reflect a blank ceiling), and will see things before him. He is then instructed to describe exactly what he sees.

In this connection, it is interesting to note that *imaginative aids are often more effective than material procedures.* Indeed, it has been found that on numerous occasions, when a patient has been instructed to imagine himself or visualize himself looking into a crystal ball or mirror, much better results were obtained.

This technique can be extremely successful in recovering buried memories. The patient may be able to reconstruct scenes from his past life by hallucinating them exactly as they occurred. These arise more readily since the patient is dissociating himself from them and describing events as if he were watching actors on a stage. Nevertheless, intense emotional reactions are often associated with the recall of such material, and a considerable degree of abreaction can sometimes be produced.

Experimental Conflicts:

Many patients have so rationalized their behaviour that they are unwilling to admit that anything can influence their conduct outside of awareness. They greatly resent the fact that they have impulses of which they are ashamed. Consequently, no matter how convincing the evidence may be, they firmly refuse to admit it. In these cases, the induction of an experimental conflict will often succeed in demonstrating to the patient the influence exerted by his own unconscious mind, and enable him to gain insight when every other method has failed.

The object is to show the patient how unconscious impulses and emotions can actually cause his symptoms to arise. For instance, situations may occur from time to time that cause the patient to feel hostility which his circumstances forbid him to express. He consequently turns this hostility inwards and this will cause symptoms to develop. During his treatment he may become aware of the fact that he feels hostile, and yet be quite incapable of realizing that this suppressed hostility is actually producing his symptom.

The technique involves the creation of an experimental conflict during the hypnotic state, which must be deep enough to ensure post-hypnotic amnesia. An entirely fictitious situation is suggested to him that will arouse hostility that he will be unable to express, possibly one in which he has been unfairly treated. He will feel this emotion acutely, but will be unable to give vent to it and will have to suppress it. The patient is then told that when he has awakened, this situation will come to mind. He will not consciously know what it is, but it will still be on his mind. It will worry him and influence his actions and his speech, but he will be quite unaware that it is doing so. When he wakens the unconscious conflict that is thus provoked will produce the same psychosomatic symptoms that arise whenever he spontaneously feels hostility. In this way, it becomes possible to demonstrate to the patient how certain emotions are responsible for his symptoms. Finally, an explanation may be given to the patient, in a further trance state, of the meaning of this experimental conflict. Directions to recall it in the waking state will often give him considerable insight into his problem.

PRINCIPLES UNDERLYING SPECIAL HYPNOANALYTICAL TECHNIQUES

Hypnosis is a state which easily lends itself to the production of 'dissociative' phenomena even in normal subjects, and these can be employed very effectively in exploratory, in confronting, and in therapeutic ways in hypnotherapy and hypnoanalysis. Erika Fromm[3] gives a clear account of the principles involved. She points out that the major areas of dissociation commonly used for this purpose are:

1. Dissociating the 'observing' ego from the 'experiencing' ego.
2. De-egotizing parts of the body to express unconscious wishes, thoughts and feelings—as in automatic writing, hypnotic drawing and painting.
3. Dissociating various ego-states, processes and functions and helping the patient to re-integrate them in healthier ways.

In any kind of psychotherapy, particularly psychoanalysis, the patient has to learn to observe himself while he experiences affect. In hypnosis, this occurs spontaneously. The patient experiences strong affects, thoughts and hypermnesia and is aware that he does so. He has thus dissociated the 'observing' part of the ego from the 'experiencing' or 'behaving' part. For instance, in hypnoanalysis, the patient can be told to watch himself making a decision, or to hallucinate a person who looks exactly like him and who feels just as angry as he unconsciously does, come into the room and act exactly as he wants to, without feeling fear or guilt. In fact, in a deep somnambulistic trance, a patient who has to undergo surgery can even be told that another man who looks just like him, steps out of him and lies on the operating table whilst he, himself, sits over there in a chair in the corner of the theatre and watches that other man being operated upon. The patient's 'observing' ego in this case retains 'ego-cathexis' whilst the 'experiencing' ego is de-cathected. Because the 'observing' ego is separated from the 'experiencing' ego, and because the 'observing' ego alone retains the ego-cathexis—*that man, not I*—the patient does not feel any pain and can be operated upon without any anaesthetic. This technique is reminiscent of Hilgard's concept of the 'hidden observer'[4].

Then again, in hypnosis we can often 'de-egotize' certain parts of the body to enable them to express unconscious wishes, thoughts and feelings. One of the easiest ways of producing automatic writing is to induce a 'glove-anaesthesia' in the patient's hand. He is then told that his hand is separating from his body, that it is beginning to experience a life of its own, and that it knows the patient's unconscious thoughts and wishes and can write them down. In this case, the 'conscious' ego has become separated from the 'unconscious' ego, and has afforded the latter a direct means of expression. If such a patient is asked a question, he may answer verbally with a 'yes' or a 'no', according to what he consciously feels. Simultaneously, his hand will write the real or unconscious answer, often a 'no' when the answer verbally given is 'yes'. The hand can also write events, thoughts and feelings that have been repressed and are unavailable to the conscious memory. Drawing and painting can be similarly used in hypnotherapy, and it may be noted that the same principle underlies the 'ideomotor finger-signalling technique' which was earlier described. Thus, it may reasonably be concluded that in the trance state the patient is in a state of regression in the service of the ego.

HYPNOANALYTICAL METHODS AND GENERAL PRACTICE

Before discussing this question it is necessary to refer briefly to the transference situation, which plays such an important part in psychoanalysis, and to the resistances that are frequently encountered.

Freud noticed that when a patient had been freely associating for some time he began to display emotional attitudes towards the analyst. These emotions might be either love or hate, but although they were never expressed in so many words they became more or less obvious from the patient's behaviour. The patient who wished to express love would often forget something—possibly his gloves or umbrella—at the end of his consultation so that he had an excuse to return, or he would become increasingly solicitous in his attitude toward the analyst. On the other hand, if he began to feel hatred, he would show his hostility indirectly by praising some other psychiatrist, by forgetting to pay for his consultation, or by speaking disparagingly of the analyst.

Eventually Freud made the surprising discovery that his patients were behaving towards him as if he were someone they had loved or hated in the past, usually a parent. The patient was therefore 'transferring' to Freud emotional attitudes toward the parents that had actually been repressed in childhood. Freud called this manifestation of emotion the *transference,* and the analyst can only deal with it by continually referring it back to its source. Thus there is positive transference, a negative transference and also counter-transference in which the feelings of the therapist are involved. Whatever it is, it always must be strictly controlled, and this calls for a great deal of psychiatric knowledge and experience. The analyst who allows the transference to get out of hand will deserve what he gets. If the patient's love for the analyst remains unchecked, the analysis will get nowhere. If he hates the analyst too much, he may even become provoked to physical violence.

Transference is a most valuable instrument in psychoanalysis. Since the analyst is unconsciously identified by the patient with someone from the past towards whom he felt strong emotions that had to be repressed at the time, he becomes able to project these upon the analyst without feelings of guilt, thereby releasing much material that would otherwise have remained inaccessible. This has to be interpreted most carefully and handled with extreme delicacy until its true meaning can be accepted by the patient.

In hypnoanalysis, as in psychoanalysis, two patterns of resistance are commonly encountered. The first revolves around the patient's unwillingness to acknowledge unconscious drives and impulses and repressed traumatic memories and experiences; the second arises from the transference itself.

In the first type, the patient is either too afraid or too ashamed of his inner conflicts and memories to allow them to enter consciousness. Tension and panic cause him to erect barriers which succeed in blocking his train of thought whenever he approaches painful material. Sometimes he will even seek refuge in amnesia. Since hypnosis renders the unconscious mind of the individual much more accessible, it can help greatly in resolving such resistances.

Resistance arising from the transference situation is not so easily dealt with. The patient may become so frightened of his unconscious impulses that he seeks not only reassurance and support, but also affection from the analyst. In order to secure this he will adopt an attitude of helplessness to enlist sympathy, and will often refuse to work out his own problems until the analyst has first removed his symptoms. Alternatively, resistance may show itself in the form of hostility. If he finds it impossible to express his feelings of aggression, he may conceal them by becoming depressed and discouraged and will often wish to terminate his treatment. On the other hand, if he is able to display his hostile feelings openly, he may become critical or defiant, ridiculing the explanations and interpretations the analyst makes. Transference resistance may manifest itself in many other ways, details of which may be found in many authors' writings. They can only be dealt with by analysing them and interpreting them to the patient, showing him their purpose and how they are affecting his relationships with the analyst and with other people. This is often a long and tedious task which can only be undertaken by those with the necessary psychoanalytical training and experience.

In view of these difficulties and complications, the mishandling of which may easily lead to grave repercussions, it is best to avoid the use of most of the hypnoanalytical techniques in general practice. Indeed, they should normally only be undertaken when the doctor is sufficiently well versed in abnormal psychology to be able to deal effectively with any situations that may arise. The patients who can achieve a sufficiently deep trance state to secure the release of highly charged emotions will certainly require a fully trained psychotherapist to interpret the material produced, and to deal promptly with any acute anxieties or fears that may follow in its train.

The therapeutic use of hypnoanalysis *always* demands a specialized training in psychiatric techniques in order to cope with transference situations and resistances. But when hypnoanalytical methods are restricted to the recovery of buried memories and experiences, as in the treatment of war or traumatic neuroses, this kind of training is less essential. One or two of the simpler techniques can prove exceptionally valuable in uncovering the superficial conflicts that underlie many psychosomatic symptoms. These can then be resolved and treated by the general psychotherapeutic measures already decribed. *The safest course to adopt in general practice is to restrict the use of hypnoanalytical techniques to diagnostic purposes only, and to shun them altogether as therapeutic instruments.* How long treatment is likely to take or how successful it will be depends entirely on the nature of the emotional problems involved. Generally speaking, psychosomatic conditions are much more easily influenced than character disorders, and it is largely with the former that we are concerned here as the latter come within the realm of the psychiatrist.

When questioning under hypnosis fails to shed light upon the superficial conflicts and emotional attitudes underlying the patient's illness, one or two of the simpler hypnoanalytical methods may help to resolve the problem.

Some patients respond readily to the direct suggestion that they will be able to recall forgotten events and experiences: 'When I place my hand on your forehead you will be able to remember what was happening when you first began to suffer from your symptom.' Even if nothing is remembered in detail, a clue will often emerge that can be used as the starting point for free association under hypnosis. This will sometimes yield further valuable information. But once the general pattern of the patient's difficulties becomes clear, it is best to discontinue this and to proceed with treatment on the nonanalytical psychotherapeutic lines already described.

Should these direct methods fail to overcome the patient's resistance, an indirect technique may prove more successful:

> In a few moments, I am going to count up to five. When I have reached the count of five, a number will come into your mind. This number will be the number of letters in an important word that is closely connected with your trouble. Through this word you will be

able to remember many things that you have completely forgotten.
One...two...three...four...five!
What number are you thinking of?
Now I am going to count up to five several times, and each time
I reach the count of five, a letter will come into your mind. Each
letter will be one of the letters in that significant word. They
will probably be jumbled up at first and you may not be able to
understand them, but don't let that worry you.
Now I am going to count up to five several times more, and this
time at each count of five, the letters will come into your mind in
their correct order in that important word.

Once the word is obtained, it should be followed immediately by
free association without awakening the patient. He should be told
to concentrate upon the word, and that as he does so many
thoughts and recollections will come into his mind. He is not to
withhold anything, and is to report each consecutive thought or
memory, however trivial or irrelevant it may seem, the moment
it enters his mind. In many instances, this technique will prove
invaluable in providing the missing key to the problem as the following case well illustrates.

The patient was an ex-service man, aged 34. He was unable to
travel either by bus or motor car without becoming panic stricken.
Since his discharge from the army, he had been quite incapable
of resuming his peace-time occupation as a driver. He was unmar-
ried, and living in lodgings. In the course of taking his history it
emerged that on one occasion, during his service in Italy, he and
his section were fired upon by a German Tiger tank which appeared unexpectedly from an adjoining wood. This was his last
recollection until he awoke 24 hours later to find himself in bed
in hospital, well behind the lines. He had no idea of how he got
there.

It seemed impossible to fill this vital gap in his memory since
not only did all routine methods of investigation fail, but even age-
regression was unable to penetrate the barrier. He readily entered a somnambulistic trance, during which he could easily be
regressed to any age *except* 28, the age at which this incident occurred.

Eventually the technique just described was adopted. The number of letters in the word was 7. They first appeared as follows:

EQSSRIU. When arranged in their correct order they spelt: SQUIRES, and subsequent association to this key word produced the following story.

Squires was the name of a young soldier in the same platoon as the patient. He was aged 19 and had a wife and a young baby that he had never seen. He was not of the stuff of which heroes are made and became terrified when under fire. On one occasion he ran away from the firing-line, and his company commander ordered the patient to fetch him back. This was extremely risky as it involved crossing a stretch of ground which was under heavy bombardment at the time. Since he fought and struggled when caught, the patient stunned him with the butt of his rifle and carried him back to his lines.

Being incensed at having had to risk his own life, the patient set himself out to make this lad's life a misery, taunting him, bullying him and even hitting him whenever he could get away with it. Then came the explosion of the shell from the Tiger tank. When the patient regained consciousness, he found that he was the only survivor of his section and that the mangled remains of the lad lay almost at his feet. He felt overcome with guilt and remorse but even now his ordeal was not ended, for on the journey back to hospital the ambulance in which he was travelling was blown off the road by a shell-burst. He once again became unconscious and woke up about 24 hours later without the slightest recollection of what had occurred.

Wolberg's 'Theatre Visualization' Technique

Another useful indirect technique may prove equally effective in giving a lead, even in the more frequently encountered non-traumatic type of case. This consists of dream or fantasy induction in the hypnotic state. Wolberg[1,5] gives many interesting examples of this method and the way in which it is employed, and it is one which is most valuable and informative.

The patient is told to imagine that he is sitting in the stalls at a theatre. As soon as he can picture himself quite clearly sitting there watching the closed curtains, waiting for the performance to begin, he is to raise his right hand. When this occurs, he is told that he can see a man (or woman) standing on the side of the stage, and peeping behind the closed curtains. He can see what is taking place on the stage behind the closed curtains—the patient cannot—and what this man sees is making him look very frightened or unhappy. As the patient watches, the curtains open and he can now see what is actually causing the man to look unhappy and frightened. As soon as the patient can see the little play that is occurring on the stage, he is to raise his hand. As soon as this happens, he is told to describe the action that is taking place on the stage.

Almost always, the situation that the patient describes will be one that is connected either with childhood memories, or with the difficulties of which he is consciously unaware. This technique is successful in enabling him to recover them because, in fantasy, he is dissociating himself from them and describing them as if they were applicable to other people and not to himself.

The patient is then told that he will see the curtains close, and that what the man at the side of the stage can see behind the curtain is now making him look extremely happy, as if his dearest wishes had been fulfilled. The patient will wonder what it is that is making this man feel so happy, and as the curtains open once more, he will be able to see the action on the stage that is causing this. As soon as he can see this, he is to raise his hand. He is then asked to describe exactly what he can see.

The 'Jigsaw Puzzle Visualization' Technique

Another investigatory technique is that known as the 'jigsaw puzzle visualization technique'. The effectiveness and simplicity of this method renders it of great value, not only to the psychiatrist but also to the general medical practitioner and dental surgeon. Moreover, deep trances are certainly not essential (though naturally desirable whenever possible) and in the average adult, a medium-depth trance is usually all that is required.

Since the success of the technique depends upon the patient's capacity for visual imagery, it is always wise to test this, immediately after the induction and deepening of the trance. Say to him:

> I am going to test your powers of imagination...so, whilst you are lying comfortably relaxed in the chair...I want you to try to imagine that you can see a pair of shoes.

> Just visualize them...and try to picture them quite clearly in
> your mind's eye.
> Tell me...what colour are those shoes?
> What material are they made of?
> What kind of heels have they?
> Do they fasten up...and if so...how?

Most patients seem to have no difficulty at all in answering these questions. Therefore, you can feel quite confident that they possess a sufficient capacity for visual imagery to justify proceeding with the technique itself. If they fail in this test, however, it will be prudent to select some alternative method of investigation that does *not* depend upon visual imagery. On the other hand, when the test succeeds, proceed in the following manner:

> I want you to sit upright in the chair...and picture a small table
> standing in front of you. On that table...there are several coloured
> boxes...red...green...yellow...and blue. Each of these contains the
> pieces of a separate jigsaw puzzle.
> As soon as you can see yourself sitting at this table...with its
> different coloured boxes...your right hand will rise.
> That's fine.
> Now...I want you to choose one of those boxes...any colour that
> you prefer...and turn out the pieces of the jigsaw puzzle on the
> table.
> You will notice that there is no picture on the lid of the box.
> I don't know what picture will eventually emerge...neither do
> you...but it will be the picture of a scene or incident that is
> closely connected with your present illness.
> Your unconscious mind knows...and will help you to fit those
> pieces of the jigsaw puzzle together...so that we shall be able to
> see what this picture is.
> Now...start fitting the pieces together...you will be able to do so
> much more quickly than when you are wide awake...and tell me
> what you can see...as the picture gradually builds up.

You will note that in the above description, the kind of picture that is to be produced may be specified but this is not always necessary or even advisable. It may be better at first to leave the choice of the picture to the patient himself, until he has become familiar with the technique. If desired, the picture suggested may be one that will cause either distress or pleasure, as in the 'theatre visualization' technique.

It may well be also that the colour of the box selected is not entirely without significance. Four boxes are generally specified—red, green, yellow and blue. Some therapists believe that when the red box is chosen, it not infrequently happens that the picture, together with the patient's associations to it, reveals the presence of unconscious dangers, phobias and even aggressive sexual conflicts. The green box is often connected with conflicts in which jealousy (particularly sibling rivalry) plays an important part, the yellow one with cowardice and feelings of inadequacy, and the blue box with conflicts centred around problems of frigidity and lack of feeling. Extensive use and considerable experience of the technique will be necessary before arriving at any definite conclusions.

Should the patient achieve a deep or somnambulistic trance, it may be noted that he will enact the whole process of picking up the pieces of the puzzle and fitting them together. This, however, is certainly not essential. All that is really required is that the patient should be able to *imagine himself doing the appointed task,* and to describe whatever he sees. This is the more usual reaction.

If at any stage the patient says he can see nothing more, he can be told that the picture is not yet complete, and that as he continues to fit more of the pieces together he will be able to describe what else he sees.

Patients usually begin by describing scenes containing meadows, water, trees and houses (that is when the choice of picture has been left to them) and seem curiously hesitant at first to include people or animals. In this case, a discreet question such as 'Can you see any people or children there?' will generally stimulate them to open up with little difficulty. One then asks whether they can remember having seen this before, whether it reminds them of certain places, people, etc., whether they have any idea as to what is going on, and what the people are thinking or doing.

At this point, the patient often drifts off into free association, which can be followed up very advantageously. In special instances it may be wise to suggest to the patient that there is no need for him to acquaint you with the content of the picture as long as he takes a good look at it himself, and works out its significance.

When using this technique, you will notice that the patient sometimes produces a spontaneous abreaction to the content of the picture he is describing, without any stimulation whatever on the part of the therapist. This can prove both informative and helpful, and there is no danger of it getting out of hand provided that it is very carefully observed and since it can be terminated immediately by telling the patient to break up the picture and restore the pieces to the box.

On one occasion, this happened quite suddenly and unexpectedly when this technique was being demonstrated by one of us (J.H.), upon a previously unknown volunteer subject before an audience of doctors and dental surgeons, the choice of picture being left entirely to the subject. When asked to describe what she could see, she surprised everybody by abreacting violently, shrieking out 'Cats...cats...I hate them'. She was told immediately to break up the picture and to put the pieces back in the box, whereupon she calmed down almost instantaneously. She was then told to select a different box which would contain a picture which would give her pleasure, and the demonstration proceeded successfully without further difficulty.

Whether an abreaction occurs or not, it is usually wise to tell the patient that after he awakens, he will be able to remember just as much as he wishes of what has transpired, but that anything that he does not wish to remember, will be forgotten.

In a further reference to Wolberg[2], the following must be emphasized. 'Regression and revivification do not invariably uproot buried memories. Furthermore, the recovery of forgotten traumatic events and experiences does not always produce therapeutic change.'

It should also be remembered that the patient does not always tell the truth. He may confabulate or lie purposefully—even under hypnosis. But what we are interested in is why the patient says what he does.

REFERENCES

1. Wolberg L.R., 1948. *Medical Hypnosis,* Vol. 1. Grune and Stratton, New York.
2. Wolberg L.R., 1946. *Hypnoanalysis.* Heinemann, London.

3. Fromm E., 1968. Dissociative and integrative processes in hypnoanalysis. *Am. J. Clin. Hypnosis*, **10,** 174.
4. Hilgard E.R. and Hilgard J.R., 1975. *Hypnosis in the Relief of Pain.* Kaufmann, Los Altos, California.
5. Wolberg L.R., 1948. *Medical Hypnosis,* Vol. 11. Grune and Stratton, New York.

CHAPTER 13

Ericksonian Hypnosis and Neurolinguistic Programming

ERICKSONIAN HYPNOSIS

No description of the techniques of hypnosis could be complete without particular reference to Milton H. Erickson. Generally acknowledged to have been the foremost authority on hypnotherapy, his induction techniques and original methods of treatment, his extensive writings and the very considerable folklore which built up around him were a legend in his own time.

A great innovator, he developed and utilized resources which are and have always been available to any therapist with the vision to recognize them. As Mesmer was to hypnosis in the eighteenth century or as Freud was in the nineteenth, so Erickson was in the twentieth century.

He taught and treated by an indirect approach and relied upon unconscious learning, rather than by a formalized process of analysis and insight or unlearning and relearning. He used hypnosis for 60 years until his death in 1980.

Ericksonian hypnotherapy is unique in its mode of induction and treatment. Perhaps so unique that the very word 'hypnosis' assumes a new dimension. Here the familiar rituals of eye fixation and deepening no longer apply. Hypnotherapy has become a particular form of communication between the patient and the doctor. It is no longer some divine or magical experience or a transference or a psychological or a neurophysiological state. It is a very special interaction between two people in which the one gives expression by his attitudes and demeanour, by his physical and verbal messages and by every nuance of his behaviour, whilst the other observes, listens and utilizes what is being imparted.

Erickson used his own especially developed style, representations, language and metaphors as a means of communication with the patient. His approach was oblique, he made frequent use of anecdotes, with the occasional induction of 'trance' indirectly, in which essentially, the attention of the subject was positive and productively focussed. In this way changes would take place unconsciously. His metaphors were non-restrictive in that they were a signpost to the general direction of change so that the patient could find his own way. His early method was particularly indirect using a phraseology with which he was able to communicate with many therapeutic levels at the same time. This also helped the process of empathy and the eventual response. In this way, Erickson demonstrated the most important facet of his technique, namely that all patients have within themselves the necessary storehouse and reserves to permit change. It was up to the therapist to recognize this and to utilize those resources for the benefit of the patient. Yet so wide was his understanding that every therapy was individual to that particular patient and could be tailored to his specific needs.

The cornerstones of Ericksonian hypnotherapy are his confusional and utilization techniques. 'The Confusion Technique in Hypnosis' was described by him in 1964[1]. It is primarily a verbal method which is based upon a play of words which, when written,are perfectly straightforward,but when heard, are confusing and hold the attention, for example, 'write right right, not wright or write', or 'a man has lost his left hand in an accident and his right is left.' The next item in the confusion technique is the employment of irrelevancies and non sequiturs 'each of which taken out of context appears to be a sound and sensible communication' stated Erickson. Each can be completely meaningful in itself but has no bearing except as an interruption upon the original situation. In context therefore they are confusing, distracting and inhibiting and the perplexity which results causes a suppression of natural responses. Originally introduced for the purposes of hypnotic age-regression, the technique was later employed to induce hypnosis itself or in order to elicit other specific phenomena.

It is a prolonged and complex procedure and not for the amateur but, Erickson added, 'once one has learned to recognize the fundamental processes involved, there can then be a very easy, comfortable and rapid trance induction' (even under unfavourable conditions). It is nevertheless a technqiue which can only be learned by attending specific teaching courses, workshops and demonstrations, by observing and listening, by practice and by developing one's individual modification of the method. There was only one Milton Erickson. There can never be another.

Erickson's interspersal technique[2] basically is the interspersal of suggestions as disguised therapy within an anecdote in order to help bring about change.

Zeig[3] described as follows how anecdotes may be used during any phase of the treatment process in order to achieve the goals of therapy.

1. To make or illustrate a point.
2. To suggest solutions.
3. To get people to recognize themselves.
4. To seed ideas and increase motivation.
5. To control the relationship therapeutically.
6. To embed directives.
7. To decrease resistance.
8. To reframe and redefine a problem.

The utilization approach involves the wording of suggestions so that the subject is able to feel that he is responding according to the direction of the therapist. To 'accept and utilize'. Erickson himself stated[2] that he had been asked on innumerable occasions to commit to print in detail the hypnotic technique which he employed to alleviate intolerable pain and correct various problems. He asserted that the technique itself serves no other purpose than that of securing and fixating the patient's attention, creating in him a receptive and responsive mental state and thereby enabling him to benefit from unrealized or only partially realized potentials for behaviour of various types. This could be aided by suggestions and guidance.

Resistances may also be utilized but again they must first be recognized and accepted. A situation may then be suggested in which the resistance itself becomes part of the induction technique so that the therapist is working all the time *with* the patient and never against him.

Continued repetition of the therapeutic suggestions are of the utmost importance so that one can feel that they have been adequately absorbed.

Perhaps the greatest tribute that has been paid to Milton Erickson is in the number of seminars, lectures and courses of instruction which have been given in his methods, in the learned papers and the innumerable books which have been written to commemorate his work and in the very considerable following which posthumously still is growing in numbers. Yet with all this, Ericksonian techniques remain essentially the technique of the late Milton Erickson. Nobody can really emulate him. We can only follow his teachings in a general sort of way and hopefully perhaps achieve more for a greater number of people than by relying solely upon the narrow and limited approach of conventional methods.

An important observation was made by Haley[4] that although considerable research is being carried out 'to demonstrate that hypnosis does not exist or rather that no more can be accomplished in trance than when awake...such research is largely irrelevant for clinicians, since hypnosis in research and hypnosis in therapy are two different orders of phenomenon'. Much of the latter is the result of the work and teaching of the late Doctor Erickson.

NEUROLINGUISTIC PROGRAMMING

By a deep and intuitive understanding of the needs and thinking of his patients, Erickson translated the science of hypnosis into a language which the unconscious could interpret and follow. It was directly as a result of his work and skills, particularly in the area of observation and communication, that the ideas of neurolinguistic programming or N.L.P. were to evolve.

In their discussion of Ericksonian hypnosis, Grinder and Bandler[5] defined this as meaning 'developing the skills of a hypnotist so well that you can put someone into a trance in a conversation in which the word hypnosis is never mentioned'. They added that 'neither resistance nor co-operation is a demonstration of anything except the ability of people to respond. Everybody who is living can respond, but how and to what? Your job when you do hypnosis is to notice what people respond to naturally.' This is the essence of N.L.P.

Neurolinguistic programming was originally called 'The Study of Subjective Reality', then latterly, Dennis Chong[6], author, teacher and exponent of Grinder and Bandler described N.L.P. as 'the study of the nature and form of those implicate structures and the forms of language in which they are coded that determine human behaviour'. 'This definition', he continued 'assumes that we agree that, notwithstanding the apparent unpredictability of human beings, for one specific human individual, however, it is not random phenomenology. Behaviour, for every given person, is patterned and, therefore, pre-determined. It is true for our linguistic behaviour. It is also true for our non-verbal behaviour whether one is a smoker and cannot give it up or a depressive who cannot be otherwise.'

In the use of verbal and non-verbal feedback from patient to therapist to patient, it allows the patient to find his own direction and in so doing to arrive at his own solution to his problems.

N.L.P. is 'a model of human behaviour and cognition, which describes how people represent their world, how they interact and communicate with it and with one another, how it can be that they can experience distress and disappointment in these interactions, and how they can be helped to change their representation of the world to alleviate their distress and cope with life more effectively and with greater fulfilment' (Heap[7]).

Thus another important factor is how, having observed that representation, it may be utilized and modified to guide a patient in the direction of altering a behaviour which may be unacceptable to him. This, the protagonists of N.L.P. maintain, can be achieved by a modelling on this 'primary representational system' of the patient. By accepting and by utilizing that which the patient presents, by watching, pacing and leading the patient's behaviour and by permissiveness, that is allowing the patient a choice of response to suggestions.

This primary representational system is identified by observation of the various sensory signals; visual, auditory, kinaesthetic, olfactory and gustatory used by the patient. Taking the first three, which are the more common, does the patient indicate his world in some pictorial way, is it through sounds and words or is it through touch and feeling? Perhaps it is through the less common forms of smell or taste.

In exploring the relevant system, the manner of speaking and in particular of the use of predicates or words a person chooses to describe their situation, should first be noted. A person may say 'I could *see* what he was getting at', 'I liked the *sound* of his voice', 'He's got the right *touch*', 'I can *smell* a rat', or 'It's not to my *taste*', and so on. The direction of gaze is also important. Looking upwards indicates the accessing of visual information (recall to the left, constructed to the right). Looking horizontally will be accessing auditory information (recall to the left, constructed to the right). Looking down and to the left is also the accessing of auditory information. Looking downwards and to the right is accessing kinaesthetic information. If the gaze is not focussed but looking into the distance, the subject is considered to be accessing visual information or cues.

Eye movements and the predicates which are employed may indicate that certain information is accessed in one guise and expressed in another but Bandler and Grinder[8] claim that this is not particularly unusual. It is the system which predominates which is relevant. Having ascertained the primary representational system, this may now be matched by the therapist by pacing or mirroring the observed behaviour, his gestures, movements and other idiosyncracies displayed at the interview. In this way, it is claimed, there is a 'tuning-up' in this representational system and by the use of identical predicates, rapport and understanding are encouraged and enhanced and treatment will be simplified. A negative effect will inevitably result if these systems and predicates fail to be in harmony.

So it may be seen that N.L.P. is in a way, an extension of the Ericksonian technique of hypnotic induction. Efferent signals are received from the patient. Then using as it were a two-tiered system of communication, afferent messages are conveyed verbally and also at the unconscious level by tone, emphasis and movement.

Use is made of numerous other modalities of induction and deepening and of extending the trance state, along the route of treatment and of change within the larger framework of N.L.P. For example 'anchoring' refers to a specific element of an experience, such as of a particular tune, causing the recall of that entire experience. It is essentially an extension of the 'stimulus–response' idea of animal behaviour. Such anchors therefore may be identified in any single or combination of sensory signals. 'Analogue marking' implies the placing of especial emphasis on certain words or phrases. By repetition of both word or phrase coupled to that particular emphasis, then the message is conveyed far more effectively.

The technique of 'reframing' is basically symptom substitution by 'talking' to the affected part through the unconscious. Grinder and Bandler[5] describe conversion symptoms as being 'people's friends' not their problems, since they serve a purpose (of which the patient is consciously unaware) and are a channel for communication. Albeit the meaning may be lost en route, it is the need to rediscover the meaning which is important. The need is to show the patient that meaning and to teach him that the symptom is no longer required and indeed that it can be 'talked' away.

Other techniques for treatment, for dealing with both physical and emotional problems and for effecting behavioural modification may be introduced and utilized within the altered state of awareness produced by N.L.P. Those students who are interested should study the authors to whom reference is made in this chapter in order to gain an understanding of the facilities and effectiveness of this relatively new form of hypnosis. It could well be the beginnings of a new era in psychotherapy.

REFERENCES

1. Erickson M.H., 1964. The confusion technique in hypnosis. *Am.J. Clin Hypnosis,* **VI,** 183–207

2. Erickson M.H., 1966. The interspersal hypnotic technique for symptom correction and pain control. *Am. J. Clin. Hypnosis,* **VIII,** 198–209.
3. Zeig J.K., 1980. *Teaching Seminar with Milton H. Erickson.* Brunner/Mazel, New York.
4. Haley J., 1973. *Uncommon Therapy.* Norton, New York.
5. Grinder J. and Bandler R., 1981. *Trance Formations.* Real People Press, Moab, Utah.
6. Chong D.K., 1987. Personal Communication.
7. Heap M., 1987. Neurolinguistic programming — what is the evidence? Paper read at 4th Congress of Hypnosis in Psychotherapy and Psychosomatic Medicine, Oxford.
8. Bandler R. and Grinder J., 1979. *Frogs into Princes.* Real People Press, Moab, Utah.

PART THREE

THE CLINICAL APPLICATIONS OF HYPNOSIS

CHAPTER 14

General Considerations and Uses of Hypnotherapy

Every illness with which the general practitioner has to deal is primarily organic, functional or psychosomatic in origin. In the last two instances, the importance of mental and emotional attitudes is fully recognized, but in the case of physical complaints too little notice is apt to be taken of the extent to which they can be aggravated and prolonged by psychological factors. Mind and body can never be separated. Each reacts on the other, and consequently needs to be taken into account in every case.

Physical disease may be accompanied by pain, discomfort or impairment of function, sometimes all three. But these will invariably be associated with some disturbance of emotional balance and harmony. The patient who is suffering pain cannot help worrying about the significance of his symptom. He constantly asks himself, 'Is it a sign of cancer?' or 'Am I having a heart attack?' or 'How long am I likely to be ill and unable to earn my living?' In the first two cases, his fear may be so great that he cannot summon up the courage to seek advice. And when he eventually does so, he may be quite unable to convince himself that the doctor, being human, may not be mistaken in his opinion. In the third instance, he may be afraid to resume his work for fear of breaking down again, and destroying all hope of being able to earn his living in the future. This is particularly prone to occur when he has a wife and family to support. Furthermore, such fears and anxieties are far from being the only emotions that can be aroused by illness. The patient may feel bitter resentment at his ill-luck or even depressed as to his prospects, all the more if he has previously enjoyed good health. And then, there is another aspect of the picture which strikes us even more forcibly, namely the problem of gain through illness, the individual who seems to 'enjoy' bad health. Some people often receive so much more consideration, kindness and attention when ill than when they are well that it is hardly surprising that they are so reluctant to give up these advantages. They consequently make very little effort to recover. Additionally, the illness may be a means of manipulating the spouse or family, or may achieve some other important advantage for the patient. This is not necessarily a conscious objective. Yet when examined closely, the message may be all too clear. Now this is extremely important, for without the co-operation of the patient, there are few illnesses from which recovery can be made either quickly or completely.

Every single case, medical, surgical or psychiatric, needs to be approached from three angles—the physical, the psychological and the environmental. Indeed, the importance of viewing every illness against the background of the various stresses and strains to which the patient has been subjected cannot be overemphasized. This is particularly essential when hypnotic treatment is considered, for lack of success can often be traced to an insufficient knowledge of the patient's personality and life history. Both the choice of the best method of induction and the approach to treatment may well depend upon these factors.

In each case, the problem must be explored in depth and with painstaking care. The questions must be asked systematically and as much information as possible must be elicited in order to arrive at a firm decision. The diagnosis should be unequivocal.

In order to achieve this a full medical and psychiatric history must be taken. This should include the basic questionnaire in which every doctor has been trained, i.e. history of present complaint, past illnesses including any previous psychiatric illness (better referred to in discussions with the patient as 'nervous illness'). Personal history with particular note of anxiety symptoms, biological symptoms of depression or evidence of other possible psychiatric symptoms, alcohol consumption, smoking or other addictions and current use of psychotropic medication as well as activities and interest must all be known. Also family history with particular regard to any similar illness amongst close relatives. Family relationships and attitudes to the patient's illness should all be explored. Finally, investigation of early childhood and childhood relationships, possible nervous traits, schooling, academic and sporting achievements, university or further education if applicable, employment history, present status in society and ambitions. Friendships, relationships with the opposite sex, psychosexual history and marital status. Relationship with spouse if married, or with common law partner and children must all be known. Details of previous treatment and results must be enquired into. When all this information is obtained the therapist should be in a position to assess the condition with some accuracy, make a positive diagnosis and formulate the line of treatment to be followed.

Where the patient is currently taking some form of medication there is no need whatsoever to discontinue this, unless it is obviously contraindicated. Antidepressant and anxiolytic drugs including night sedation should always be phased out slowly if and when the patient's condition indicates that this is a safe and correct procedure.

Where the patient is found to be suffering from depression whatever the aetiology, antidepressant medication must first be prescribed and hypnotherapy should not be commenced until the drug is beginning to take effect.

Young children usually above the age of seven and where there is some understanding of what is being undertaken, usually prove good subjects as already stated and old age is no contraindication to hypnosis provided there is no evidence of cerebrovascular change and concentration and hearing are unimpaired.

Patients suffering from any of the conditions listed under 'Contraindications to the use of hypnosis' should never be hypnotized (p.276).

In proceeding along the lines indicated, the information obtained should be sufficiently comprehensive to enable any medical practitioner to undertake the hypnotic treatment of the milder forms of psychosomatic or nervous conditions, should he wish to do so. It should, moreover, help him to be able to discriminate between the cases which are likely to fall within his province, and those which would be best referred to a therapist with psychiatric training or the appropriate specialist.

But in the course of his everyday work he will encounter a large number of medical conditions in which the taking of such a comprehensive history will seem neither necessary nor desirable. Yet, even in these cases it is equally essential to take a full history and this should always be insisted upon. Important information relevant to the condition and treatment of the patient might otherwise inadvertently be withheld. Although much of such detailed case history taking appears to belong more to psychological than general medicine, we are invariably dealing with conditions in which psychological, emotional and environmental factors are involved. Everything that it is possible to know about the patient must be known, whatever the presenting symptom may be.

The reassurance and encouragement that can be given under hypnosis to patients with any complaint, functional or organic, should not be underestimated. Although hypnosis can be extremely useful in many organic illnesses, it will always prove most effective in those conditions accompanied by strong emotional components. In any disturbance, which is physically determined by the presence of organic disease, hypnosis can help considerably in the alleviation of the patient's symptoms. It will do this by modifying his reactions to such symptoms, by lowering emotional tension and by reducing his fears, particularly the fear of death. Physical disturbances that originate from emotional disturbances or psychological stress and not from organic disease should yield much more easily to hypnotic treatment. It is necessary to inculcate in the patient a strong faith in his ability to recover, and to try to teach him to readjust to himself, to reality and to his environment. In talks such as these, hypnotic suggestion can be of the greatest possible assistance.

In addition, hypnosis can be used to afford symptomatic relief in certain chronic physical diseases. It does this partly by reducing tension, anxiety and apprehension, and partly by exercising a direct influence on the patient's attitude to the symptoms and to the illness itself.

Treatment by hypnosis emerged from the forces of magnetism through 'imitation and imagination' into the nineteenth century and then for almost one hundred years the techniques used were by suggestion only.

With the work of Joseph Breuer and Sigmund Freud[1] and by the chance discovery made by one patient, Bertha Pappenheim, hypnotism became hypnotherapy. In her spontaneous regression she was able to talk about her problems and to liberate the 'strangulated affects', the suppressed emotions of those painful memories which had been repressed below the level of conscious awareness and which had precipitated her symptoms. Thus the new technique of treatment, by dynamic exploration (later also called hypnoanalysis), i.e. by discovering the cause of the illness, was evolved. With the abreaction which followed, the symptoms disappeared. At least, so they were expected to do, but unfortunately this did not always happen (see Chapter 1). Freud went on to discover other methods of treatment by using the transference, by dream interpretation and by free association. This latter method has been revived as a useful addition to dynamic hypnotherapy. There occur many instances when a patient is unable to go back in memory to specific instances suggested by the therapist. He may then be allowed to freely associate—that is to report any thoughts or ideas that come to mind, without reservation. Since resistance is minimized by relaxation, free association in hypnosis is more likely to lead towards what is significant and in this way, useful unconscious material may more likely be recalled.

The somewhat more recent development with the use of a behavioural desentitization technique was described in Chapter 1. After every *relearned* response the patient must practise what he or she has newly discovered can be achieved, without experiencing the previously unacceptable symptoms. The patient must therefore practise going into that earlier situation in order to prove that the original symptoms no longer exist and to reinforce that belief as frequently as possible.

Another technique originated by one of us (D.W.) and previously described[2] is that of 'retrospective desensitization'. The patient is asked, in the waking state, to describe one or more earlier experiences in which symptoms had occurred. He is next put into hypnosis and is taken back in imagination, in place and in time to that situation and shown that he can experience it just as it then was (the therapist repeats the description in full) and yet remain completely calm and relaxed and symptom free. An ideomotor signal is requested at the end of the description confirming the patient's newly learned response. Other unacceptable experiences are similarly dealt with. This technique considerably reinforces the routine of 'prospective desensitization' usually practised. Similarly, aversion methods are used by some therapists, particularly for the addictions. The patient is told that he will respond with adverse symptoms (recalling some previous unpleasant effects such as nausea and vomiting) whilst indulging in the unwanted behaviour and demonstrates that the symptoms actually occur! Finally whatever treatment methods are adopted, ego-assertive retraining and self-hypnosis have proven valuable adjuncts to recovery and are used by most experienced clinical therapists.

Below is a summary of the methods available for treatment of the patient in the hypnotic state.

Summary of Hypnotherapeutic Techniques
  1. Dynamic (or psychodynamic) techniques

    (i)   Regression and recall
    (ii) Ventilation and abreaction
    (iii) Interpretation and insight psychotherapy
    (iv) Free association

  2. Behavioural techniques

    (i)   Prospective desensitization (followed by practical retraining)
    (ii) Retrospective desensitization
    (iii) Hypnoaversion

  3. Supportive techniques

    (i)   Ego-strengthening

(ii)   Ego-assertive retraining
(iii) Self-hypnosis

Whatever form of treatment is undertaken must depend entirely upon the history which the patient has presented, the interpretation of that history and the expertise of the therapist. Freudian or dynamic techniques should not be attempted by the amateur. The therapist must always be in control of the treatment and able to contain any adverse symptoms which may arise. In the final analysis the treatment which is judged to be the best for the patient is that which should be prescribed not that which he, the therapist is able to do or thinks he would like to try. If he feels that any case is beyond his capabilities, then the patient should be referred to the appropriate specialist.

There remain many advocates of simple symptom removal by direct suggestion and the first author was a firm believer in this method. It must be understood, however, that the symptom is saying something. An attempt *must* be made to understand the message rather than to ignore it. Every reader will agree that in general medicine one does not treat the symptoms in order to effect a cure. It is the problem that causes that symptom which must first be exposed. If this is then satisfactorily dealt with, the symptom may well subside without further damage to the patient.

Unfortunately, again as in general medicine, the origin of the problem may remain obscure or in doubt. In such cases a palliative may sometimes be given but the search for the aetiology of the symptoms must continue.

Perhaps the only occasions in which symptom removal by suggestion is justified are in obstetrics, dentistry and surgery, when pain relief is the main objective. Without doubt also it may be the method of preference for the relief of pain in the terminally ill.

The notorious lack of success which may be experienced by any therapist in attempting symptom removal is exactly for the reasons given. The symptom is saying something and *will* be heard. Therefore that symptom is defended until it is heard, until the repressed memory, by some means, will appear at the surface and no longer require to be held incognito below the level of conscious awareness. Unless of course, the patient is shown in some other way, that the symptom is no longer required.

It was precisely this problem which was met with by Freud, a hundred years ago. He eventually found that he was unable to penetrate the defences of most of his patients in order to reveal the hidden memories, events and emotions which were the cause of their problems. It was precisely for this reason that he abandoned hypnosis and concentrated on his newly discovered technique of free association.

It may be argued that his patients went into hypnosis nevertheless. For who could resist so to do, when lying on that famous couch, in the chambers of the Herr Professor himself. And when the master laid his hand upon the brow of the now highly suggestible patient and said—'close your eyes, concentrate and tell me the first thing that comes into your mind', was that patient in hypnosis? The answer may be left to the imagination of the reader.

Today, few of us have the charisma of our great predecessor. Moreover and perhaps because of his teachings we know better than to try to *penetrate* the defences of any patient. Rather do we encourage him slowly to remove them himself, brick by brick as they are no longer required.

It is a sad reflection of the needs of society today that many people look upon hypnosis as a cure for smoking or as a means of treating obesity. It is none of those things.

Others consider that it is a way of penetrating the unconscious, of revealing the skeletons in the cupboard or of some dramatic experience or encounter in early life, which was the cause of all the trouble. It is rarely any of these things.

Or perhaps it is some power by means of which we are able to *make* people do things that they would not or could not normally do in the waking state. Well, fortunately, hypnosis cannot achieve even this.

The hypnotic state is a very particular form of relaxation, in which, possibly as a result of certain neurophysiological features inherent in its use, various psychological and behavioural responses and changes may take place. It should be recognized that hypnotherapy is certainly not the panacea for all ills. Neither is it merely an adjunct or complementary form of treatment used to supplement physical methods. It is frequently and quite unequivocally the most suitable form of treatment available and specific in its own right.

Hypnosis is used essentially in the treatment of certain mental illness. Stengel[3] divided the latter into four main categories. These are the neuroses, in which the patient remains in touch with reality, the psychoses which are a group of severe disorders in which there is a distinct break with reality, the abnormal personalities and the mentally subnormal or deficient. Of these it must be emphasized that *the only group of disorders in which hypnosis may be safely used are the neuroses.* There are many additional problems which do not come under the heading of mental illness but in which hypnotherapy may be the treatment of choice. Most of these conditions will sometime or other present to the medical practitioner and these are listed as follows:

1. *The neuroses*
Anxiety.
Psychosomatic responses.
Phobic illness.
Obsessive–compulsive disorders.
Hysterical–conversion symptoms.

2. *Problems of personality*
Alcohol and drug addiction including smoking.
Problems of body image (anorexia, bulimia, dysmorphobia).
Social disabilities (stammering, blushing, habit spasms or tics and unacceptable mannerisms etc.).
Immature personalities.

3. *Psychosexual problems*
In Men:
　Erectile impotence.
　Premature ejaculation.
In Women:
　Vaginismus.
　Frigidity.
In Men or Women:
　Anorgasmia.
　Loss of libido.
　Some sexual variations.

4. *Miscellaneous problems*
The alleviation of pain.
Obstetrics.
Surgery.
Sports medicine.
Dentistry.
Terminal care.
Forensic hypnosis.

5. *Reactive depression*
Must be treated with antidepressents. When under control hypnotherapy may be used for the anxiety component and as an exploratory procedure.

Other uses of hypnosis will present themsevles from time to time. Some of these are mentioned in the text. Any treatment must be according to the general guidelines.

Contraindications to the Use of Hypnosis

It cannot be stated often enough, that hypnosis is not the panacea. The interests of the patient are paramount and the treatment must be made to fit the patient and not the patient to the treatment. It would seem to be superfluous to advise any physician to be certain of the diagnosis before offering a remedy. But in mental illness, perhaps more than in any other discipline of medicine, an error in judgement and an error in treatment could lead to disaster. One must not be 'trigger happy' about the use of hypnosis and shoot down every possible complaint with this newly acquired magic bullet. As with every problem, history taking must be extensive and the diagnosis accurate.

There are certain conditions in which hypnotherapy is definitely contraindicated. These are mainly as follows:
1. Depression (endogenous or bipolar).
2. Schizophrenia.
3. Senile, anteriosclerotic or organic psychosis.
4. Alcohol or drug psychosis.
5. Pathological personalities.
6. Mentally subnormal or deficient patients.

7. In certain physical disorders including thyroid dysfunction, hypoglycaemia and cerebral tumours.

(The treatment of patients suffering from various neurological problems requires especial expertise.)

Problems inherent in the treatment of those conditions which may arise with the use of hypnosis are obvious. It has been emphasized that since the hypnotic state is essentially one in which the subject is calmed and non-anxious, the use of hypnosis in a depresssed person should never be undertaken until that depression has been effectively treated by drugs. This applies especially to chronic endogenous and manic depression. Where a psychotic illness exists this could well be in remission at the time of treatment and the use of imagery in hypnosis could well result in a relapse. Schizophrenia, however, has been treated by hypnosis but there is little justification for this since there are today very adequate drugs with which the condition may be contained.

Additionally, hypnotherapy should never be attempted if the patient is poorly motivated or objects to treatment by this method. If it is to be used as the treatment of choice, hypnosis must be applied with care and with confidence and only for the conditions which have been described. In this way the physician will find that he has a most valuable additional instrument in his therapeutic armamentarium for the treatment of a considerable range of disorders which could otherwise defy relief.

REFERENCES

1. Breuer J. and Freud S., 1955. Studies on hysteria. In: *Standard Edition of the Complete Psychological Works of Sigmund Freud* (ed. Strachey), Vol. 11. Hogarth, London.
2. Waxman D., 1981. *Hypnosis: A Guide for Patients and Practitioners.* George Allen and Unwin, London.
3. Stengel E., 1964. *Suicide and Attempted Suicide.* Penguin, Harmondsworth.

CHAPTER 15

The Treatment of the Neuroses

The problems which fall into this category and their treatment through the use of hypnosis will now be considered.

1. Anxiety

This in its turn may be subdivided as follows:

(a) Normal Healthy and Frequently Protective Anxiety
Am I going to be late for that appointment?
Perhaps I should take an umbrella, it looks like rain.
Hold that child's hand whilst you cross the road.

This type of anxiety may be no more than natural concern and thus the person is symptom free. Should the stimulus become more acute then the response will vary accordingly, so that in the extreme it will be 'stand and fight' or 'turn and run for your life'. As the stimulus decreases or disappears so does the response and the anxiety level settles at normal for that particular person. No treatment is indicated.

(b) Reactive Anxiety
The condition is a response to a stimulus that produces symptoms, both psychic and somatic. They are transitory but none the less may be incapacitating and can result in general nervousness, an irrational preoccupation with the problem, minor physical ail-

ments and sleep difficulties.

Hypnosis should be induced by a permissive technique ensuring that the patient is completely calmed by the induction.

The precipitating cause is researched and discussed in detail, stopping at frequent intervals to ensure that there is no increase in the level of anxiety at any stage. Confirmation that the feeling of calmness persists should be requested by an ideomotor signal.

The extent of particular stressful experiences or anticipated fears may be exaggerated slightly in order to allow a wider margin for possible anxiety responses to occur, emhasizing calmness if they do so and again confirming the calmed response with an ideomotor signal.

Instruction in self-hypnosis and regular twice daily application is essential. The subject is shown that he can think about his problems whilst in self-induced hypnosis and remain perfectly calm and symptom free. The effect will persist on opening the eyes, for a half hour or so in the early stages, the time gradually extending. Self-hypnosis should additionally be used when in bed at night in the event of sleep difficulties. The subject should allow himself to drift into sleep without dwelling on any specific anxiety.

(c) Chronic Anxiety and 'Endogenous' Anxiety

Although the latter term is not usually applied to anxiety it is in fact relevant to the type of anxiety which originates from within, which is part of the make-up of the patient. That anxiety in which the patient lives a life of fear. In which these fears take over, affecting every thought and every response. Anxiety in which psychic and somatic symptoms dominate every action, which is irrational and which is totally out of context to the needs of the situation.

This is the type of patient who will readily become dependent upon tranquillizer drugs. In addition it is not uncommon for symptoms of depression to supervene. This can easily be missed by the physician and would account for many difficulties arising in treatment unless the appropriate antidepressant medication is prescribed.

This type of anxiety, which is built-in to the personality, will require long-term treatment. Since he is always anxious, the patient will more readily respond to situations of stress with anxiety symptoms. However, those situations which the patient may find stressful may be an accepted part of everyday life to others. Psychosomatic responses, sleep problems and depression may already be additional features and require more specific treatment. Before the latter develop however, the anxiety level of the patient can be reduced by regular sessions of hypnotherapy involving the technique utilized in reactive anxiety and additionally the more traditional method of dynamic exploration may be introduced. It is best to leave most of the talking to the patient. In this way he will more likely recall events from the past which he considers to be to blame for his symptoms. Many practitioners will call this regression. It is not regression at all. It is usually simply remembering. The patient, in hypnosis, is asked to go back to events earlier in life and to talk about them. He will usually commence with the words 'I remember etc. ...'. If instructed specifically to be a certain age again or to relive a particular event, then in true regression *he will be there* and will speak in the present tense. An example is as follows:

> Now Mr Smith, you will remain very deeply relaxed in this state of hypnosis and follow carefully what I am saying to you. I want you to go back in your thoughts to the earliest memory you can recall. Some people can remember far, far back into early childhood. Others remember events only as far back as eight or ten years, whilst others remember nothing of their childhood. This is not important at this point. Think back as far as you can and when you have that memory in your mind, tell me about it. Although you are in hypnosis, you are able to hear every word that I say and you can certainly speak to me. So when you are ready—talk to me about that memory Mr Smith.

There is a pause whilst the patient is obviously considering your question. He then mouths a few words and gradually realizing he can speak will say...

> I remember when I was about five years old my father bought me a bicycle.

This therefore is remembering. Often, with the anxiety which fills his mind temporarily lifted by the hypnosis which preceded, he is able to think more clearly and to recall events which were clouded by the passage of time but certainly existed within his conscious memory. Recall allows the patient to 'get things off his chest', specific events and responses may be explained and this may often have a salutary effect.

Where it is felt that regression is indicated with ventilation of repressed memories and possible abreaction, then the hypnosis is deepeneed and the approach is as follows:

> Now Mr Smith, I want you to go back in your mind, in place...in time...and in memory to events earlier in your life. It isn't yesterday or the day before or last week or last year...go back...deeply deeply relaxed...you are not twenty...you are not fifteen...you are not ten...you are five years old...it is your birthday...be that little boy again...it's your fifth birthday...be where you were at that time...see the clothes you are wearing...see how you look, how your hair is brushed...you are five today...What is happening Johnny?"

There is a pause. The patient begins to show some signs of distress.

> Daddy won't let me have a birthday party.
> Why not Johnny?
> Because I'm a naughty boy.

This is true regression. The patient is there, he is reliving the situation and memories of events which have been repressed are more likely to surface. Not only may the memories be recalled but also might the emotional effects of that particular event and which *might* be responsible for the presenting symptoms. This could involve a classical catharsis or abreaction after the manner described by Breuer and Freud[1], to the ultimate benefit of the patient.

The therapist must be warned however, that this is not a technique for the amateur, nor is it lightly to be embarked upon. He must be prepared for a distressing scene and ready and able to follow it up and deal with the problems which may arise. The patient must never be left wondering what to do next. The therapist must also be warned however that a true abreaction is a rare occurrence and that the patient does not necessarily tell the facts about the particular event uncovered. He may well be saying what he believes to have been the facts. But whether fact or fiction it is what he says that is important. The value of that information and what can be done with that information will depend upon the therapist.

In the treatment of general anxiety it should be remembered that arousal and associated performance can only reach a certain level. That level or ceiling differs with every person. If pressed beyond that level then the ceiling will begin to crack, performance will deteriorate and symptoms will appear[2].

2. Psychosomatic Responses

Psyche was the Greek goddess of the soul or the mind, who gave her name to that part of us within which our neuroticism is hidden. The soma is the body, the physical site at which the neurotic symptom manifests itself.

A psychosomatic response is the psychic effect resulting from an external situation, real, imagined or anticipated, which the patient interprets as stressful, which causes severe anxiety and which produces an autonomic response to that anxiety.

Psychosomatic responses may be experienced in any system of the body and there does appear to be a prediliction in individuals, for one particular organ. This is known as 'organ inferiority'. This expression was coined by that great psychologist Alfred Adler[3]

(a) The Central Nervous System

Migraine *type* headaches are a familiar response to anxiety. Notwithstanding, classical vascular migraine may be precipitated by tension and anxiety. Many people are acquainted with some of the common symptoms of migraine such as unilateral headache and vomiting and these are physical responses which may readily occur at times of stress. The problem must be thoroughly researched in extensive history taking including, of course, learning of the types of situation which trigger an attack. Nervous patients will invariably fear a cerebral tumour if attacks are persistent and this fear will not be relinquished until a full neurological examination, including X-rays and brain scan have been undertaken. Unless the patient is reassured about this problem, no progress can be made in treatment. Treatment by hypnosis with instruction in self-hypnosis to be used regularly twice daily, as well as before or following situations of stress, usually gives excellent results. In hetero-hypnosis, discussion of the origin of attacks if known, of personal problems and fears, of family problems, not forgetting sexual difficulties, are a necessary adjunct. Specific anxieties are dealt with by visualization of these situations in the relaxed state of hypnosis and showing the patient that symptoms do not appear. Particular attention is paid to the customary focus of the symptoms—for example tension ascending from the back of the neck and into the head.

It is most essential to try to understand what the symptom is saying. Is it to manipulate the family or the environment, to avoid responsibility, sexual intercourse or work? All these questions must be answered if therapy is to be successful.

Hypnotic treatment of migraine has been well researched and its value is established[4,5].

Vasovagal attacks may also occur as a psychosomatic response. Fainting with fear is a well-known phenomenon which may readily become paired to situations which invoke memories of the previous attack. Such attacks have at times been mistaken for petit mal or even erroneously thought to be cardiovascular in origin.

One patient had been treated with barbiturates and other antiepileptic drugs for seven years even though neurological examination had revealed no abnormality. History taking revealed that this first attack occurred during military service. He was on parade together with other members of his unit awaiting inspection by the brigadier. As the great man approached patient 'fainted' and was subsequently put on a charge of falling out without permission. He continued to fall out in similar threatening situations, was labelled epileptic and the label stuck!

Full discussion of his fears, under the relaxed state of hypnosis and insistence on regular self-hypnosis relieved him of his attacks and of his need to take medication. He was followed up for several years and has been totally symptom free.

There is no doubt also that grand mal epilepsy sometimes may be triggered by anxiety, whatever neurological or organic pathology may exist, and the reduction of anxiety through hypnotherapy can be most beneficial.

(b) The Cardiovascular System

Stress, personality and cardiovascular disease are a triad of features familiar to every physician and research into the relationship of these factors has been ongoing for many years. There is no doubt that the reduction of the anxiety response to stress can do much to reduce and even to cancel out the physical effects. Early studies showed that the risk of coronary heart disease appeared to be twice as high in type A individuals compared to their type B counterparts[6] and the more recent Western Collaborative Group[7] and Framingham Projects[8] confirmed the original findings, albeit there remains some dispute about the matter. Although hypnotherapy makes no pretence that it can alter the personality of the individual, it can certainly reduce his level of anxiety.

The regular use of self-hypnosis can be of considerable benefit to patients suffering from anginal pains induced by stress and from essential hypertension.

One can well imagine the benefit to a patient with labile hypertension if he can take a deep breath, think of the word 'calm' and allow its full meaning and experience to take over in situations which would otherwise send his blood pressure soaring.

Brief Hypnosis   This is the technique which is intended to teach the patient to attain 'instant' calmness (see Chapter 11).

A deep state of hypnosis is not always attainable in some patients, the striving, assertive type being reluctant to relinquish what he may see as his control. This trait is exploited as follows. A hierarchy is constructed of stressful and competitive situations anticipated for the week ahead. The patient is put into hypnosis and asked to visualize the first item in the hierarchy. As he experiences his anxiety level rising he is told to take a deep breath, hold for a moment and then allow the air to go from his lungs and the tension from his chest. Simultaneously as he breathes out, to see the word 'CALM' in his thoughts, to say the word silently to himself and as the tension goes from his mind and from his body, he feels completely calm, more alert and wide awake and ready to tackle whatever problem with which he may be confronted. The response should be monitored by the ideomotor signal throughout.

The hierarchy is completed and the patient is seen again one week later when a further programme is constructed for the days that follow.

With this technique the patient is assured that control is not given into the hands of the doctor but remains with him as something he can use and extend for his own benefit.

The type B personality who certainly does not show his anxiety in the same assertive manner as his type A counterpart may equally be helped with the use of hypnotherapy and self-hypnosis, to explore and 'externalize' his problems, reduce his general level of anxiety and improve his attitude by ego-assertive retraining.

(c) The Respiratory System

The main symptoms in this area are hyperventilation and anxiety-induced asthma. 'Panting with fear' is a phrase which requires no explanation and this response may be noted in many individuals. The respiratory rate is generally increased or the occasional, or sometimes even frequent 'need to take a deep breath' or 'I can't get enough air in my lungs' is a well-recognized complaint.

Relaxation in hypnosis, exploration and discussion of anxiety-related problems, desensitization and self-hypnosis will bring relief to this often incapacitating symptom.

Equally well known is 'nervous asthma'. The attack which is triggered is a direct response to anxiety-anticipated situations. Monday morning—back to school is a classical example—the 'Pavlov-like' conditioning resulting in the symptom was described by Maher-Loughnan and Kinsley[9] who reported the successful results of a clinical trial of hypnosis in asthma. The advantage of this technique over the use of drugs, particularly steroids, in 'psychogenic' asthma is obvious. Again, the emotional events which trigger an attack must be explored. Loss, separation and suppressed anger. The initiating event which may be revealed by questioning before or under hypnosis must be discussed and in particular, the regular use of self hypnosis is an important factor in reducing the frequency of attacks. Hypnotherapy has been shown to be of considerable help in patients who are generally not progressing well with other treatments.[10]

However, it should never be used in acute asthma when standard emergency procedures should be instigated. Hypnosis is suitable for mild to moderate asthma only.

(d) The Gastrointestinal System

The effect of anxiety upon the gut is equally well known. Complaints of 'butterflies', feeling 'sick with fear', 'my stomach turned upside down' are commonly used descriptions of symptoms which may readily pre-empt an attack of peptic ulcer-like symptoms. In addition there must be very few who have not experienced the response of the lower bowel at some time or other. It is extraordinary to think that some experts still consider the irritable bowel syndrome to be an organic condition and a vast amount of research is still ongoing to investigate this problem[11]. This syndrome was discussed by one of us (D.W.) in a paper presented to the 4th European Congress of Hypnosis in Psychotherapy and Psychosomatic Medicine[12]. The basis of treatment is relaxation in hypnosis, exploration, ventilation, discussion and desensitization with ongoing self-hypnosis as a continuing means of lowering the level of anxiety. The problem of suppressed anger, expressed via the bowel is sufficiently common to be very well understood by most patients and early parental attitudes may be of considerable relevance.

(e) The Genito-urinary System

In spite of the physical proximity, these two systems may be psychologically separated. Anxiety will frequently express itself through the genital system in the female and the emotional difficulties associated with dysmenorrhoea, amenorrhoea and menorrhagia are only too well known to every gynaecologist. In the absence of any organic pathology these symptoms may be researched under hypnosis and treated accordingly. Much can be done to alleviate distress but many factors must be borne in mind. These include early sexual education (or lack of education) and subsequent experiences, family and marital problems, the general environment and the personality of the subject. The condition known as the pre-menstrual syndrome needs especial care as this is most certainly endocrine induced although associated with a considerable emotional overlay. It should be remembered that depression is frequently a feature of this distressing and cyclical problem and must be treated accordingly. It must also be borne in mind that the regular monthly appearance of the symptoms may serve a purpose. The reason for this may surface during the phase of dynamic exploration. Nevertheless it is essential that a very comprehensive evaluation not only of the symptoms, but of all the medical, psychological, environmental and social factors that may affect them be embarked upon before treatment is decided.

The urinary system too, is frequently affected by emotional difficulties. The problems of nocturnal enuresis is one which is common in children and may also occur in adults. It is frustrating to parents and paediatricians alike but it must not be forgotten that the effect on the child is degrading and demoralizing. Numerous methods have invariably been used before the unfortunate patient reaches the hypnotherapist. Drug treatment including antidepressants and the amphetamines as well as psychotherapy and conditioning by the use of the enuresis alarm have invariably been attempted and failed. The child has often been punished for this 'misdemeanour' and defiance may be an added factor. Anger, guilt and confusion compound the problem.

The further treatment of enuresis in children is discussed in the chapter dealing with paediatric hypnosis.

Nocturnal enuresis in adults may respond to a relaxation and ego-strengthening technique, suitably adapted, but resistance to treatment will indicate the need for an analytic approach.

Another and perhaps directly opposite symptom to the above is the inability to relax sufficiently say in a public toilet, in order to empty the bladder. This is typically an anxiety response and may occur in males or females. Treatment consists essentially in teaching the patient to relax through hypnosis and the use of self-hypnosis followed by desensitization to a hierarchy of anxiety-provoking stimuli in hypnosis such as imagining being in the toilet and emptying the bladder whilst other people are within earshot. Practical retraining should take place if possible in the doctor's premises where for example, a secretary or receptionist can be strategically placed near the toilet door, the patient being aware of her presence there.

Hypnosis has also been used for incontinence caused by 'idiopathic' detrusor muscle instability and one paper reported good results in 50 women with this conditon. Twelve sessions of symptom removal by direct suggestion and ego-strengthening were completed with treatment continued at home on cassette[13]. Unfortunatley however there was no control group but this could be one of those rare instances where direct symptom removal may be suggested without other difficulties arising.

(f) The Musculo-skeletal System

Muscular tension is invariably a concomitant of anxiety states and pain may frequently result. Tension symptoms in the back of the neck and extending upwards into the head have already been discussed under the heading of 'migraine'. Similarly, chronic backache may occur in other parts of the spine possibly originally triggered by some minor strain or injury. This is without doubt one of the commonest causes of absence from work and results in considerable sums being paid out in sickness benefit. In the absence of other pathology, hypnosis can be used to treat the problem but positive motivation is of prime importance. The therapist must be certain that the patient is not using the symptom either deliberately or unconsciously to obtain some gain. The usual five stages of hypnosis, analysis, explanation and desensitization may be used, with of course self-hypnosis for self-treatment between sessions. Hypnosis may also be used in order to increase relaxation during physiotherapy and manipulative treatment and proves a useful means of aiding recovery.

(g) The Skin

Many dermatological conditions are aggravated by anxiety or may even be triggered by the neurosis. Pruritis, urticaria, eczema and psoriasis are amongst those which are most common. Dermatologists will frequently prescribe some tranquillizer drug where the problem is severe[14] and antidepressant medication may often be indicated. Psychotherapy certainly has a place where the condition seems intractable and in this respect hypnotherapy may be useful for uncovering early memories which could be responsible for the condition[15].

Hypnotherapists frequently are requested to treat warts and are often successful. The rationale of their disappearance remains a mystery but doubtless is related to the powerful belief of the subject in a cure.

A patient of 22 attended one of us (D.W.) for the treatment of a stammer which was particularly associated with situations creating anxiety. After two sessions he suddenly held out his hands turning them from side to side. 'Why are you showing me your hands' he was asked. 'Well', he replied, 'both of my hands were smothered with warts but I was too embarrassed to tell you about them. I knew that hypnosis could cure them and hoped that whilst you treated my stammer they would disappear'. They had done so. The skin of his hands was as clear as a new born babe's!

The skin has been called the mirror to the mind and may well be the visible manifestation of some internal conflict. Emotions of anger and aggression, perhaps of frustration or guilt. Is the patient telling the world something in this way? Is this some self-inflicted and visible punishment?

A man of 38 was referred to the second author on account of severe and generalized pruritis. The skin was reddened and excoriated as a result of scratching. It was always worse when warm and was particularly so when in bed at night. As a result sexual intercourse was impossible. In fact exploration of his problem under hypnosis revealed the more likely reason, that because intercourse was impossible his pruritis provided an ideal excuse for abstinence. The patient had been impotent for at least a year before the rash appeared. Frank discussion of the problem and treatment of his impotence by desensitization under hypnosis resolved the dermatological condition and the need for any gain through the symptom disappeared.

3. Phobic Illness

It is interesting to consider two descriptions of phobias:

(a) as a learned maladaptive habit, which is aquired by the rules of conditioning and learning (Marks[16]) and

(b) as a disproportionate, obsessive and unrealistic fear of an external situation or object, symbolically taking the place of an internal unconscious conflict (Blakiston's Medical Dictionary[17]).

A phobia is an irrational fear, the experience of which may produce any simple psychosomatic response—such as tachycardia, or a massive response in which all systems may be involved. So common are these symptoms that their description is in everyday usage. Sweating with fear, panting with fear, paralysed with fear—butterflies in the stomach, thumping in the chest, etc. We have all experienced one or more of these symptoms at some time but when they become a 'learned habit of reaction', when they occur repeatedly in specific situations, when they are maladaptive and are unacceptable to the patient, then the phobia has become pathological and must be treated.

The word phobia itself derives from antiquity having originated from the deity of ancient Greece—Phobos the god of fear. It appears first to have been clinically described by Westphal in 1871 in an account of patients suffering from what we now know as agoraphobia. An excellent definition of the condition is also given by Marks[16] as follows:

A phobia is a special form of fear which is (1) out of proportion to demands of the situation, (2) cannot be explained or reasoned away, (3) is beyond voluntary control and (4) leads to avoidance of the feared situation.

Symptoms may be monophobic, that is related to one particular fear such as the fear of heights, or they may be multiphobic and very resistant to treatment.

The phobic patient is an anxious patient but that patient may additionally be depressed. As already mentioned it is of the utmost importance to determine whether that depression is primary or secondary to the anxiety. If the former, then the appropriate antidepressant medication *must* be instituted without delay and before hypnotherapy is commenced. Antidepressants will also facilitate treatment if a reactive depression exists.

That a phobia may be a conditioned response there is no doubt. From the days of Pavlov through the researches of J. B. Watson and Mary Cover Jones experiments have been deliberately conducted to produce such a behaviour. Equally that the patient may be deconditioned there is also no doubt and a considerable array of techniques have been devised for this purpose. Yet there may also be a dynamic origin to the problem and it could well be that many patients in whom the phobia resists extinction would occasionally respond to exploration along those lines. Through the use of hypnosis both channels of treatment may be exploited for the benefit of the sufferer.

We may assume that the appropriate history taking is completed and that it has been established whether in addition to the specific fear or fears, anxiety, depression or symptoms of both are present. In the event of depression being present with or without anxiety it is essential to prescribe antidepressant medication. The most suitable drug is clomipramine, this having been shown to possess additionally valuable antiphobic properties (Waxman[18]). Many hypnotherapists would equally resist the prescription of any form of chemotherapy but in the interests of the patient, an eclectic approach is essential. Moreover, depressed mood is probably one of the commonest causes of resistance to hypnotic treatment and the removal of this problem will more likely facilitate its success. Psychodynamic exploration under hypnosis may sometimes contribute to symptom relief. The technique is based upon the Freudian premise that our neuroses are buried in the unconscious and that a phobia is but a facade behind which lie other deep-rooted fears and conflicts. It would seem to follow therefore that uncovering these will resolve the immediate symptoms. Unfortunately this is not always as simple as it sounds, nor is it as successful. Freud himself was soon to discover this even after working on a single case with Dr Breuer[1].

Although origins must be explored, desensitization is the method of choice with most phobic patients.

Let us take as an example the treatment of a patient suffering from a case of the modern epidemic, a flying phobia. The origin has been determined. Perhaps a prolonged delay at the airport when the patient was already tired and depressed. Perhaps some incident on the plane itself, engine trouble or a forced landing. The patient knows this and it does not help to remind him of it. Perhaps even something in the personality of the patient himself. Maybe he feels insecure being transplanted several thousand feet above the earth by this vast machine and in this most unnatural habitat and develops symptoms of panic. There is overall, the fear of death. The objective in treatment is to show the patient that he can think about the journey, make preparations for the journey, travel to the airport, board the aeroplane, experience take-off, the ascent, bumps and air pockets and the subsequent descent and throughout remain calm and relaxed. Each stage of the journey is considered as one step along the hierarchy and the patient, in hypnosis, is asked to visualize them, one at each session whilst remaining totally calm and relaxed. There are four essentials attached to the desensitization of the flying phobia in hypnosis and these are as follows:

1. Systematic desensitization to the objectives mentioned above.

2. Self-hypnosis must be used twice daily to bring down the level of anxiety and to repeat the therapeutic session.

3. There must be a target. The patient must have air flight prearranged for the end of the treatment for practical desensitization.

4. The therapist is strongly advised to acquire or to make a tape recording of air travel sounds, e.g. in the departure lounge, various flight announcements; in the plane, engine and passenger sounds, stewardess and pilot announcements, etc, for use in desensitization. Also preferably a tape for self-hypnosis on the journey itself to eliminate other sounds and distractions (earphones must be used).

Similar treatment may be adapted for a wide range of phibias.

Finally, no patient will ever be desensitized if he or she is entering into the contract against his or her will or if there is an absence of any real positive motivation.

The therapist should never forget in the treatment of a flying phobia to *get the patient back home* otherwise the outcome is likely to be somewhat embarrassing.

One should never be surprised at the type of phobia presented. Blakiston's Medical Dictionary[17] lists some 250 but there must be at least an equal number that are unrecorded.

The Hypnotic Treatment of Lack of Confidence and Stage Fright
This is usually characterized by an outbreak of acute anxiety
whenever the individual has to perform, make a speech or deliver
a lecture in front of an audience and so may be included under
the heading of phobic illness. Under such circumstances he always undervalues and depreciates himself, expects disapproval
and fears adverse criticism. He may be neurotic with strong obsessional traits who sets himself far too high a standard. In everyday life he is likely to feel uncomfortable and ill at ease in the
presence of people in authority, or those he believes to be superior to himself. It is a problem which is common in solo musicians
for example, who are frequently supplied with benzodiazepenes
or beta-blockers to help them overcome the symptoms. Unfortunately this will often result in drug dependency and will do nothing to eliminate the condition.

It is a 'focus of attention' anxiety, similar to the problem of blushing and may be dealt with in the same way.

However, when lack of confidence arises as the result of deep-
seated personality defects, nothing less than the analytical approach is likely to be successful, but if the patient has a reasonably
well-integrated personality a more direct and persuasive hypnotic approach will often produce remarkable results. The restoration of self-confidence is one of the easiest and most rapid
results that can be achieved by hypnotherapy. The full ego-
strengthening routine, suitably reinforced by specific suggestions
appropriate to each individual case, has proved invaluable in the
treatment of this condition. Begin with this, then proceed in the
following manner:

> As you become...*more relaxed* and *less tense,* each day...*so*...you will
> remain *more relaxed*...and *less tense*...when you are in the presence
> of other people...no matter whether they be few or many...no
> matter whether they be friends or strangers.
> You will be able to meet them on equal terms...and you will feel
> much more at ease in their presence...*without* the slightest
> feeling of inferiority...*without* becoming self-conscious...*without*
> becoming embarrassed or confused...*without* feeling that you are
> making yourself conspicuous in any way.

You will become...so deeply interested...so deeply absorbed in
what you are saying...that you will concentrate entirely upon this
to the complete exclusion of everything else.
Because of this...*you will remain perfectly relaxed...perfectly*
calm and self-confident...and you will become much less
conscious of yourself and your own feelings.
You will consequently be able to talk quite freely and
naturally...without being worried in the slightest by the presence
of your audience.
If you should begin to think about yourself...you will immediately
shift your attention back to your conversation...and will no longer
experience the slightest nervousness...discomfort...or uneasiness.

When the patient is likely to be called upon to appear upon the
stage, to make a speech or to deliver a lecture, the above may well
be modified in the following manner.

The moment you get up to speak...all your nervousness will
*disappear completely...*and you will feel...*completely*
*relaxed...completely at your ease...*and *completely confident.*
You will become so deeply interested in what you have to
say...that the presence of an audience will no longer bother you in
*the slightest...*and you will *no longer feel uncertain...confused...or*
conspicuous in any way.
Your mind will become so fully occupied with what you have to
say...that you will no longer worry at all as to how to say it.
You will no longer feel nervous...self-conscious...or
embarrassed...and you will remain throughout...perfectly
calm...perfectly confident...and self-assured.

Whenever a speech or talk has to be given, or a stage appearance made, the patient must be impressed with the importance
of making thorough preparation. The feeling that he has mastered his subject or become word perfect in his lines will help him
enormously. It is always essential to rehearse it thoroughly before the actual performance. He should be instructed to speak
slowly, clearly and deliberately, and to concentrate entirely upon
what he is saying.

At every session, following the ego-strengthening phase, the
subject is desensitized, as in other phobic problems, to the next
situation along the hierarchy in which he is liable to feel the focus
of attention.

The teaching of self-hypnosis, whenever possible, can prove invaluable in these cases. Not only can the patient be taught to visualize himself addressing an audience without difficulty, but he can also suggest to himself, during hypnosis, that he will gradually be able to do this without nervousness, self-consciousness or apprehension *in real life*. 'Brief hypnosis' (see Chapter 11) is also taught to the subject for emergency use.

Some Problems Arising in the Academic Field

Hypnosis can often be used most effectively to help students to gain more efficiency in their studies. Many fail to realize all their natural capabilities because so many factors tend to interfere with the efficient use of the mind. Lack of attention, distraction, the inability to concentrate sufficiently and even a dislike for the subject to be studied, can all cause the student to fall behind with his work, and become over-anxious and discouraged.

When hypnotic treatment is contemplated, the first step to be taken is to discuss the situation fully with the student himself, to discover the precise nature and, if possible, the cause of the difficulties he is experiencing. He should be closely questioned about his home life, his working conditions, his habits, his interpersonal relationships, his attitude to his teachers and his particular worries and anxieties. As a result of this, disturbing emotional factors (which are seldom deeply seated) may often be brought to light, and appropriate advice may be given both in the waking and in the hypnotic state which will help him in coping with these. Further treatment of such cases by desensitization and ego-strengthening proves an effective combination for symptom relief.

School phobia. In the case of school children, it is always essential to talk to the parents as well. Only too often they are so over-anxious for their children to succeed that they unconsciously press them too hard or, with the best of intentions, repeatedly stress the importance of passing an examination and the disastrous results of failure; the child becomes resentful and develops a feeling of inferiority with excessive anxiety, a complete lack of confidence, and may even become depressed. Truanting is a common result. Stomach ache or various gastro-intestinal upsets or nervous asthma are frequent complaints and often the real cause may be overlooked. The parents must be encouraged to alter their own attitudes and behaviour if a successful result is to be obtained. Where the child has become disheartened in its efforts to keep up with the others, or when its difficulties seem to arise as a result of disturbed relationships with certain teachers, a change of class or even of school may sometimes be necessary as a preliminary step. Each individual case must be carefully considered on its merits.

Although full discussion of the problem with the parents is essential, it is important to treat the child as an equal and as a person. If treatment through the use of hypnosis is to be undertaken, a simple explanation of the method should be given. Most patients will respond rapidly to a classical desensitization technique with practical retraining carried out involving full co-operation of parents and teachers. An ego-strengthening routine should additionally be employed with suggestions given as follows:

> Every day...(at such and such a time)...you will get into the habit of working for at least two hours or so...without fail.
> You will be able to *think more clearly*...you will be able to *concentrate much more easily.*
> You will become...*so deeply interested and absorbed in what you are studying* that you will be able to *give your whole attention to what you are doing*...to the complete exclusion of everything else. Because of this...you will be able to *grasp things and understand them more quickly...more easily...and they will impress themselves so deeply upon your memory that you will not forget them.*
> With every treatment that you have...*your memory will improve enormously...and your work will become easier and easier.*
> *You will not only be able to remember what you have learned...but you will be able to recall it without difficulty...whenever you need to do so.*

Examination phobia.   Many students and school children fail to do themselves justice during examinations. No matter how thoroughly they may be prepared, they become so nervous and apprehensive that their minds seem to go blank and they are unable to remember things that they know quite well. They consequently put up a much poorer performance than might reasonably have been expected from them, and fail examinations which they ought to have passed without difficulty. In such cases hypnosis can be of the greatest possible assistance.

> *The moment you enter the examination room and pick up your paper to read the questions...you will become completely calm and relaxed...and all your nervousness and apprehension will disappear completely.*
> No matter how difficult the questions may seem at first sight...or how little you seem to know...*you will not panic*...because you will find that things are not as bad as they seem.
> You will *read all the questions carefully and deliberately...you will decide upon the one that you can tackle best...and answer that one as fully as you can...without worrying about the others until you have completed it.*
> As you do this...*you will find that you will actually remember far more than you originally thought you would.*
> When you have put down all you know about this first question...*choose the next easiest to answer...and tackle that in exactly the same way.*
> Continue in this way with the rest of the questions until you have written all that you can remember...or until the time is up.

When you have finished...you will find that you have remembered far more that you thought possible when you first read the questions.

The combination of the two techniques, of desensitization and ego-strengthening, will usually be found to be successful. However, in all cases one must be certain that there is no other underlying neurosis or personality problem.

Other neuroses occurring in young children are further discussed in the chapter in paediatric hypnotherapy.

4. Obsessive–Compulsive Disorders

Minor obsessions which are not particularly incapacitating or even inconvenient may frequently occur. Obsessions may become pathological when they are persistent and intrusive. They include recurrent thoughts, ideas, doubts, fears, images and various miscellaneous obsessions and impulses which involuntarily invade consciousness and are experienced by the subject as useless, unreasonable and sometimes even repugnant. The sufferer will invariably make unsuccessful attempts to ignore or suppress them. Compulsions are repetitive behaviours which the subject performs in accordance with rules which he has developed and which he feels compelled to carry out, perhaps in order to prevent some future catastrophe or undesired event. The fact that the activity is needless or stupid is recognized by the subject but cannot be resisted. Attempts at resistance will in fact increase anxiety, whilst carrying out the compulsive behaviour will reduce the anxiety, but at the same time will reinforce the compulsion.

These behaviours are seen in children at play and in the superstitions of adults as well as in the ritualistic religious behaviours of certain societies. They may also occur in manic depressive illness and in chronic schizophrenia where the patient may feel himself under some external influence. It is essential that any additional psychopathology be excluded and that the degree of anxiety and/or depression which accompanies the condition be thoroughly assessed. Obsessive compulsive disorders, fortunately relatively rare, are amongst the most difficult of all psychiatric conditions to treat.

Drug therapy has been used extensively as also have various forms of behavioural treatment (Marks et al.[19]) and both have been found to produce some significant improvement. Hypnotherapy offers itself as an additional form of treatment although by no means can it be claimed to be superior.

Hypnosis may be used: (1) to induce feelings of calmness and composure and by regular application, including the use of self-hypnosis if the patient will co-operate, to reduce the level of anxiety and with it the obsessive–compulsive component; (2) as an exploratory modality; (3) as a technique for desensitization.

Genetic or early environmental experiences have been shown to have a bearing on the problem and the latter may be revealed during hypnoanalysis. Attention to compliance with the rigid and obsessive behaviour of parents will also reinforce what may already be a rigid and inflexible personality. As time passes some particular psychological stress may then actually percipitate the neurosis. A common problem is a morbid fear of dirt or germs resulting in excessive hand-washing activities. These may be conducted to some form of ritual and occupy endless hours of each day. Extensive discussion under hypnosis of the precipitating problems are essential and may offer the patient a 'way out' of the compulsion if for example, someone else was to blame for it all. Desensitization may be utilized by setting time limits. For example reducing washing time by five minutes each day. First of all this is imagined. Then it is visualized as happening whilst in hypnosis. Finally the ritual is actually carried out '*in vivo*', but within the specified time limit—whilst remaining totally calm and relaxed. This form of treatment may be applied to a wide variety of obsessive–compulsive symptoms but must really be extended over a very considerable time.

5. Hysterical–Conversion Symptoms

Hysteria is not an illness as was long considered but a symptom of that ubiquitous problem, anxiety. Such symptoms frequently mimic some organic condition and Mesmer's Marie-Thérèse Paradis and her 'hysterical' blindness is immediately brought to mind. The use of hypnosis for the treatment of hysterical conditions reached its height of popularity in the late eighteenth and late nineteenth centuries when the 'disease' and the diagnosis was extremely common. Charcot's demonstrations of hysteria treated by hypnosis were a well-known feature of the Salpêtrière and many of Freud's early cases exhibited symptoms which were diagnosed as hysteria. It was because of the prevalence of this condition that Freud was able to make a special study of his cases. It was he who discovered that if the emotional response of a particular situation was too great for the patient to tolerate, that response could be 'converted' to a physical symptom. Hence the more appropriate term 'conversion neurosis' should be applied.

Overall, the condition lends itself ideally to hypnotherapy. The therapist must resist all temptation to treat by suggestion of symptom removal since in this problem more than in any other, the *cause* of the symptom must be treated. In this condition more than any other, dynamic exploration is essential.

A typical example was that of a young girl of 14 who was referred to one of us (D.W.) with a history of aphonia of two years duration. Extensive E.N.T. and neurological examinations and investigations revealed no abnormality and a diagnosis of 'hysteria' was eventually made. She had exhibited various nervous traits in childhood, had been a poor sleeper and nail biter but there was nothing else of relevance. Her mother had died when she was aged 11. Her father remarried one year later and she had two elder brothers aged 15 and 17. Under the relaxed state of hypnosis she ventilated her feelings of rejection in the family heirarchy. She felt that her stepmother hated her and her father's attitude towards her had changed. The brothers appeared to withdraw within their own peer group, adopted an aggressive attitude towards her and when she attempted to intrude into this group, they largely ignored her or told her to 'belt up'. In the end she did 'belt up'. Her anxiety now was so great that she could tolerate the situation no longer. To paraphrase a well-known remark, the girl's silence spoke volumes. She was able to speak quite freely under hypnosis and the cathartic effect of these discussions and some sessions of desensitization to resist the family attitudes was sufficient to restore her voice and her speech within five sessions. In addition, a number of sessions were held with all the other members of the family, counselling, them in their future attitudes to this highly anxious young lady. Follow up over two years revealed no recurrence of the symptoms.

The use of Hypnosis in Sleep Difficulties

Since hypnosis is commonly considered by the general public to be some form of sleep, it might appear that it would not be a big step to bridge the gap between hypnotic 'sleep' and normal healthy night time sleep. This is far from the case however and simply to suggest to the insomniac that the use of self-hypnosis at night would overcome his sleeplessness would be quite misleading.

The problem must not be taken out of context to the make up and life situation of the individual sufferer. It must be regarded as a symptom of a condition rather than as an illness in itself. It is essential to take a complete and searching history in every case and the reason for the sleep difficulty must be fully explored.

A possible physical cause should be eliminated. The patient may be taking some artificial stimulant such as coffee or tea before bed. There are additionally certain drugs which have an alerting effect and these must be considered. These include many substances from the amphetamine type of cerebral stimulants to certain antidepressants which could have activating properties. Disturbed sleep may also accompany some neurological disorders and pain or pruritis may be precipitating causes.

Emotional problems must be openly discussed. Life events, financial or business worries, family problems, matrimonial or sexual difficulties may cause anxiety which weigh heavily upon the mind. Illness and death fears are not uncommon. In the still of the night these anxieties appear to magnify and gain proportions often out of context to the reality of the situation and sleep becomes impossible.

The nature of sleep difficulty may help to establish the cause and any possible psychogenic origin of the problem. Patients commonly claim that they 'don't sleep a wink all night' but when specific questions are asked, sleep difficulties can usually be divided into three phases. There are:

1. Initial sleep difficulties.
2. Intermediate sleep difficulties.
3. Early morning waking.

Initial and intermediate sleep difficulties are commonly associated with anxiety, the subject being too preoccupied with his worries to allow himself to drift off to sleep, or he might awaken during the night with the worry on his mind. He will often get out of bed, pace the room, try to read or make himself a hot drink to little avail, eventually returning exhausted to his bed. Early morning waking was long regarded as a typical symptom of a depressive illness but this is certainly not always the case. Other features should be present such as loss of appetite, loss of weight, loss of interest, depressed mood and so on and a firm diagnosis must be established to determine whether the patient is anxious, depressed or both. There can be considerable overlap in the type of sleep difficulties experienced. Anxious patients may also awaken early and depressed patients may have difficulty in getting off to sleep. Additionally, manic depression and various psychotic states may all contribute to the problem and it is essential to exclude these conditions before deciding to use hypnosis. The appropriate antidepressant or antipsychotic medication should be prescribed as required and when effective, then other measures to procure sleep, such as hypnotherapy may be considered if the sleep difficulty has not disappeared.

If the patient is taking tranquillizer drugs it may be necessary to substitute a sedating antidepressant for night-time use if any symptoms of depression are also present. This drug should be slowly introduced as the tranquillizer is slowly withdrawn. When such medication is used, it is advisable to prescribe the smallest dose necessary to produce a therapeutic effect as this will render the eventual withdrawal of the drug simpler to achieve and reduce the possibility of side effects.

Most of us are aware that sleeplessness is notoriously self-reinforcing. One or two bad nights will lead to the fear that another will follow and often that fear will become a fact. In behavioural terms the fear has resulted in a learned response. Patients will often claim that they fall asleep in the armchair after dinner in the evening but 'as soon as my head touches the pillow doctor, I'm wide awake'. In fact the bed, the pillow, the darkened room and even saying 'good night' have all become that combined stimulus which results in the alerting response and sleeplessness is the result. Once the patient begins to resort to tranquillizer drugs and sleeping pills the problems really begin.

If anxiety has been diagnosed as the cause of the sleeplessness then hypnotherapy may be commenced without delay. Where there is depression, hypnosis may be used if required but only when the antidepressant medication has begun to have the desired effect.

Where hypnotherapy is decided upon, the procedure should be as follows:

1. The induction and deepening of the hypnotic state using a gently and permissive technique. The consulting room couch should be used and not a chair. The patient should lie in the position in which he would feel most comfortable when in bed. All feelings of physical arousal should be reduced and any anxiety produced by the fear of sleeplessness must be eliminated.

2. Exploration and explanation of the origin of the problem, giving the patient as much insight as possible.

3. Desensitization to specific anxiety situations revealed in routine history taking. Relearning the new response to sleep, to the environment of the bedroom and the stimulus of the pillow etc.

4. Instruction in self-hypnosis with positive suggestions of deep, relaxed sleep from which he will awaken in the morning, refreshed and invigorated.

Instruction in Self-hypnosis
Early in treatment the patient should be taught self-hypnosis for regular morning use, for the purpose of reducing his general level of anxiety and for visualizing his intended daytime activities, seeing himself, when self-hypnotized, doing the things that he intends to be doing, being with whosoever he thinks he will be and remaining calm and composed throughout.

Special instruction is given for the night-time use of hypnosis and this is as follows:

The patient is lying on the consulting room couch and is put into hypnosis using an essentially permissive technique. He is then told to imagine himself at home or wherever he may be staying. He has gone to bed, said good night, put out the lights and turned on to his side or the position in which he feels most comfortable. He is then asked to 'see' himself looking into the darkness and then proceed...

> You are looking ahead of you but see yourself as if you are here
> in my room, looking at what you would be looking at here. I will
> continue talking to you but you now talk with me, saying the
> words that I say, but silently and to yourself as I say them
> aloud, so that my words are coming from your mind.

Then continue with the permissive technique which the patient has been taught but using the first person so that the patient is instructing himself. He has now put himself into hypnosis and in his imagination is lying on his bed, head on the pillow, eyes closed and very relaxed. Emphasize this. Now say quietly...

Continue talking silently in your mind, with me, as I talk aloud
counting...
One, relaxing deeper, two deeper, three deeper, four deeper, five
deeper...
Six deeper...
Seven deeper...
Eight deeper...
Nine deeper...
Ten deeply, deeply relaxed and calmer and calmer...(now
emphasize)
Ten times deeper and calmer and calmer...
Twenty times deeper and calmer and more composed...
Thirty times deeper and deeper and more and more composed...
Forty times deeper and calmer and more and more composed...
Fifty times...deeper...and drowsier...and drowsier...
Sixty times...drowsier and dreamier...and dreamier...
Seventy times...dreamier...and sleepier...and sleepier...
Eighty times...sleepier...and ready to switch off...
Ninety times...switch off...and into sleep...
One hundred...GO TO SLEEP...

Wait a few minutes. If you have taken all matters into account
and proceeded as instructed, the patient will be asleep. Allow him
to sleep on for a while then alert him by saying in a loud and cheer-
ful voice...

It's morning time, time to get up...eyes open, awake, alert and
ready to get on with the day.

This technique is repeated at every session until the patient is
sleeping without difficulty. In the case of those who had been taking tranquillizer drugs, these must never be discontinued suddenly since there may be a withdrawal and rebound effect of
greater anxiety and increased sleep difficulties. These preparations must be *very* gradually reduced in dosage. For example, two
milligrams of diazepam should be reduced to one and three quarters of a milligram for at least a week until the patient is stabilized on this dose. Then by a further quarter to one and a half
milligrams for a week and so on until the dependency is completely eliminated. In this way there will be no rebound effect at all.
The patient must take several weeks before the dosage is com-

pletely discontinued and in the meantime the perfectly safe procedure of self-hypnosis is being substituted in its place. By a natural process, the patient has learned to avoid sleeplessness, by losing his fear of sleep.

Antidepressant medication, if used, must be continued for as long as it is required and for weeks or even months after the depression has lifted. The patient must be kept under surveillance and the dosage monitored throughout. The dosage should eventually be tapered off but only when certain that the patient is no longer depressed and is sleeping well.

REFERENCES

1. Breuer J. and Freud S., 1955. Studies on hysteria. In: *Standard Edition of the Complete Works of Sigmund Freud* (ed. Strachey), Vol. 11. Hogarth, London.
2. Nixon P.G.F., 1976. The human function curve with special reference to cardiac disorders. *Practitioner* **217,** 765–770.
3. Adler A., 1917. Study of organ inferiority and its psychical compensations. *Nervous and Mental Disease Monograph Series,* No. 24, New York.
4. Anderson, J.A.D., Basker M.A. and Dalton R., 1975. Migraine and hypnotherapy. *Int. J. Clin. Exp. Hypnosis* **XXII,** 48–58
5. Graham G.W., 1975. Hypnotic treatment for migraine headaches. *Int. J. Clin. Exp. Hypnosis* **XXIII,** 165–171
6. Friedman M. and Rosenman R.H., 1959. Association of specific overt behaviour pattern with blood and cardiovascular findings. *JAMA,* **169,** 1286–1296.
7. Rosenman R.H., Brand R.J., Jenkins C.D. *et al.,* 1975. Coronary heart disease in the western collaborative group study: final follow-up experience of 8.5 years. *JAMA,* **233,** 872–877.
8. Haynes S.G., Feinleib M. and Kannel W.B., 1980. The relationship of psychosocial factors to coronary heart disease in the Framingham study. *Am. J. Epidemiol.* **III,** 37–58.
9. Maher-Loughnan G.P. and Kinsley B.J., 1968. Hypnosis for asthma—a controlled trial. *Br. Med. J.* **4,** 71–76.
10. Freeman L.J., Conway A. and Nixon P.G.F., 1986. Physiological responses to psychological challenge under hypnosis in patients considered to have the hyperventilation syndrome: implications for diagnosis and therapy. *J.R.S.M.,* **79,** 76–83.

11. Read N.W. (ed.), 1985. *Irritable Bowel Syndrome.* Grune and Stratton, London.
12. Waxman D., 1987. The mythopathology of the irritable bowel. Paper presented at the 4th European Congress of Hypnosis in Psychotherapy and Psychosomatic Medicine, Oxford.
13. Freeman R.M. and Baxby K., 1982. Hypnotherapy for incontinence caused by the unstable detrusor, Br. Med. J., 284, 1831–1834.
14. Lester E.P., Wittkower E.D., Kalz F., *et al.*, 1962. 'Phrenotropic drugs in psychosomatic disorders (skin). *Am. J. Psychiat.,* **119,**136–143.
15. Ambrose G. and Newbold G., 1980. *A Handbook of Medical Hypnosis.* Baillière Tindall, London.
16. Marks I.M., 1969. *Fears and Phobias.* Heinemann, London.
17. *Blakiston's Gould Medical Dictionary,* 1972 (ed. Osol). McGraw Hill, New York.
18. Waxman D., 1977. The management of phobic disorders using clomipramine. *J. Int. Med. Res.* **5**(suppl 1.) 24–31.
19. Marks I.M., Hodgson R. and Rachman S., 1975. Treatment of chronic obsessive compulsive neurosis by *in vivo* exposure. A two year follow-up and issues in treatment. *Br. J. Psychiat.,* **127,**349–364.

CHAPTER 16

Hypnosis in the Treatment of Problems of Personality

Certain difficulties which may result from how one sees one-self as a person and the effect on behaviour as a consequence are included under this somewhat all-embracing heading. As a result of this perception, perhaps some minor, common and persistent response pattern may be established which is unacceptable to the patient and indicates a need for treatment. Other and more serious symptoms may be caused by more severe problems of self-image, which will respond to hypnotherapy. Some of these are discussed below.

1. The Addictions

The suffering and unhappiness which is caused by smoking, alcoholism and drug abuse in general is only too widely known. Equally known is the difficulty in treatment. Recognizing the problems which exist, many doctors will readily accept a compromise solution. Patients are encouraged to change from cigarettes to cigars or a pipe, and to permit 'social' drinking, perhaps a sherry instead of spirits, a little wine with the meal or in more severe problems prescribing chlormethiazole as short term therapy. In the far more severe problem of heroin addiction, methadone may be substituted with the hope of reducing the dependency.

The main features of an addiction are recognized as twofold.

(a) The psychological dependency, i.e. there is an emotional need for the drug which decreases feelings of tension and other unpleasant symptoms.

(b) The physical dependency. There are certain physiological changes which take place as a result of the drug. Withdrawal symptoms are experienced as the effect of the drug wears off.

Before there is any attempt at treatment, a full medical, psychiatric and psychosocial assessment must be made. The latter may appear to be irrelevant in the smoker, this form of addiction being so common it would hardly appear to warrant such inclusive and perhaps intrusive, investigation. Yet this is particularly necessary, since the nature of employment, general daily activities, domestic life, personal and marital relationships and peer group habits have a direct bearing on our emotional responses and coping abilities.

In all cases of addiction, whatever the drug, it is essential for an eclectic approach to treatment *in addition* to hypnotherapy, if the latter is to be considered. Any or all of the following measures may have to be adopted.

1. Removal from the drug culture environment.

2. Mobilization of the appropriate social services (health visitors, social workers, Alcoholics Anonymous etc).

3. Treatment of the physical condition.

4. Treatment of the psychological condition. Is the patient depressed? (a possible cause or accompaniment of alcoholism).

5. Other therapy, e.g. drug replacement.

Hypnotherapy

It is essential to know whether the patient is sincerely motivated to overcome the problem. If attendance is merely to satisfy the spouse or parents or doctor then the likelihood of recovery is remote. The simply question 'why do you want to give up the habit?' should be sufficient to supply the answer. If the therapist is satisfied with the reply, then treatment may be commenced. Initially most addictions will begin as a response to anxiety.

'Everybody is smoking and I don't want to feel different.'
'It's grown-up to have a drink.'
  'All my mates are doing it, it will make me feel better to be like one of them.'

Weekly sessions of hypnosis will usually prove insufficient and twice weekly sessions at the least should be instigated at the outset.

As deep a trance as possible should be attempted and very positive suggestions of well being and calmness are emphasized. Ideally the patient should be encouraged to depend on the effect of hypnosis rather than the drug. Self-hypnosis should be taught and its regular use insisted upon at an early stage. Addicts unfortunately are most unreliable because of the power of the addiction and will easily default and so the support and encouragement of family and friends is important.

It is customary, although the value of this is variable, to emphasize whilst the patient is in hypnosis, the considerable dangers of the addiction. It should be remembered that when in hypnosis the patient is in a particularly suggestible state and repitition of the problems that may result does not go amiss. For example, in the smoker, the furring-up of the arteries, the dangers of a coronary thrombosis, suddenly dropping dead at work etc. No fabrication is necessary—simply an emphasis on the truth. Point out the horrific picture that carcinoma of the lung will really present to the victim and his family and an idyllic picture of what the money could be spent on instead. This latter is always worthwhile.

However the main thrusts of treatment must be desensitization and aversion.

Let us take the problem of smoking as a typical example. Smoking usually commences in adolescence (apart from the schoolboy clandestinely experimenting with a cigarette). He smokes because everybody else is doing it. It makes him feel grown up, an adult. Thus he feels less anxious about himself and will subsequently take a cigarette each time he is in the company of his friends and so gradually the habit generalizes into other situations where he may feel perhaps a little threatened. The habit soon becomes an addiction and the addiction reinforces the habit.

Desensitization.   The patient is put into hypnosis by any of the methods preferred and taught self-hypnosis. Twice daily practice of the latter is essential. Provocative desensitization by the method of brief hypnosis is then made use of.

> Now just see yourself in your office. You're sitting at your desk and longing for a cigarette. Just feel the need right now...feel the desire right now...you must have a cigarette...tell me when you feel the craving...you must have a cigarette...tell me when you can wait no longer...just send the message down to your right index finger...it will give a little twitch when you can wait no longer...

After a few moments the right index finger will respond with the ideomotor signal as suggested.

> Now, when I give you the signal, I want you to take a deep breath in, hold it for a moment, then let the air from your lungs and the tension from your body just as you regularly practice here. As you slowly breathe out, see the word CALM in your thoughts, say the word CALM silently to yourself and all the tension goes and all desire to smoke, disappears with the tension.
> Tell me when all the tension is gone and you no longer desire to smoke.

After a few moments the right index finger will give the desired movement.

This technique is practised over and over again in as wide an area of situations as can be devised. In the home, after a meal, at various social occasions, whilst relaxing in the evenings, etc.

A hierarchy of anticipated events is constructed for the few days between each treatment session and brief hypnosis is practised against this list. This usually produces a good response and the smoking will be reduced accordingly.

In addition, targets should be set for a gradual reduction of total daily smoking. Initially to reduce by ten before the next session, then by five and then by one less each day until the patient has become a non-smoker.

It therefore is useful to set a date by which the patient is expected to become a non-smoker and working towards this target will often be helpful.

Aversion.   This technique is only effective in highly hypnotizable and highly suggestible subjects but is most rewarding.

When in the deep trance state, the patient is told that he is no longer a smoker. That he is revolted at the sight, the smell and the taste of cigarettes. That this feeling is so intense that he knows he will never smoke again. That should he perchance be tempted to light a cigarette he will immediately be aware of the foul smell of the smoke and the disgusting taste in his mouth, that he will feel sick and dizzy and will vomit if he does not take the cigatette from his mouth immediately and put it out.

This is repeated several times, the words being strongly emphasized, then continue as follows.

> Now *you are a non-smoker.* You will *never* smoke again. The sight and the smell and the taste of cigarettes is poisonous to you....
> You are in your office. Somebody near you is smoking. Note the horrid smell of the smoke as it drifts over towards you.
> Nevertheless you are tempted...
> Perhaps one won't hurt...
> Is there an old pack left in your desk?
> Have a look...
> Ah, there's one...open it...there are a couple of cigarettes and the box of matches is still there.
> Now take a cigarette...
> Put it between your lips...
> Feels a bit strange...
> Never mind, light up...
> Now immediately as the smoke enters your mouth, feel a horrid and filthy taste, like bad eggs, rotting fish, all the filth in your dustbin. A stench in your nostrils, in your mouth, in your lungs, you feel sick, you feel dizzy, you want to vomit...you *will* vomit if you don't take that cigarette from your mouth right away...take it out...
> Take a deep breath to clear your lungs. The word is CALM as you breathe out and you will never smoke again.

The contortions of the patient's face are interesting to watch and very often, the patient will appear to be on the verge of vomiting, as your suggestions are reinforced.

This process is repeated at least three times with increasing positive suggestions of vomiting in embarrassing places, e.g. at work, in a restaurant, etc. The patient is then told that he will *never* smoke again. That if perchance he should, perhaps at a weak moment, at a time of stress, or even just out of curiosity, ever take a cigarette again and light it, it will immediately have the same effect as he has just experienced.

The use of hypnosis in the treatment of the addictions is no new idea and the many directions it has taken only confirms the difficulties that exist. Moll in 1890[1] listed six European authorities as having used hypnotherapy for alcoholism. Kraft in 1968[2] treated a young man addicted to 'drinamyl'. He had many social difficulties which he overcame by taking this drug and the hypnotic session was mainly directed at helping the patient communicate with others without feeling anxious. Miller in 1976[3] treated alcoholic patients by suggesting that each time they took a drink they would relive the worst hangover they had ever experienced. He claimed a considerable success rate. The use of group hypnosis for smokers in general practice is a popular idea. It is claimed that the spirit of competition will enhance the effect. Poor results have been reported for this method however, but this may be due to the fact that the same technique does not suit all the participants and different emotional problems may be involved (Watkins[4]; Barkley *et al.*[5]).

An excellent survey of methods and details of a three year follow-up of treatment of smokers by hypnosis is reported by Barabasz *et al.*[6]. They point to the important finding that the occurrence of depression was significantly higher for clients who failed to achieve smoking abstinence.

Additionally however, many patients who have been strongly addicted for many years may become agitated and/or depressed, even on successfully relinquishing an addiction. The possibility of this problem occurring must be closely watched for and the appropriate medical treatment instigated as soon as such adverse effects are noted.

All cases of addiction successfully treated must be followed up for a considerable period. It should be noted that the word 'cured' may not always be applied even when patients have achieved abstinence for a number of years. 'Cured' addicts should perhaps more accurately be described as 'non-smoking nicotine addicts', or non-drinking alcoholics and so on.

The Minor Tranquillizers

A very great number of people unwittingly become dependent upon this type of drug which fortunately has largely replaced the barbiturates. These patients are usually the anxious, facing the challenges of the day, or the sleepless even more fearful of the challenges of the night. Benzodiazepenes have become the drugs of preference, the very wide variety available offering considerable choice to the doctor and his patient.

With the best of intentions 'try these' very soon leads to 'may I have some more please?' The prescription is repeated and the patient becomes dependent. Any attempt to discontinue the use of the drug results in withdrawal symptoms often mistaken for a recurrence of the original anxiety which prompted the request for drug treatment in the first place. The prescription is again repeated and the dependency is reinforced.

Patients will frequently resent the implication of the term 'addiction'. They would prefer to hear the word 'habit', 'habituation' or 'dependency'. Oswald and Lewis[7] made the point that addiction should be the correct word, there being no distinction between one or the other. This being the case, patients should be made aware of the real seriousness of the problem, that this type of drug use does result in an addiction and early discontinuance is essential. Tolerance would otherwise develop with the consequent escalation in dosage as the original symptoms increase.

In such cases the use of hypnosis lends itself admirably for treatment. The history might reveal that the patient was primarily depressed or may be depressed as a result of the continued anxiety or lack of sleep. It cannot be emphasized often enough that untreated depression will prevent the resolution of the original complaint and may even increase if tranquillizer drugs or hypnosis is used. If symptoms are evident an antidepressant must be prescribed, the most suitable type being one which additionally has partially sedating properties and which may therefore be given as a night-time dose. Initially a fraction of the minimum recommended dose is prescribed, simultaneous with the removal of just a fraction of the tranquillizer drug. This new dosage is maintained for a few days (or nights) and a further increase of the one and decrease of the other follows. The gradual substitution is continued until after several weeks the minimum therapeutic dose of the antidepressant is being used and the tranquillizer has been discontinued.

Simultaneous with all this, the level of anxiety is reduced by regular sessions of hypnosis and early instruction in self-hypnosis. Exploration may have revealed specific fears and problems and these are dealt with by discussion and desensitization. If an antidepressant has been used, this may be very slowly withdrawn when indicated but the use of self-hypnosis should be continued indefinitely, it being remembered that such patients are usually rather vulnerable individuals.

Other Drug Abuse

The problem of smoking is rapidly losing its attraction as a social attribute but alcohol remains a persistent need in most cultures and in a very wide area of relationships. The use of more potent drugs, however, including the opiates, although on the increase, appears to be confined to individuals and peer groups, no doubt because of the type of person involved, the legal restrictions on their use and the consequent limited availability. These drugs may be divided into various classes. There are the narcotics and sedatives (morphine type and barbiturates), the stimulants (amphetamine and cocaine types), cannabis, hallucinogenic and khat type drugs (khat is a stimulant drug rarely encountered in the U.K.) as well as various other modifications which are appearing from the illicit laboratories.

In treating this problem, extensive history taking is an essential prerequisite. A family history of alcoholism, mental illness, personality difficulties or antisocial behaviour may emerge but fashion, culture and the environment play a larger part and socioeconomic status can no longer identify the possible victim.

The hypnotherapist may be called upon to treat such addictions but it must at once be said that this should rather be left to the experts. Removal from the drug culture environment and institutional treatment is often imperative. Drug replacement therapy may additionally be needed. If hypnotherapy is additionally to be employed, relaxation, self-hypnosis, insight-directed psychotherapy, ego-strengthening and possibly aversion therapy may all be required.

In spite of the multidisciplinary techniques available for the treatment of the addictions, if hypnosis is used, it must be noted that there is very little evidence from the many published papers that it may be the treatment of choice or that it is generally successful.

2. Problems of Body Image

The concept that one has of oneself as a person will greatly influence one's behaviour in the world. When, as a result, this perception is disturbed, many distressing and serious neurotic disorders may occur. Amongst these, eating problems such as anorexia and bulimia are not unusual. Unfortunately, both of these disabilities are extremely resistant to the many psychological and other therapeutic approaches that are offered. It may readily be seen however that they are not unrelated to anxiety and so perhaps hypnosis has a part to play in treatment.

(a) Anorexia Nervosa

This condition commonly occurs in young women below the age of 30 but may also occur in men. The main characteristics are fear of obesity to the extent that they will 'feel fat' even though they may be well below normal weight. In addition there is an obsessional preoccupation with the quantity and type of food eaten. Deliberate vomiting and purging carried out in a secretive manner are fairly typical and when the illness is well established, loss of appetite becomes a serious problem. In the female, amenorrhoea is a diagnostic feature.

Family relationships are frequently blamed for the condition. Discussion with the patient may indicate that the starvation represents a rebellion against a dominating or over-solicitous mother or a weapon with which to manipulate the parents. This must not be assumed to be the fact of every case however but full discussion and co-operation with the entire family is an essential ingredient of any treatment.

In addition to the anxiety, the patient is also frequently depressed and antidepressant medication must not be withheld. The possibility of hospital admission should be seriously considered before it becomes a matter of urgency.

In the hypnotic treatment of the patient, any attempt at reason and logic is useless since the condition is not amenable to suggestion of this type even when in the hypnotic state. Therapy must be intrusive and directed towards a lowering of the level of anxiety and dynamic exploration of the patient's early memories, particularly as regards family relationships. Possible unresolved guilt feelings must be dealt with and increasing feelings of self-esteem and feelings of general well being should be emphasized. Any attempt at post-hypnotic suggestions of increase of appetite and of eating more are useless and should be avoided.

(b) Over-eating and Bulimia Nervosa

It is well known that eating relieves anxiety. From early history and from our earliest childhood the offering of food has been the great consoler—'sit down and have your dinner and you will feel better!' Patients will often complain of compulsive eating and will request hypnosis to stop them from eating. First of all it must be emphasized once more that hypnosis does not stop anyone from doing anything. However, if that person is really well motivated then one can begin to consider treatment in this way. But then one must ask of these so-called 'compulsive' eaters—who is compelling whom? The question cannot be answered, since apart from outright greed, any compulsion to eat is unconscious. Thus it is this area which has to be explored, and it is the anxiety which is at the root of the problem, which has to be discussed and treated. In this way, hypnotherapy can supply the answer and the answer may not be one which is acceptable to the patient. She knows that by over-eating she is making herself fat, she knows that fat ladies have certain difficulties, difficulties with clothes, difficulties with sunbathing, difficulties in being attractive to the opposite sex. Why then is she making herself unattractive and unwanted? Is there a sexual origin to the problem? Sadly, few women will face up to the realities of 'compulsive eating'. As a result, 'even hypnosis' will not supply instant cure.

The problem of bulimia is far more severe however. This includes over-eating but in addition, repeated episodes of 'bingeing' are often followed by deliberate vomiting and purging. The condition was well described by Russell[8] and presents a difficult and a dangerous problem. The patient will often sit down and consume half a loaf of bread or eat slice after slice of cake protesting that she wasn't even hungry. Or perhaps, go down to the kitchen during the night and raid the larder. Considerable feelings of guilt will follow and once again, depression will appear almost inevitably as an additional symptom. The episodes of bingeing may settle down giving way to periods of anorexia together with the continued pre-occupation with weight.

One lady of 29 (treated by D.W.), attributed her symptoms to guilt feelings following the death of a friend as a result of a street accident. Nevertheless, she had tended to over-eat throughout her adult life, although the bouts of bingeing were of more recent origin. 'Often' she said 'it was as if a swarm of locusts had been through my kitchen.' Following such an episode she would put a finger into her throat in order to make herself vomit and would take a powerful laxative. She appeared to be happily married, her husband who was interviewed was concerned and understanding and there were two children aged five and seven upon whom she doted.

Further exploration revealed a very unhappy childhood. She was the youngest of three sisters. Her father was an ex-regular army sergeant, strict and unapproachable and her mother was totally under his influence. 'The entire family had to march to his orders.' She recalled frequent punishment by beating. Her parents had separated when she was six years of age but her memory for the following three years was a complete blank. She was unable to recall where or with whom she lived.

Treatment was by relaxation by hypnosis, instruction in self-hypnosis and regression to her earlier childhood. Information obtained from this latter technqiue was sparse until one day she was asked to allow her memories to 'float freely' through her early days. Suddenly she appeared startled, became agitated and wept proclaiming 'there's that horrible smell again'. She continued weeping but was gradually calmed and gently awakened. After she had settled she was questioned about this incident. 'I now remember it all' she said, 'the smell was the horrible smell of carbolic which I can't abide to this day. I was in this children's home after my parents split up. The aunts wouldn't have me because I was my mother's illegitimate daughter but my "father" adopted me. In the home, the food was sparse and what there was, was inedible. Many of us were often sick. They used to swab down the tables and the floors with this horrible carbolic stuff and I was there again and smelled it all over again before you woke me up.'

Her parents had been reunited when she was about eight but the unhappy experience of the children's home had produced its effect. She became withdrawn and had several episodes of enuresis. Discipline was even more severe and at the age of 15 she was 'thrown out' to live with a distant relative. Although always being aware that she was overweight her eating problems now really escalated. The death of her friend was merely the event which precipitated the more severe bulimic attacks.

It was after this revelation that her condition settled. Continued exploration revealed no further problem of her childhood and early adult life. Although she was allowed to ventilate her earlier memories and associated emotions on several occasions the abreaction which she had previously experienced was not repeated. Her eating habits and her weight stabilized and she continued to attend at monthly and then three monthly intervals for surveillance and reinforcement of her self-hypnosis.

This patient's history emphasizes the difficulties in treating this very vexing problem. Unfortunately not all cases have such a happy ending.

(c) Dysmorphophobia

This is a condition which may be ascribed to 'Problems of Body Image'. Hay[9] described the disorder in which there is an excessive concern with some imagined defective appearance, usually referred to one particular bodily feature. Again, the sufferer does not see himself as a real and positive person in the world. 'I know why nobody likes me—it's because my nose is too long.' Extensive investigation and expensive and damaging cosmetic surgery has often already been experienced, but to little avail. The problem in fact may be due to more than just anxiety. It may be part of a more serious personality disorder or a symptom of schizophrenia or of some neurological condition. Again, the patient may be depressed. Hypnosis can usually only be used as an adjunct to more intensive treatment.

Several such cases have been referred to the writer (D.W.) including anxiety directed to the size and shape of the ears, the forehead, nose and to the left thigh. Hypnotherapy was of little help initially and antidepressant medication and neuroleptic drugs were subsequently employed. Hypnosis was then used as an adjunct to lowering the general level of anxiety and increasing feelings of self-esteem.

3. Social Disabilities

Once again, many of these problems are related to anxiety. A situation which causes one person to 'stammer with fright' may cause another to 'flush with fright' or the two may occur simultaneously in the same individual. These and many other responses such as tics and various habits may become quite unacceptable. Anxiety increases and confidence decreases so that the person will tend to withdraw from society or avoid any situation in which he might be the focus of attention. Depressed mood will often result and treatment becomes more difficult.

(a) Stammering

When problems of speech are purely functional in character, the normal speech rhythm becomes both inhibited and interrupted. This is particularly likely to occur in certain social situations which tend to produce shyness, embarrassment and uneasiness. The patient dreads having to speak in the presence of other people, and seems to look upon speech as an act through which he is bound to reveal himself and his own shortcomings. Most stammerers are of the dependent type, lacking in self-assurance to an extent that makes it extremely difficult to assert themselves in the company of others. Curiously enough, they are usually able to sing without difficulty and this fact can be made use of in treatment.

Stammering is sometimes precipitated by a shock or traumatic experience. In children, especially, it may be connected with emotional conflicts centred upon the parents, brothers, sisters or school, which, if treatment is to succeed, will often have to be revealed and explored. Le Cron and Bordeaux[10] stated that 80 per cent of cases appear before the age of 6 years, and that the incidence in boys is approximately nine or ten times greater than in girls. They consider stammering to be a neurosis, possibly of the compulsive type, and emphasize the difficulty of cure after the age of 30. It is generally acknowledged that a stammer *must* be treated as early as possible, since once a deep-seated habit pattern and conditioning has been established it is exceedingly hard to break and cure not only becomes difficult, but the treatment becomes tedious and is often ineffective. Indeed the shorter the duration of the stammer the greater will be the prospect of success. The prognosis also tends to be more favourable when the stammer is associated with subjective feelings of anxiety, for individuals who stammer badly, without becoming unduly anxious or embarrassed, rarely seem to improve to any marked extent. The prospect is also much worse in the case of children who have never learned to speak properly. Those who once spoke normally and subsequently developed a stammer, usually show greater improvement under treatment.

Stammering varies greatly in its intensity and may be mild or exceedingly severe, accompanied by spasms of various muscles, twitching or facial contortions. Nervousness, shyness, embarrassment and fear lead to tension, which usually affects the muscles of the larynx, throat, face, tongue and lips. Even the diaphragm and respiratory muscles may become involved. The harder the patient tries to overcome the speech defect, the more muscular incoordination seems to occur, with the result that the spasm becomes greatly intensified.

It is not always realized what agonies of mind the stammerer experiences, especially when the difficulty threatens to prejudice his career or prospects of advancement. His feeling of inferiority becomes greater, talking becomes more and more associated with anxiety, his speech mechanism becomes temporarily paralysed, and his uncertainty is manifested in increased stammering. He dreads having to speak to other people. He becomes more and more self-conscious and embarrassed, increasingly afraid of failure, of being criticized and of appearing conspicuous. He is unable to think clearly, whilst he is talking to others, since he is constantly on the look-out for words which he thinks he will be unable to pronounce. He tends to develop excuses designed to extricate himself from difficult situations, and to withdraw from people more and more as a result of his difficulty and this leads to a progressive loss of self-esteem. His speech defect will be less marked when he is amongst friends or acquaintances who are aware of it, and much more pronounced when he is with strangers. He is likely to be much worse when he is in the presence of people in authority, and upon occasions which are of some importance to him. He may experience difficulty and hesitation in starting to speak, or his speech may become interrupted by his inability to pronounce certain words or consonants. He will often substitute other words for those which he originally intended if experience has taught him that he will stammer with their use. The harder he tries, the worse his stammer becomes. In many cases, stammerers tend to think faster than they can speak, and their attempts to catch up only lead to increased difficulty.

Treatment, particulary under hypnosis, is likely to be of great value in children and young adults. In older people results are inconsistent. In cases which fail to show any material improvement, hypnosis may be more effective when combined with speech therapy by a recognized speech therapist.

Schneck[11] pointed out that the treatment should be aimed at the underlying neurosis. From the general practitioner's point of view, this is the line that should be followed. Some patients can talk quite easily in the hypnotic state, without the slightest suspicion of a stammer, whereas others continue to stammer however deeply hypnotized they may be.

Ambrose[12] found that children who stammer are usually tense, anxious and dependent, and that they are often both highly strung and difficult before the onset of the complaint although it must be remembered that this is invariably an assessment made by the parents and may not be the complete picture. He emphasized the importance of investigating, and if necessary correcting, the parents' attitude towards the difficulty. Sometimes, simple questioning under hypnosis will reveal some emotional incident in early life which precipitated the onset of the stammer. In more obstinate cases, age-regression under hypnosis may be required provided that the necessary depth can be achieved.

In planning systematic therapy, certain fundamental principles should be borne in mind, and some important explanations given, both in the waking and in the hypnotic state:

1. Where it is suspected, emotional trauma should be investigated and any relevant conflicts explained and resolved.

2. Environmental disturbances must be dealt with and, in the case of children, parental attitudes and those of school teachers etc., explored and adjusted.

3. General suggestions of calmness, physical and mental relaxation, increased confidence and reassurance should be given.

4. Feelings of equality should be encouraged, and any sense of inferiority removed.

5. The patient should be told that he will become so deeply interested in what he has to say, that he will develop complete confidence in his ability to say it.

6. It should be explained to him that he pays far too little attention to what he has to say, and far too much to how he says it.

7. He must face the fact that he has this difficulty, and be prepared to admit it, not only to himself, but to others, who will take far less notice of it than he thinks.

8. He must be told that, in everyday life, he will form the habit of speaking more slowly and more deliberately, and this will help considerably with his speech.

As deep a hypnotic state as possible is always desirable, and when this can be obtained, certain desensitization techniques can be most advantageously employed. It must be emphasized to the patient, if of an age to understand it, that self-hypnosis is an essential part of the treatment and must be practised regularly in order to reduce the level of anxiety. In self-hypnosis, the patient visualizes what he anticipates will be happening during the rest of the day, with whom he will be, etc., and hears himself in fluent and relaxed conversation with the person or persons.

But the real basis of treatment lies in re-education, whereby the patient learns to display more tolerance towards himself and others, and to adopt a more relaxed attitude to life in general.

Wolberg[13] holds the opinion that some forms of speech training do as much harm as they do good, and often have a bad psychological effect. He considers that through emphasizing will-power and control, they concentrate the attention too much on the mechanics of speech, rather than upon what is said. Because of this, the patient becomes more and more conscious of his difficulty. This is correct. Too much attention to this aspect without the simultaneous and continued reduction in anxiety will do little to improve matters.

A young man of 24 presented (to D.W.), with a history of a stammer since the age of five. There was nothing of relevance in his past, personal or family history and in spite of his disability he had numerous friends. His parents, sister and brother were understanding and rarely commented upon his speech. His early schooling and later education was unremarkable and he worked in an insurance office with reasonable chances of improving his position. However, he felt that his speech was hopeless with people in authority as well as with clients and he was terrified of speaking on the telephone. To achieve any promotion at all he knew he really had to do something positive about his stammer.

His motivation was excellent and he proved a deep hypnotic subject. At the session following the initial induction he was taught self-hypnosis and carried out the exercises regularly. Whilst in hypnosis it was pointed out to him that he would still be able to chat or make comments—and yet remain in hypnosis and so we casually discussed various topics. His speech was virtually impeccable and his attention was immediately drawn to this fact as well as to the reason for this—namely that any anxieties that he possessed in the waking state were completely reduced during hypnosis. He was told that on waking he would read aloud passages from the newspaper handed to him—and that since he would continue to remain non-anxious, then his speech would continue to remain fluent. He was awakened and proved the point. This exercise was repeated for three sessions.

At the next session he was instructed whilst in hypnosis, in the technique of brief hypnosis by taking a deep breath and saying the word CALM, silently to himself whilst exhaling. The successful effect of this exercise was confirmed by an ideomotor signal.

Whilst remaining in the waking state, he was once more given some reading material, brief hypnosis was again demonstrated and he was told that he could then proceed with reading without the need of the preliminary full hypnotic session. He was instructed to practise this technqiue as frequently as possible and in his own time with reading aloud or chatting to members of the family or friends.

At the fifth session, ego-assertive retraining was commenced. The therapist (D.W.), adopting the role of a wealthy and aggressive client, plied the patient—in hypnosis, with questions, relating to some complicated insurance negotiations. Instructions were given as follows:

> Before you reply, take a deep breath, hold it for a second and then as you breathe out you release all the tension from your body and from your mind, you release the tension which inhibits your speech and your words flow quietly and fluently without any difficulty. Your speech will be slow and clear. Each word will be distinct and have a meaning. Each word will be separated from that which it follows and that which it precedes by the slightest pause. Take a deep breath...hold it...let go...calm...speak now.

These exercises were repeated with the therapist adopting the role of various people with whom the patient usually experienced difficulties and with whom he anticipated meeting and experiencing difficulties in the intervals between sessions. Voice control was emphasized. He was shown that he can add different tones to his voice so that it will sound musical and pleasing.

A total of 46 sessions were given—almost half a year of therapy. Perhaps it seems quite a lot. But with a well-reinforced background of nearly 20 years of a crippling speech disorder it was worth all the effort. His speech had made a very considerable improvement, he was no longer afraid to speak on the telephone and subjectively he no longer felt that he had a problem. Follow-up and reinforcement has been given over a period of two years.

Summary of treatment.   1. Full history taking and discussion with the patient of his problem and the intended process of treatment.

2. Regular induction of hypnosis with emphasis on feelings of calmness, composure, control and confidence.

3. Instruction in self-hypnosis and regular twice daily use.

4. Casual discussions whilst in hypnosis with the therapist.

5. Practice in reading aloud immediately after the hypnotic session.

6. Instruction in achieving feelings of immediate calmness by brief hypnosis.

7. Ego-assertive retraining.

8. Full and repeated instruction in voice control.

9. Good motivation and dedication to all stages of treatment.

10. Follow-up and reinforcement of self-hypnosis over prolonged period.

Patients should always be advised that any treatment must be persistent and prolonged. Much depends upon the age and the underlying personality of the subject. It also depends particularly upon his regular and assiduous application of self-hypnosis. Curiously enough, however, although some patients may improve only slightly, many of these same patients will maintain also that their speech is very much better. The reason for this is that with many situations previously interpreted as threatening, the patient's subjective feelings have so much improved that although he continues to stammer in the presence of other people, it no longer bothers or distresses him.

(b) Blushing

This is an anxiety response which, when well established can bring untold distress to the sufferer. Although a common occurrence and one which would appear very trivial, in certain highly anxious personalities, it may become a major social disability. It is more common in women and it is interesting that in any particularly anxious situation where one is actually seen by others, that blush will also appear where it may be seen, that is on the face and usually at the area of skin made visible by the wearing of an open-necked shirt or blouse. What is this blush saying to the world? In psychodynamic terms the interpretations could be endless.

Anxiety does not necessarily indicate that the person may be in an overtly frightening situation. Feelings of embarrassment, humiliation or guilt, or of being the focus of attention are anxieties which may also trigger a blush.

Most people blush at some time or other particularly when young. Others blush more frequently and as a result, the problem may become a conditioned and maladaptive situational response. In severe cases it is accompanied by other familiar fear responses, such as dry mouth, stammering, tachycardia and 'butterflies' in the stomach, etc. In other words the patient experiences a phobic attack which becomes paired to other similar situations and in the highly anxious will generalize to encompass a wide area of activities. The patient now has what may be known as a social phobia.

Most patients soon begin to rely heavily on regular and large doses of tranquillizer drugs or alcohol.

One lady of 37 described her feelings as 'being very frightened of people, more especially a lot of people. I think everyone is looking at me and my face goes bright red. I feel sick and trembly and my heart thumps so much I'm sure everyone can hear it.' As a consequence she developed a well-defined social phobia or 'people' phobia. She could entertain in a very modest way in her own home where she felt secure but would only visit friends whom she knew well with her husband and would only eat in restaurants with which she was familiar and which were especially dimly lighted. She was also very much worse in the presence of the opposite sex. She worked alone in a small office and daily dreaded the intrusion of anyone but familiar staff. In addition she regularly consumed considerable quantities of benzodiazepenes.

Extensive exploration revealed only a highly anxious personality. There was no unresolved guilt nor any overt sexual fears nor was any precipitating cause revealed and there was no biological evidence of depression. The problem was attributed only to her own particular response to anxiety and was treated accordingly as follows:

1. Relaxation in hypnosis at weekly sessions.
2. Instruction in self-hypnosis for use twice daily.
3. Desensitization to a hierarchy of anxiety-producing situations from walking down the street and meeting a neighbour to

that situation which could cause the greatest anxiety, i.e. the annual office party.

4. Practical retraining at every step along the hierarchy.

5. Gradual weaning from the benzodiazepenes and substituting the 'deep breath and calm' method of brief hypnosis.

6. Some ego-assertive retraining.

After nine sessions the patient was able to enter into the entire hierarchy of one-to-one and social situations which had earlier paralysed her activities. Her self-image had greatly improved and she no longer depended upon benzodiazepenes, although, she added, she was addicted to self-hypnosis!

(c) The Habit Spasm or Tic

This is a disorder which is characterized by involuntary, rapid, spasmodic, purposeless and often repetitive muscle contractions. The movements frequently occur in the face and shoulders and are invariably aggravated by stress. The pattern of these individual tics varies. Commonly seen are blepharospasm, twitching, sniffing movements, clearing of the throat and shoulder shrugging. Spasmodic torticollis may occur and when well established the muscles may become painful and the spasm in a fixed position.

The tic may be the result of some suppressed emotion or may commence as an automatic or voluntary reaction to a local stimulus or external situation and may subsequently develop into a habit. It affords relief to the sufferer but if resisted may increase the emotional stress. The patient is fully aware of the movement and this could aggravate his feelings of inadequacy. An interesting observation was made by Mawdsley[14], namely, that everyone has a ritualized movement which comforts him during stress.

The twitching movements must be distinguished from the side effects of certain drugs such as amphetamines or phenothiazines or from organic disease. It is considered that some malfunction of the basal ganglia may result in various dystonic spasms and postures and this possibility must be investigated. Nevertheless whether purely psychological or neurological there is no doubt that situations which increase anxiety will certainly exaggerate the spasm and in either case the problem is reinforced and becomes steadily worse. Although haloperidol is sometimes prescribed there is really no satisfactory drug treatment and tranquillizers are generally useless.

Tics may occur in either sex. They are seen commonly in children frequently between the ages of seven and twelve years. Such children are usually normal in all other respects and intelligence is unimpaired. They commonly have other nervous traits however and the problem itself may be imitative. Some conditions such as conjunctivitis may initiate blinking which may persist as a tic long after the local condition has subsided. If persistent in children, they should not be dismissed as unimportant and a psychiatric assessment should always be carried out. In the absence of any other abnormality, many children recover completely with the passage of time and often the condition is better ignored. If psychological in origin the symptom will always disappear under hypnosis and if the anxiety level can be reduced with persistent treatment the prognosis is good.

The longer the period of time that the tic has been present, the worse the outlook. However, results again depend on the motivation of the patient, the regularity with which he will attend for treatment and the effectiveness of his use of self-hypnosis. It has also been said that the older the patient the less likely is he to respond but this is not necessarily the case.

A professional man of 75 was referred to the second author for treatment of a facial tic involving prolonged and repeated blinking of the right eyelid accompanied by a somewhat grotesque distortion of the nose and cheeks. It had been present for three years. He had noted that the condition was always worse when he was upset, if trying to read or to concentrate and in the presence of certain visitors. Neurological investigation had revealed no abnormality. He was otherwise an active but rather anxious man. He also revealed an extra-marital relationship which was discovered by his wife two years before the tic developed, subsequent to which the marriage had been under considerable strain. With the passage of time his sexual potency diminished and this compounded his guilt feelings.

In view of his age no attempt was made to investigate further by hypnoanalysis. Treatment was by straightforward discussion of his problem followed by relaxation in hypnosis and desensitization to an extended list of anxiety-producing situations. This was reinforced by a self-hypnosis tape. The patient responded well and was relieved of his symptom after seven sessions. He attended follow-up and six months later, after a trip to the USA, described his improvement as 'terrific'.

Another and possibly related problem, although fortunately rare, is that known as the Gilles de la Tourette syndrome. This involves multiple twitches, convulsive noises, coughing, barking sounds and in some cases echolalia and coprolalia. There is no known cause but the differential diagnosis may include obsessive–compulsive neurosis or hysteria. An early history may be obtained of transient tics in childhood. No organic pathology has been demonstrated and the condition is often labelled psychogenic. Indeed the syndrome has been considered to be the severest form of tic known. Drug treatment includes the use of tranquillizers and particularly of haloperidol but the side effects may be severe. Numerous psychological techniques have been attempted but the response is equivocal.

A young man of 18 was referred for treatment of the Tourette syndrome. The parents felt that the condition had commenced at about the age of five with a twitching of the head which fluctuated in intensity over the years. He then developed a blink, followed by a twitching of the shoulders. At almost twelve years he started to make sudden noises in the classroom to the dismay of the teacher and so not surprisingly this was encouraged by the other pupils. The condition became well established, his attendance at school eventually became impossible and his employment prospects extremely poor. When seen however he was holding down a job as a clerk, working alone in an office where he was generally left to his own devices.

Yates[15] applied learning theory to the treatment of tics and considered that they could be treated with behaviour therapy. He hypothesized that some tics may be drive-reducing, conditioned, avoidance responses, originally evoked in a highly traumatic situation. In this situation, he maintained that intense fear is aroused and a movement of withdrawal or aggression is made. If the fear-inducing stimulus ceases then the movement is reinforced. The same tic comes to be elicited by a variety of stimuli and as a result develops into a powerful habit. Just as the tic becomes a learned response, so (theoretically at least), it can be unlearned. The ideal method for this unlearning would therefore be as practised, with the use of hypnosis. When the patient is sufficiently becalmed, he can visualize entering into a hierarchy of anxiety-provoking stimuli, whilst remaining calm and no longer responding with the tic.

Thus it was reasonable to hope that behaviour therapy under hypnosis might be effective in the treatment of the Tourette syndrome. In fact with this patient this proved to be the case. The spasms and the vocal tics entirely disappeared under hypnosis. Desensitization to general life events was commenced and treatment was continued for two years. A self-hypnosis tape was made early in treatment and updated as necessary. However, the condition lapsed whenever the patient failed to attend for any reason and finally the intervals between sessions increased until he abandoned treatment completely. This was an unsuccessful outcome, but emphasizes that hypnotherapy does have a place in the treatment of this most distressing and unfortunate condition.

(d) Nail Biting

This is an extremely common and often isolated habit which occurs most frequently during childhood and adolescence and usually remits spontaneously. Whilst in itself it is of no great importance, it often serves as an outlet for tension. In psychoanalytic terms it might be interpreted as a fixation at the oral level or a regression to that stage. In many instances it is an anxiety response, associated with feelings of insecurity and sometimes of repressed hostility directed against an over-dominant parent. It consequently represents a combination not only of oral gratification but also of self-punishment, the aggression being masochistically turned back on the child's own body. The oral satisfaction is identical with that gained by the baby from its comforter, or later on, perhaps the adult from the pipe, cigarette or cigar.

Nail biting is generally much more distressing to the parents than it is to the child itself. Nevertheless if persistent, it should always be regarded as an indication for enquiring into the child's emotional problems. Observant parents can often tell exactly when the habit started and may even be able to suggest the possible cause. The birth of another child—going to school for the first time—an illness—or admission to hospital may all be instrumental in starting the habit. Sometimes it has been known to start after only a few days' separation from the parents, and in such cases it usually responds to discussion of the resulting problems, the reduction of anxiety under hypnosis and strong suggestions that the habit will cease as a consequence. Ego-strengthening additionally is essential. However, when nail biting is associated with continuing emotional conflicts or maladjustments, hypnosis must also be used to resolve the conflicts, to relieve the tension, to re-establish a feeling of security and to re-educate the child.

Occasionally, if the habit can be completely controlled for a continuous period of 48 hours, this will prove quite sufficient to break the conditioning. In every case, however, an attempt should be made to discover the cause and to deal with the root of the trouble, despite the fact that symptomatic treatment will often be successful.

Adults and adolescents generally seek relief solely from the embarrassment of their habit. They cannot understand the persistence of the urge to bite their nails, and have no idea that they may be helped by psychotherapy. Whenever children are concerned, it is essential to interview the parent, usually the mother. She must be told that her own attitude will greatly influence the success or failure of the treatment. She must try to ignore the habit altogether since constant nagging will only result in the prolongation of the trouble. Sympathy and constant reassurance to the effect that it really doesn't matter, because presently the habit will cease, may even induce the child to reveal the nature of its worries.

One of the most important factors in successful treatment is to be found in strengthening the patient's desire and motivation to stop the habit. This is equally necessary in child, adolescent or adult, first in the waking state, and subsequently repeated during hypnosis. Once again, the deeper the trance, the more rapid and effective treatment is likely to be. The procedure seems to be particularly successful when the patient is female:

> As you grow up...you will become more amd more attractive.
> You will not want your appearance to be spoilt by ugly hands.
> Nice hands and shapely nails will make you even more
> attractive...and you will want to make every effort to stop biting
> your nails, and spoiling them.
> With my help...you will be able to stop biting them altogether...and
> then they will soon begin to grow.

Commence treatment with the routine ego-strengthening and then proceed in the following manner:

> As your nerves become stronger and steadier...as you become
> calmer and more relaxed, each day...so, there will be no reason for
> you to go on biting your nails.
> You will no longer *want* to bite them...you will *stop* biting them.
> If at any time you do start to bite them, without realizing what
> you are doing...*the moment your fingers touch your mouth...you
> will know immediately what you are doing...and you will be able
> to stop yourself right away...before you have done any damage at
> all.*
> From now on...you will stop biting your nails...they will begin to
> grow...and you will feel proud of your hands.

Strong, authoritative, direct suggestions under hypnosis will often succeed in stopping the habit altogether. Where a very deep trance or somnambulism can be obtained, the prohibition may be rendered much more effective by telling the patient that he will experience a strong feeling of distaste whenever he puts his fingers in his mouth:

> Whenever you start biting your nails...the moment you put your
> fingers in your mouth...you will get a horrible bitter, nasty taste
> in your mouth. This will become stronger and nastier...and will
> make you feel sick.

Conditioning a feeling of nausea to the habit in this way may help greatly in establishing control. When this particular method is used, however, fairly frequent sessions will be necessary, and even when the nails begin to grow the suggestions may need to be reinforced about once a fortnight, for a time. Increasing motivation is a much superior method and the results are likely to be more effective.

An alternative method is to *permit the biting of one or two nails, whilst allowing the others to grow.* Once this succeeds, it is surprising how often and rapidly the habit is abandoned altogether.

Whilst the patient has actually stopped biting her nails after one or two sessions, she may substitute a habit of picking them instead. This occurs more in adults and adolescents than in the case of children. It is not difficult to deal with, since the inclusion of specific suggestions prohibiting this as well will usually cause it to stop.

(e) Thumb Sucking

This is a very common childish habit which seems to provide comfort through oral gratification in much the same way as nail biting. It is usually harmless and generally should be ignored. If it persists into adolescence however, it may well result in deformity of the palate and mal-occlusion of the teeth. The parents usually become very worried about the prospect of the child developing unsightly teeth. In most cases it seems to continue simply as a habit which is not as frequently associated with emotional conflicts as in nail biting, but when it is, an antagonistic child–parent relationship may be the cause and greatly reduces the chance of successful treatment.

The parents should always be interviewed and warned not to discuss treatment with the child. They must do their best to disregard the habit completely, and refrain from scolding or nagging. It may be of interest to learn whether the child was breast fed but such information is not particularly helpful in so far as treatment is concerned.

As deep a trance as possible is always desirable, and the approach should be persuasive. Once again, the establishment of adequate motivation is of the greatest importance.

> When you grow up...you want your teeth to look nice and attractive, don't you?
> If you do...you will have to do your best, with my help, to stop sucking your thumbs and fingers.
> I can help you to stop.
> If you go on sucking your thumb, your teeth will become crooked

and ugly as they grow.
This won't happen if you stop sucking your thumb now...and I am
going to help you to stop.

As in nail biting, in deep-trance subjects it is possible to condition a bitter, unpleasant taste to the act of sucking the thumb or
fingers, and this may accelerate the breaking of the habit. In this
case the fingers and thumbs of *both* hands should always be included.

An interesting and original approach was that of Erickson. After
insisting that the parents did not interfere with his treatment of
the child in any way, he proceeded to obtain co-operation by
saying that he would under no circumstances consider stopping
the child from sucking his thumb. He obtained his agreement,
however, that one of the most important lessons he had to learn
when he went to school was that of sharing things with other
children. Erickson then pointed out that, in sucking one thumb
only, he is hardly being fair to his other thumb and eight fingers,
each of which is entitled to a share. He proceeded to get the child
to promise that every time he sucks his thumb, he will not only
suck the other one as well, but also each individual finger. In carrying this out, the child soon tended to give up the habit altogether
since, instead of continuing to give him pleasure, it had become
converted into a intolerable nuisance!

The therapist may be called upon to treat many other unacceptable mannerisms and habits. Some of them are extremely difficult, may involve considerable expertise and application and
before embarking upon any form of therapy, the patient should
be fully aware of the commitment.

(f) Trichotillomania

This is the name given to compulsive plucking of the hair. It occurs more commonly in young girls and may involve not only the
hair of the head but also of the eyebrows and eyelashes. Many
girls attending for treatment show a considerable thinning of the
hair as a result and may already wear a wig. The patient may also
exhibit other artificial dermatoses and it is considered that the
condition is a sign of serious emotional problems.

If hypnotherapy is used, insistence on the use of self-hypnosis is essential in order to reduce the level of anxiety. Counselling as regards her appearance is usually a waste of time since the patient is intellectually only too aware of this aspect of the problem. Any attempt at symptom removal by suggestion is useless and may result in symptom substitution but desensitization will be of help after hypnoanalysis and extensive exploration of any underlying emotional problems.

A wide range of behavioural techniques have been applied. Barabasz[16], in a brief review of methods used, emphasized the fact that treatment failures and relapses were frequently due to compliance problems. She described a method in which patients were treated in a special chamber from which sound had been excluded as far as possible. They were relaxed in a comfortable chair and given post-hypnotic instructions targetting hair-pulling behaviour as follows:

> You will be acutely aware whenever you put your hand to your
> head, then it is entirely up to you, you have the power, the
> control, no-one else, no habit controls you. You can pull your
> hair if you want to or you can choose to control the habit.

Since earlier clinical reports indicated that only highly hypnotizable clients responded successfully, Barabasz proposed that this 'restricted environmental stimulation technique' (REST), which enhanced the hypnosis, might therefore extend treatment to a much wider range of patients.

(g) Acne Excoriae

Pustules, bleeding spots and scratch marks sometimes seen around every acne spot or suspected spot on the faces of young girls was known as 'acne excoriée des jeunes filles'. Perhaps the young ladies of France were more concerned about their features than were those in other parts of Europe. The anxious adolescent only too aware of her complexion sees every spot on her face as disfiguring and herself therefore as unacceptable in the presence of her friends and other acquaintances. She becomes even more anxious and indulges in regular, extensive and time consuming examination of her skin, squeezing and picking at every suspicious spot, often using a needle to extract real or imaginary comedos. Consequently the skin is damaged and becomes inflamed and the underlying tissues even more infected. Treatment consists of extensive discussion of what she thinks of herself as a person, how she sees herself with other people and what she believes other people think about her. Regular twice daily self-hypnosis is essential and repeated ego-strengthening must be given at weekly sessions of hetero-hypnosis to improve the self-image. Emphasis is placed on her good features. For example, shape of nose, pretty eyes, colour of hair and so on. All the patient's attractive characteristics may be emphasized and even exaggerated, but no attempt should ever be made to tell an untruth as this will certainly be counter-productive.

In the absence of other pathology such cases respond well to treatment.

One lady of 29 had suffered from acne since her adolescence. She was referred to the second author on account of continuous picking and squeezing of her spots for as long as they had been present. She was rather a tall person and highly anxious. She had been brought up in an unhappy environment, frequently beaten by a dominating father and bullied by her two older brothers. She was always teased at school, on account of her height and noted that her picking had become worse when worried or bored. For example she had developed a (benign) lump in her breast about one year after a pregnancy and her picking became much worse at that time. The relationship with her husband was poor and she found herself picking excessively every time they had a quarrel. She would sit in front of a mirror squeezing every spot on her face and chest that she could discover. Her skin was a mass of scratch marks and small infected areas. When asked why she did this she said 'to get out the bad'. Bad girl as a child, bad figure as a teenager, bad wife to her husband? We had a long talk about that. Following several sessions of discussion she was hypnotized and then taught self-hypnosis. She was then treated by desensitization, seeing herself whilst in hypnosis in every conceivably anxious situation that we could list, remaining calm and relaxed in that situation and not picking or squeezing her spots. Subsequently, gradually learning to ignore her skin, whilst ego-strengthening was used to enhance her self-image emphasizing her height as a positive feature, her smooth skin and her fine complexion. The patient responded well and treatment was phased out after ten sessions. She was finally discharged after 15 sessions and followed up for two years. There was no recurrence of the picking although the acneous lesions appeared spontaneously from time to time. These were treated when necessary by a short course of antibiotics.

4. The Immature Personalities

This type of problem implies that the person has characteristics and traits which are less developed than expected for his age, irrespective of physical maturity. Additional problems may co-exist. Realization of inadequacy in certain areas may result in many symptoms, neurotic or otherwise. Anxiety, anger and aggressive feelings may all be present and dependency is often a feature. This may become particularly so when hypnosis is used. The subject readily learns to lean heavily upon the therapist.

Before embarking upon any attempt at treatment it is essential that a full psychiatric and psychological assessment be undertaken. It must also be understood that as with any form of psychotherapy, a powerful transference may develop and any ensuing problems must be recognized, understood and appropriately dealt with.

The objectives of hypnotherapy must be as follows:

1. To reduce the patient's anxiety with which he regards himself as a person and his consequent role in the world.

2. To explore, identify and encourage his potential.

3. To develop his ego-structure and increase confidence in himself.

Patients should be allowed to verbalize their experiences, memories and emotional feelings by *recall* under hypnosis. Regression to specific periods in early life is not particularly indicated. The therapist should simply commence by asking.

> Now I want you to go back in time to your very earliest memory.
> Think back as far as you can go...and when you have that
> memory in your mind just tell me about it...but you will remain
> relaxed, with your eyes closed as you speak to me. Go
> back...back...back and talk to me when you have that memory.

The patient will remain silent for a few minutes and then begin to speak. However trivial the recall may appear to be, there may be some significant material which will give a lead to further questions and the development of a particular area for discussion. Once a start has been made the patient will usually feel more comfortable to continue.

However, there may be a tendency for him to take over and try to control the session. This should be watched for and he should be gently steered back on course. Otherwise the therapist may find himself involved in long 'intellectual' discussions that take on the nature of debates. Wolberg[17] explained this very succinctly. 'Words' he said, 'replace experiences and constitute a defense against feelings.'

At each session ample time must be allowed for relaxation in hypnosis, recall, discussion and insight-directed psychotherapy followed by ego-strengthening. The therapist should never undertake to treat such cases if he is not prepared to give continuity of treatment over a considerable period of time. He must be supportive, understanding and firm in his guidance. Ideally any treatment should commence as early as possible and should continue at least until the patient is deemed to have emerged from adolescence. Every patient, and the family where appropriate, must be warned of the inevitable period of time over which therapy must be extended if any positive results are to be seen.

REFERENCES

1. Moll A., 1890. *Hypnotism.* Walter Scott, London.
2. Kraft T., 1968. Successful treatment of a case of drinamyl addiction. *Br. J. Psychiat.,* **114,**1363–1364.
3. Miller M.M., 1976. Hypnoaversion treatment in alcoholism, nicotinism, and weight control. *J. Natn. Med. Assoc.,* **68,** 129–130.
4. Watkins H.H., 1976. Hypnosis and smoking: a five session approach. *Int. J. Clin. Exp. Hypnosis,* **XXIV,** 381–390.
5. Barklay R.A., Hastings J.E. and Jackson T.L. Jr., 1977. The effects of rapid smoking and hypnosis in the treatment of smoking behaviour. *Int. J. Clin. Exp. Hypnosis,* **XXV,** 7–17.
6. Barabasz A.F., Baer L., Sheehan D.V. *et al.,* 1986. A three year follow-up of hypnosis and restricted environmental stimulation ther-

apy for smoking. *Int. J. Clin. Exp. Hypnosis,* **XXIV,** 1969–181.
7. Oswald I. and Lewis S.A., 1971. Addiction or dependance. *Br. Med. J.,* **2,** 229.
8. Russell G.F.M., 1979. Bulimia nervosa: an ominous variant of anorexia nervosa. *Psychol. Med.,* **9,** 429–448.
9. Hay G.G., 1970. Dysmorphophobia. *Br J. Psychiat.,* **116,** 399–406.
10. Le Cron L.M. and Bordeaux J., 1947. *Hypnotism Today.* Heinemann, London.
11. Schneck J.M., 1953. *Autogenic Training.* Grune and Stratton, New York.
12. Ambrose G., 1961. *Hypnotherapy with Children.* Staples, London.
13. Wolberg L.R., 1948. *Medical Hypnosis,* Vol. 1. Grune and Stratton, New York.
14. Mawdsley C., 1975. Diseases of the central nervous system: involuntary movements. *Br. Med. J.,* **4,** 572–574.
15. Yates A.J., 1958. The application of learning theory to the treatment of tics. *J. Abnorm. Soc. Psychol.,* **56,** 175–182.
16. Barabasz M., 1987. Trichotillomania: a new treatment. *Int J. Clin. Exp. Hypnosis,* **XXXV,** 146–154.
17. Wolberg L.R., 1946. *Hypnoanalysis.* Heinmann, London.

CHAPTER 17

The Treatment of Psychosexual Problems

Man's preoccupation with his sexual prowess has existed since the creation. Equally known no doubt, have been the problems of sexual dysfunction, fears of which have been expressed in contemporary writings from time immemorial. More latterly, in addition to any organic condition, somatic, dynamic and behavioural problems have all been implicated in the development of such difficulties.

The elimination of a possible physical cause of the symptoms is a priority before any form of psychological treatment is contemplated. Diseases of the genitalia are not uncommon and a physical examination should be routine whenever the diagnosis is in doubt.

Freudian ideas of the instinctional libidinous force which we possess, and the stages of growth, passing through oral, anal and genital phases may give some enlightenment to the understanding of sexual malfunction. Popular therapy was based on retracing the latter to the original emotional conflict which, once brought to the level of consciousness, should resolve the problem. Unfortunately, dynamically based treatment does not always meet with the success originally expected of it and behaviourist methods based upon the ideas of the modification of response have gained considerably in popularity. It is well to discover the emotional experiences which may be the cause of the problem but treatment should be based upon reduction of the anxiety that follows and the symptoms that the anxiety produces. As a consequence a vast industry of behavioural techniques has developed of which hypnotherapy is one of the simplest and most effective.

Nevertheless in any problem of this nature, it is essential for all early sexual experiences to be explored and discussed. The emotional conflicts caused by feelings of guilt must be resolved.

Misplaced advice given in early childhood—'sex is filthy, masturbation is a sin, don't let any man ever touch you'—can be warnings which may well have a bearing upon adult sexual responses.

Many difficulties which result therefore are those relating to anxiety. Anxiety is notorious as an inhibitor of performance and inhibition of performance may cause many psychosexual problems occurring in both men and women.

The therapist should always have in mind the very real fear of pregnancy which so many women have in spite of advances in contraceptive techniques. This still remains in a large number of cases, a considerable hindrance to healthy sexual reponses. Additionally, exceptional problems occur in females. These are related to endocrine changes which take place during the menstrual cycle, during pregnancy and the post-partum period and at the menopause. The male menopause is largely a myth, any changes which take place at this particular time of life being due rather to age. Generally speaking however, psychosexual problems in the male mainly arise from fear of failure and those in the female from fear of attack.

In all cases, where treatment by hypnosis is indicated, it is essential to establish whether the spouse or sexual partner will be willing and available to co-operate at some stage of the proceedings. This implies that he or she will take advice as to how to behave and to respond whilst treatment is in progress and subsequently. If the partner is unwilling, this does not necessarily mean that treatment will fail. It does mean however that it will probably be more prolonged.

PSYCHOSEXUAL PROBLEMS IN THE MALE

Impotence

This, as the name implies, means lack of potency, or power and includes erectile and ejaculatory problems.

1. *Primary Erectile Impotence*
In this condition there is the inability to achieve or maintain an erection sufficient for coitus ever to have taken place.

2. *Secondary Erectile Impotence*
This implies the failure to obtain an erection or to maintain an erection in the majority of occasions of attempted coitus. The condition may be acute or insidious in origin.

The cause may be organic or psychogenic or mixed. Inevitably an organic cause must first be excluded. Local conditions such as phimosis or balanitis, etc. may be eliminated by simple inspection. Hormonal deficiences, diabetic neuropathy or atherosclerosis may be present or the condition may result from prostatic surgery or the general aging process. Drugs such as barbiturates, benzodiazepenes, various antidepressants, beta blockers, hypotensive agents, nicotine, alcohol, heroin and morphine are amongst those that may be responsible for the condition. Any psychogenic origin is invariably associated with fear of failure and is often linked with some earlier experience of erectile failure. Kinsey *et al.*[1] noted other factors such as the genetic and constitutional make-up of the individual, his sexual drive and his environment as problems which must be considered. Psychogenic factors include generalized anxiety, hostility, aggression, conflicts and guilt. Easily overlooked is impotence as a symptom of depression and at the less complicated end of the scale, excessive fatigue may be the cause. Or the relationship between the sexual partners may be the real problem— and the patient must be encouraged to discuss this.

Erectile impotence is amongst the most common of the psychosexual disorders and a paper by Reid *et al.*[2] reported that about half the cases presenting to a clinic are organic in origin and the other half are psychogenic. Hypnotic treatment is most successful with deep trance subjects in which arm levitation and rigidity are used to simulate a powerful and sustained erection. Once again however, the origin of the problem should be explored and frequently retrospective desensitization will block the memory of that traumatic and perhaps even 'castrating' experience. Again, this should be followed by visualization of a hierarchy of suggested sexual situations and contact, ending in full intercourse in which the erection is maintained until mutual orgasm occurs. The ideomotor signal for successfully experiencing the suggestions should be requested at suitable intervals.

Instruction in self-hypnosis is a necessary adjunct, to help reduce the general level of anxiety and to repeat the therapeutic session in imagination, twice daily.

Ego-enhancement is equally important with suggestions of powerful and positive feelings of masculinity.

Practical retraining should be carried out in a similar graduated process, proceeding no further than has been learned at the previous hypnotherapeutic session. For example, the subject having been shown in hypnosis that he can approach the partner, first touching, then caressing, then embracing and so on, gradually achieving a strong and powerful erection and maintaining this for several minutes, then practises this regularly with his partner, reporting success before the next stage in treatment is undertaken. Both parties should be advised against any approach which might cause anxiety in the patient and the fear of failure.

Fuchs *et al*[3] used arm levitation as a powerful symbol of the erect penis rising to touch the hair and reported nine patients regaining potency by this method after one to three sessions.

3. *Premature Ejaculation (Ejaculatio Praecox)*

This is the condition in which ejaculation occurs before insertion or immediately upon insertion and where the partner is scarcely aroused. It is invariably a problem of increased anxiety and overstimulation and the partner must be warned to keep her distance and to refrain from any approach which the patient might perceive an overly erotic.

Once again treatment consists of relaxation in hypnosis, deepening and visualization of situations of love making in a hierarchial order to insertion and mutual orgasm. Instruction in self-hypnosis and ego-enhancement are essential adjuncts to treatment. In practical retraining it must be insisted upon that the subject remains within the limits set by the therapeutic session.

4. *Anorgasmia (Orgasmic Impotence)*

This, in a sense, is the opposite to premature ejaculation. The subject will achieve an erection and maintain the erection but be unable to ejaculate. Sexual feelings decrease and as the condition repeats itself, the patient believes he is no longer able to perform adequately, the sexual partner begins to doubt the subject's true feelings for her, anxiety rapidly increases and the problem is compounded. There is now a direct threat to the relationship between the parties and treatment has become a matter of urgency. This will depend upon the origin of the problem.

5. *Loss of Libido*

The term libido in this context is taken to imply loss of any sexual or erotic desire for the partner. It is a common accompaniment of depression and where the problem exists it is essential that history taking is accurate, as other biological features of change of affect will frequently be present. Anxiety will also occasionally present symptoms of loss of libido. Drugs which produce impotence may sometimes be to blame and the therapist must be alerted to this problem. Loss of desire however may be due to loss of feeling for the sexual partner, loss of interest in her, boredom, inadequate stimulation or lack of awareness by the female of the emotional and sexual needs of *her* partner. All these possibilities must be extensively investigated and if change is to occur then it is essential that marital therapy with counselling of both parties is undertaken. At this stage it may be preferable for the experts in this field to be called to advise. In the event of the patient revealing biological symptoms of depression, then antidepressant medication must be prescribed and the situation should be closely followed up for the drug itself may reinforce the loss of libido. Other than for the treatment of any concomitant anxiety manifestations, hypnotherapy would not have a place in the treatment of this condition until the cause has been identified.

Again, the origin of the problem must be thoroughly researched. Since the difficulty may be due to loss of interest or lack of sufficient stimulation by the partner, the problem should be discussed with her and she must be advised accordingly.

Reduction of anxiety under hypnosis, instruction in self-hypnosis and visualization during hypnosis and self-hypnosis, of intercourse until a climax is reached is the treatment of choice.

PSYCHOSEXUAL PROBLEMS IN THE FEMALE

1. *Vaginismus*

This is the term given to the contraction of the pelvic muscles, around the vagina and occasionally in the back and thighs, which may occur when intercourse is attempted. It can be voluntary but is also partly a spontaneous response and will result in spasm at the introitus which will prevent penetration. It could occur as a result of some organic lesion, for example an abscess or infection in that region or imperforate hymen, but otherwise is invariably psychogenic in origin. Failure of vaginal secretion, the equivalent of erection in the male and inadequate lubrication of the external genitalia, may result from lack of arousal and this alone can cause pain at the introitus on attempted insertion.

All these possibilities already discussed must be considered before treatment is commenced. A gynaecological examination is essential and this should be undertaken at an early stage since the dysparunia which results from the condition will only aggravate existing problems. Some attempt may have been made to overcome the difficulty by stretching under anaesthetic but this will scarcely solve the emotional difficulties. The subject is often ignorant of the elementary anatomy of the external genitalia and this should be explained to her by simple diagrams and illustrations. She should be directed to use a mirror for personal exploration and she should be instructed in the use of vaginal dilators in order to help her gain confidence in the accessibility of the introitus.

Frequently, sexual fears, especially in women, are the result of inadequate or incorrect sexual instruction in early life. Such fears may be learned from mother or nanny, themselves sexually ignorant. Anxiety may also result from abuse in childhood or later sexual experience. There are many women who will report sexual abuse in childhood perhaps by father or a member of the family. Freud remarked upon the frequency of the complaint and warned us that although it must be taken seriously, as this is what the child believed or wanted us to believe, it was not necessarily to be accepted as the truth. Frank and full discussion of any misunderstandings is essential. The sexual partner must be properly advised since his sexual approaches are of the utmost importance. A caring and loving approach, patience, understanding and gentle foreplay are the essentials. No attempt should be made at intercourse until the patient has been adequately prepared and is ready for practical retraining. The use of hypnosis, self-hypnosis, desensitization and ego-strengthening, particularly tailored to enhance feelings of femininity, can prove effective and rewarding therapy. Lubrication before intercourse would facilitate entry.

2. *Frigidity*

The difference between this condition and psychogenic vaginismus is really in the degree of the symptoms. But there is in addition to a lack of sexual desire or arousal, the inability to enjoy or to complete the sexual act. As well as the muscular spasm there is considerable emotional involvement resulting in a refusal of any physical involvement and certainly prohibiting any attempt at intercourse.

In this condition, there is a combination of lack of trust, hostility and fear. Fear of loss of control, fear of submission and surrender and fear of loss of independence are very considerable problems which result in an equally considerable response.

Treatment is along the lines already suggested for vaginismus but the emotional problems revealed are of far greater intensity. The hierarchy ascended must be very gradual indeed during the desensitization process, with particular emphasis upon the reduction of the general level of anxiety. Counselling of the partner is essential and he must be directed towards an approach which is totally non-threatening. At the moment that any fear is perceived in the subject, he must move away, wait and then approach in a more gentle manner.

3. *Anorgasmia (Orgasmic Dysfunction)*

The term dysfunction is preferred to impotence in the female for obvious reasons. It means the inability of the female to achieve orgasm and once again the condition may be primary or secondary. In the former, orgasm has never been achieved, whilst the latter is situational, that is when the circumstances of intercourse prevent orgasm occurring.

Occasionally the male partner will accuse the female of frigidity when anorgasmia is purely a situational response. For example, physical discomfort or fear of being overheard. Failure of the female partner to achieve orgasm precisely at the same time as the male does not imply frigidity. What it more likely will imply is a situational response, failure to be adequately sexually aroused or some degree of early ejaculation on the part of the male. Once again counselling is an essential prerequisite to any form of therapy and hypnotherapy along the lines indicated for vaginismus and frigidity should prove effective treatment.

4. *Loss of Libido*
This may follow ongoing sexual problems such as vaginismus or frigidity and is often misinterpreted as the latter. It may be due to endocrine changes occurring during the menstrual cycle, during pregnancy, in the post-partum period or at the menopause. Drugs, anxiety, depression or a preoccupation with financial or domestic problems may all be precipitating causes. Or the patient may simply not be sexually attracted to her partner. The problem must be thoroughly investigated before hypnosis or any form of psychotherapy is contemplated.

MALE AND FEMALE HOMOSEXUALITY AND THE SEXUAL DEVIATIONS

Once again, these problems *may* be due to problems in early life where such responses are learned in an inappropriate environment. The term homosexuality refers to some sort of sexual contact between persons of the same gender not necessarily leading to orgasm. The sexual deviations are varied and sometimes bizarre but in neither case should any attempt be made at treatment unless the therapist is absolutely certain of the positive motivation of the subject and of the fact that the particular sexual response is one which has been learned and is not constitutional. Hypnotherapy, other than for the reduction of anxiety, should never be undertaken if the condition is due to some genetic variation or hormonal imbalance. The problem is notoriously difficult to treat since many such patients are desperately seeking a change in their sexual preferences and often this is impossible to achieve. Hypnoaversion techniques have been attempted but they are extremely difficult and results are uncertain. Counselling to accept the situation as it is may often be the wiser decision where the condition is otherwise harmless.

Nevertheless, when the therapist is as certain as he can be of the real positive motivation of the subject, hypnotherapy may be used, and under the circumstances described has been effective in the 'conditioned' homosexual patient. It should be borne in mind however that such patients are particularly fragile personalities and considerable support is required over a prolonged period of time.

A process of sensitization or aversion and simultaneous desensitization may be used.

The technique is best illustrated in the following case history. A 24 year old girl presented to one of us (D.W.) at the department of psychiatry at a well-known London hospital. She was referred by her general practitioner as suffering from depression which had not been alleviated in spite of three separate courses of antidepressant drugs. Comprehensive case notes were taken and some hesitancy was obvious when questions relating to her psychosexual history were put to her. She eventually revealed her lesbian habits, had never established any deep interpersonal relationship with any of her sexual partners and was confused and unhappy about her lifestyle. There was no doubt that biological symptoms of depression were additionally present. Further questioning revealed that her mother had died when she was 3 years old and she was brought up in a strictly male household with a Victorian and authoritarian father who readily chose the leather belt to assert discipline. There were two older brothers who were equally aggressive towards her.

She had no one to turn to for comfort and it is not surprising that when a young school teacher showed her kindness and opened her arms to her she readily found the solace for which she yearned. Comforting rapidly led to a much closer physical relationship and it was not long before sexual advances were made and a lesbian relationship followed. Subsequent to the departure of the teacher, there were two other relationships, yet in none was there any emotional attachment. Soon a boyfriend appeared on the scene. At least, he was a friend who was also male. Kind, gentle and caring—not at all the kind of person she had grown to expect a male to be. Although a close relationship developed and she thought that she wanted to marry him, she was confused and concerned about the situation. In truth she had by then a considerable identity problem, became more anxious and depressed and eventully sought help.

Once again the patient was treated with antidepressant medication and over the next three weeks she was allowed to ventilate her problems with some therapeutic benefit. When it was clear that the depression was lifting she was relaxed in hypnosis and taught self-hypnosis for twice daily exercises in reducing her high level of anxiety. A full description had been taken of her three earlier homosexual partners and hypnoaversion therapy for the physical relationship (feelings of disgust and distaste) was commenced. At the same time, warm feelings of closeness and understanding were suggested for her male friend. She was encouraged in the appreciation of her own feminine attributes in a very specific ego-strengthening technique and after eight sessions was no longer depressed, her anxiety level had considerably decreased and she had no doubts whatsoever about her true gender orientation. When my patient discussed her earlier sexual problems with her now 'permanent' boyfriend, he asked her to marry him and so this story had a very happy ending. The patient was followed up on an informal basis for seven years and no further sexual problems had arisen.

Unfortunately few cases of sexual deviation are easily treatable nor arrive at this satisfactory conclusion. Positive motivation on the part of the patient, although perhaps expressing the true desire of the patient, does not necessarily mean that powerful sexual habits which have existed for many years can be altered. Motivation may often be the result of circumstances or due to environmental pressures. No form of psychotherapy will help in this type of patient.

REFERENCES

1. Kinsey A.C., Pomeroy W.B., Martin C.E. *et al.*, 1953. *Sexual Behaviour in the Human Female*. Saunders, Philadelphia.
2. Reid K., Morales A., Harris C. *et al.*, 1987. Double-blind trial of yohimbine in treatment of psychogenic impotence. *Lancet,* **ii**, 421–423.
3. Fuchs K., Zaidise I., Peretz B.A. *et al.*, 1985. Hypnotherapy in male impotence. In: *Modern Trends in Hypnosis* (eds Waxman, Misra, Gibson, Basker). Plenum, New York.

CHAPTER 18

Hypnosis in the Alleviation of Pain and in Surgery

Over 2000 years ago, the Greek philosopher and scientist Aristotle, excluding pain from the other five senses, maintained that it was an agony of the mind, a 'feeling state'.

This *feeling* of pain is a symptom of many conditions and illnesses, and strikes at the root of treatment. Because of the diversity of its origins, nature and site, it embraces every branch of medicine and because of its psychological meaning, hypnotherapy is often able to provide an effective respite from that most basic of all forms of suffering. The definition of pain escapes description although similes and metaphors abound. But whether that pain be organic or psychogenic in origin, it is a subjective response as well as a symptom and the problem of treatment is one which has exercised the minds of physicians since the beginning of time.

Although the question of pain relief is of such importance to so many of the healing disciplines, there is no doubt that one of the most impressive phenomena in the entire range of techniques which are employed is that of hypnotic analgesia. Because of this, its use for operative procedures was extensively exploited in the years before the introduction of ether and of chloroform.

The term analgesia refers of course to the loss of the sensation of pain whereas anaesthesia includes a total loss of sensory perception which is only rarely indicated.

The most impressive descriptions of hypnotic analgesia were those reported by Dr James Esdaile, a Scottish surgeon practising in Calcutta during the 1840s. He is reputed to have operated upon no less than 400 patients and many of his cases were published in *The Zoist*, a journal which was at that time devoted exclusively to mesmerism. His instructions to his 'anaesthetist' were brief and to the point. 'To be mesmerised for an hour and a half daily' (for five days before operation).[1] There is no doubt of the depth of trance obtained nor does there appear to be doubt of the extensive nature of the operations performed.

In his Harveian oration delivered on 25 June 1846 the famous British physician Dr John Elliotson[2] emphasized the use of mesmerism in patients undergoing surgical operations. There is, he said, 'The loss of common feeling—anaesthesia...and in it wounds give no pain.' The mesmerists had a difficult battle nevertheless, to obtain recognition for their particular skills in this area and it is only recently and in the present century that research into the nature of pain has encouraged the more widespread use of hypotherapy so that it has extended into all areas in which this distressing symptom may occur.

Practitioners are well aware of the fact that pain may be 'all in the mind'. Breuer and Freud[3] described many instances of psychogenic pain and Freud talked of pain as a conversion hysteria and emphasized the need to understand what the patient was saying by this complaint. He showed how, by the use of hypnosis, he could encourage patients to verbalize their feelings and was able at times to give direct suggestion of loss of symptoms. However, if the symptom, pain, serves a need it may well resist treatment and certainly any attempt at symptom removal under hypnosis in such cases, without regard to the cause, may well result in symptom substitution or the reinforcement of resistance to treatment.

The problem of anxiety, depression or other psychiatric illness must also be considered in the treatment of pain and there is no doubt that as in all other uses of hypnosis, extensive history taking must be a *sine qua non* before therapy is commenced. Pain may not be dismissed, or commanded to go away. If psychological in origin, it may be impervious to all forms of treatment unless the underlying problem is satisfactorily resolved. However revelation of the origin does not necessarily remove the pain and in some cases it may even not be expedient to reveal the dynamics of the symptoms to the patient.

Beecher[4] emphasized that the more anxious the individual the more intense will he report the pain. Obviously each patient must be dealt with on an individual basis before deciding upon which form treatment may take. Beecher[5] also noted that emotion, if euphoric, can block pain (for example, soldiers injured in battle and apparently oblivious to their wounds), whereas if it is depressing, would tend to enhance pain.

Without doubt, apart from any earlier changes in affect, many patients who have suffered pain for some time tend to become depressed. This symptom must be treated and the therapist should not hesitate to prescribe the appropriate antidepressant medication when required.

One should also be alerted to pain-related behaviour of patients. Facial expression, the sound of the voice, sighing or weeping, muscular tension and guarding are all significant signs in diagnosis and in treatment. The numbers and variations of analgesics and anxiolytics ingested as well as the variety of attention-seeking activities, must be observed. Organic and psychogenic pain must not be confused although the one may certainly accompany and compound the other. In addition, the subjective experience of pain depends on the recollection of previous pain experiences, on cultural differences and on personality, the site of the pain and upon the state of arousal of the individual at the time. Together with all these difficulties the motivation of the patient must be real and positive if it is hoped to achieve success through the use of hypnotherapy.

THEORIES OF PAIN AND PAIN REDUCTION

The Specificity Theory

This maintains that there is a particular set of pathways along the peripheral nerves and spinal cord which transmit pain messages to the brain.

The Pattern Theory

This denies the presence of specific pathways in the nervous system but maintains that information derived from the periphery is conveyed to the central nervous system where the interpretation is made as to whether the stimulus is painful or otherwise.

The Gate Control Theory

This theory proposed by Melzack and Wall in 1965[6] is without doubt the most important idea that has ever been devised regarding the nature of pain. They refuted the concept of any direct line of communication in the nervous system conveying pain sensations and produce clinical, psychological and physiological evidence to support their claim. The theory although complex is simple in principle. It proposes that as the brain and spinal cord are being subjected to a continuous flow of impulses from the periphery this holds open a 'gate' so that information regarding any noxious stimulus will additionally enter. These signals are modulated as they pass upwards, by other afferent impulses and by control from higher centres.

The theory was subsequently modified and in 1978 was re-examined and re-stated by Professor Wall[7]. It was summarized by him as follows:

1. Information about the presence of injury is transmitted to the central nervous system by peripheral nerves. Certain small diameter fibres respond only to injury while others with lower thresholds increase their discharge frequency if the stimulus reaches noxious levels.

2. Cells in the spinal cord or fifth nerve nucleus which are excited by those injury signals are also facilitated or inhibited by other peripheral nerve fibres which carry information about innocuous events.

3. Descending control systems originating in the brain modulate the excitability of the cells which transmit information about injury.

Therefore the brain receives messages about injury by way of a gate controlled system which is influenced by (a) injury signals,

(b) other types of afferent impulse and (c) descending control. This gate control theory has gained universal support in both the experimental and clincial field, although some of its features are still disputed.

The Endorphin Theory

This is a theory of pain relief, now largely discounted in so far as hypnosis is concerned, but which must be very much borne in mind in view of the considerable amount of research currently in progress.

In 1975 an endogenous substance with morphine-like properties was isolated from the brain at the Unit for Research in Addictive Drugs in Aberdeen by Hughes[8] and his colleagues. This substance was called enkephalin and was found to comprise two peptides, known as met-enkephalin and leu-enkephalin. The discovery stimulated future research world-wide and it is now known that these substances are only two of a larger family, the endogenous opioids. These are the morphine-like substances which appear to be the key to how pain is perceived and mediated. Hence the name endogenous morphine or 'endorphin' was adopted. Further research has shown that they may also be related to the regulation of emotional behaviour.

Not long after this discovery the proponents of acupuncture realized that here was a possible valid explanation of the action of this age-old art. It seems that the insertion of an acupuncture needle in a spot remote from the site of pain may actually stimulate the release of these endogenous opiates not only in the brain but in other parts of the body also. Subsequently the idea gained ground that perhaps hypnotically induced analgesia could have a neurochemical basis. In order to test this interesting hypothesis numerous experiments have been carried out, many using the pure opiate antagonist naloxone.

One study, by Stephenson[9] suggested that a true naloxone effect was operating and that hypnosis-induced analgesia seemed to be reversed.

Goldstein and Hilgard[10] demonstrated that contrary to expectations, the administration of naloxone following analgesia produced under hypnosis did not cancel out the analgesic state. In spite of this Guerra *et al.*[11] in their experiments noted that although hypnotically induced analgesia appeared unrelated to endorphin variations the connection with neuronal mechanisms still required further investigation.

Frid and Singer[12] found that analgesia produced under hypnosis could be partially reversed by naloxone in conditions of stress. However although some connection was thought to exist, the evidence *against* hypnotically induced analgesia being endorphin mediated is now very strong. Finer[13] drew attention to the fact that most of the research had acute pain as the experimental stimulus but since the neurophysiological mechanisms underlying acute and chronic pain are different, it may be conceivable that patients with chronic pain might yield different results. Nevertheless in his early experiments he failed to elicit any clear pattern of change in endorphin fraction.

The Concept of the Hidden Observer

Although applicable to many of the phenomena which may be produced in hypnosis it is perhaps appropriate to explore this theory particularly in any discussion on the subject of hypnotic analgesia. Nathan, commenting on the gate control theory, said that 'Ideas have to be fruitful; they do not have to be right'[14]. Ernest Hilgard's[15] original discovery of the 'hidden observer' has certainly borne copious fruit, the harvesting of which still continues. It is also generally accepted as a valid explanation of why the hypnotized subject fails to report the *suffering* of pain. Reporting on a paradox resulting from the reduction of pain under hypnosis, Ernest and Josephine Hilgard[16] stated that although felt pain may be reduced, some involuntary physiological indications of pain may persist at nearly normal levels. 'Does this mean', they asked 'that pain is registered at some level but ignored?'

A series of sophisticated experiments demonstrated this in fact to be the case. Laboratory-induced pain in the cold pressor test (by immersing a hand in ice-cold water) or by ischaemia (obtained by applying a tourniquet to the upper arm) resulted in covert reports obtained by automatic talking or writing, of normal pain, whilst the hypnotized part suffered no pain at all.

Hilgard and Hilgard later introduced 'the concept of a hidden observer as a metaphor, representing the part of the hypnotized person found to sense covert pain even when the person under hypnosis experiences no overt pain or distress at all'. In other words the pain is not taken away by the hypnotic suggestion. The subject is aware that the pain is still present but he does not experience that pain subjectively. Could this be further proof of the fact that hypnotic analgesia is not endorphin mediated? This very acceptable idea would confirm that it is in fact something totally different.

Campbell Perry[17] likened this 'neo-dissociationist' theory to the opinion of Janet who believed that particular ideas could become split off or disassociated from the main level of consciousness. Weitzenhoffer[18] however, felt that the hidden observer notion could be an artefact created by the hypnotist by the very procedure used. The evidence in favour of the hidden observer concept, nevertheless, far outweighs the opposition.

Sacerdote[19] summarized these ideas. He said dissociation 'usually requires a sufficiently deep trance so that the patient although aware at one level of his condition, at another level becomes an observer of what is happening to his body, without perceiving subjective painful sensations'. He goes on to suggest that the patient may imagine or hallucinate the self in a different pleasant setting, where he can reproduce some enjoyable experience from the past and make use of body memories to guide him into an age-regression. He may also be guided into an age-progression to a time when the pain and illness will be left behind. However, this is a sensitive area and its use must be very carefully considered especially in the case of terminally ill patients.

From this discussion it may be concluded that pain is not banished by hypnosis. It is the subjective awareness of that pain which is blocked. How then is this accomplished? Ostenasek[20] was able to show that when the fear of pain was abolished, the perception of pain was tolerable. Beecher[4] demonstrated the need to reduce the accompanying anxiety and the Hilgards[16] stressed the importance of a permissive induction technique as essential in reducing the anxiety which accompanies the experience of pain. There is no doubt that the anxiolytic effect of hypnosis is the first step in any treatment of this very considerable problem.

It must be remembered at all times that pain is a signal that something is wrong, whether that something be physical or psychological and it is essential to arrive at a correct diagnosis before attempting treatment.

SENSITIVITY TO PAIN

The pain threshold varies tremendously from individual to individual. Some people dread and anticipate pain to such an extent that the moment they are touched they translate this into a feeling of pain. This type of patient is particularly likely to be seen in the dental surgery, and is the kind of person in whom the combination of hypnosis and local analgesia is often most effective.

Most of us have seen a line of patients at a clinic waiting with their arms bared to receive an inoculation. The first feels just a normal prick, the second doesn't feel anything at all, but the third faints either immediately before or after receiving the injection. The actual injection, the method of administration, and even the size of needle are identical in each case. The difference is to be found in the individual patient, for the one who faints is usually tensed up with fear, anxiety and anticipation. This kind of patient is extremely difficult to deal with, and is probably more frequently seen by the dental surgeon than by the doctor. This is the patient who is so terrified by the thought of the dental chair that he will postpone his visit as long as he possibly can, and only turn up once in two years instead of every six months. Even then, he is quite likely to close his mouth as soon as he is approached with the dental drill. Hypnosis can be invaluable in dealing with this type of patient, for with its aid he can be taught to relax physically, and this in itself greatly reduces and relieves mental tension. Used in this way hypnosis can produce relaxed, physically comfortable, co-operative patients who are rendered much more at ease; even should no analgesia be obtained the patient will still be much easier to work upon with the use of orthodox procedures. If an anaesthetic is required, the patient will remain calm and take it without difficulty, so that much less of the anaesthetic agent is likely to be needed. On the other hand, the emotionally disturbed patient will not only require more, but even then the anaesthetic will seldom run smoothly.

Medium-trance Analgesia

In light hypnosis the appreciation of pain generally remains unaltered by suggestion and even in medium-depth hypnosis the degree of analgesia obtained may vary from slight to considerable. It is consequently in the medium-trance patient that the greatest use of hypnotic analgesia can be appreciated. Whilst no major surgery can be performed, many minor surgical procedures can be undertaken quite painlessly, probably in some 30 to 40 per cent of medium-depth patients. Pain can either be removed or greatly diminished in such procedures as the dressing of burns, lumbar or abdominal punctures, and certain painful manipulations of injured parts. Hypnotic analgesia can also be of value in conservative dental work such as painful fillings, particularly when the patient dreads the injection of a local anaesthetic, for even should the analgesia obtained be minimal it will often suffice to get him to tolerate the dreaded injection. Sometimes the pain from chronic incurable disease such as cancer can be controlled and diminished in the early stages, thus deferring the need for potent analgesic drugs. But the greatest value of hypnosis by far lies in its ability to produce both mental and physical relaxation and to rid the patient of fear and anxiety prior to an operation. Indeed the reduction of the fear–tension–expectancy syndrome renders it most useful to the general practitioner, the dental surgeon, the midwife and the nurse. Instead of becoming frightened, over-anxious and demoralized, the patient can be rendered calm, co-operative and much less apprehensive of what lies ahead.

Deep-trance Analgesia

In deep hypnosis, since the analgesia is often total and complete, major surgery can sometimes be carried out with no other form of anaesthetic. Amputation of limbs and the removal of breasts have been performed quite painlessly, and in the dental field impacted wisdom teeth have been easily and effectively dealt with. Hypnosis has an advantage over chemical anaesthetic agents that it produces no toxic effects whatever. It is consequently most useful in dealing with patients who are shocked and severely ill. Moreover, the patient's protective reflexes remain unaltered throughout, and should he vomit, the cough reflex is not abolished. He will be in no danger of being burned, for if fluids or hot-water bottles are too hot when he is back in the ward, he will be able to complain about them. He can either swallow blood or spit it out, and if he wants a drink he can safely be given one. In addition to this, post-operative pain or discomfort can readily be relieved and the patient will become ambulant more quickly, thus avoiding chest or other post-operative complications.

When limbs or joints have been operated upon, the patient can be enabled to move them more readily without pain and function is likely to be restored more rapidly. Conversely, in plastic surgery when skin-grafting has been performed, a limb can be totally immobilized in a fixed position by post-hypnotic suggestion. Indeed, such a position can be maintained with a minimum of discomfort for many days or weeks whilst the graft is taking effect. This is discussed later in this chapter.

In view of all these advantages, it is obvious that hypnosis would be the ideal anaesthetic agent were it not for the fact that less than one in every five people are capable of this degree of analgesia. Consequently the use of hypnosis in major surgery remains at present little more than a medical curiosity, and if its value were confined to this field only it might quite easily be discarded.

THE INDUCTION OF HYPNOTIC ANALGESIA

Hypnotic analgesias *never* correspond to any anatomical distribution. They always coincide with the subject's notion of function such as is seen in certain conversion symptoms and follow his own idea as to where the loss of pain should occur. Most individuals interpret the word 'arm' as signifying the whole of the upper limb, so if they are told they will lose all sensation in an arm, they will develop analgesia extending from the shoulder to the wrist. Consequently, whenever hypnotic analgesia is to be induced, the exact area that is to be rendered anaesthetic must be clearly indicated to the subject. Wherever possible it should be stroked, or even swabbed with spirit or ether to make it feel cold, so that the subject is in no doubt at all as to where the analgesia is to be produced. If this is omitted a 'glove and stocking' anaesthesia which corresponds exactly to the type that is seen in the hysterical patient will be produced. When dental analgesia is required the operator should run his finger along the gum to indicate quite clearly the exact area that is to be made analgesic.

It should never be forgotten that unless some prolongation of hypnotically induced analgesia is needed to relieve post-operative pain, in which case a time limit can be imposed, the analgesia should always be removed before the patient is awakened.

Where areas such as the abdomen are involved it is common practice to induce analgesia in the palm of a hand. When this has been achieved the patient is instructed to place that hand over the area to be rendered analgesic and in this way to 'transfer' the feeling of numbness and loss of pain to the affected part.

The induction procedure for the production of analgesia in the hand, for example, is accomplished by repeated suggestions of progressive loss of sensation as follows:

> You are now in so deep a sleep...that presently, all the feeling is going to disappear from your left hand.
> You will not be able to feel anything in your left hand...just think of your left hand becoming quite numb...as if it had gone to sleep.
> Gradually...it is becoming more and more numb...and all the feeling is going out of it.
> And as I go on talking to you...your left hand is beginning to feel colder and colder...as if it were surrounded with ice.
> Just picture your hand being packed round with ice...and as you do so...it is feeling colder and colder...more and more numb and insensitive.
> As soon as you feel your hand becoming cold and numb...please signal with the right index finger.

(After a brief interval during which these suggestions are repeated, the subject's finger rises.)

> Your hand has now become so cold and numb...that you are losing all feeling in it.
> Soon, you will not be able to feel any pain in it at all...you will feel no pain at all.
> In a moment or two...I am going to count slowly up to *three*.
> And when I reach the count of *three...your hand will be*

> *completely insensitive to pain...and you will be able to feel no*
> *pain at all in your hand.*
> *One*...Colder and colder...more and more numb and
> insensitive...losing all sensation of pain.
> *Two*...Your hand is now completely numb...there is no feeling in
> it at all...just as if it had gone to sleep.
> *Three*...Your hand is completely numb...cold...and insensitive...*you*
> *cannot feel any pain in it at all.*

The right hand, upon which the subject has *not* been told to concentrate, after a warning, is then pricked with a sterile hypodermic needle. The subject usually flinches. The left hand is then
pricked, and if the subject neither moves nor flinches some degree
of analgesia has been obtained. Further firmer pricking without
eliciting any response will establish the extent of the analgesia.
If it is complete, the needle may be firmly driven through a fold
of the skin without the slightest evidence of pain being felt. Once
this demonstration is completed, unless the analgesia is required
for therapeutic purposes, it must be removed before the subject
is awakened.

> In a few moments...your left hand will become quite normal again.
> It is becoming warmer and warmer...and all the feeling of
> numbness is leaving it...and it is now quite normal again...just
> the same as your other hand.
> All the sensation has returned...and you can now feel
> everything...just the same as with your other hand.

Wolberg[21] finds it advantageous to produce a cutaneous hyper-
aesthesia before attempting to induce analgesia. This enables the
subject to make a comparison between the hypersensitive part
and the one that is being anaesthetized. This facilitates the latter process by emphasizing the difference between them.

> Imagine you are walking down a corridor...at the end of which you
> can see a bucket of hot water.
> You know it's hot...because you can see the steam rising from
> the water.
> As soon as you can picture that bucket...as soon as you can see it
> quite clearly in your mind...please signal with your left index
> finger.

(The subject's finger slowly rises.)

Put your finger down again.
Now, you wonder how hot the water is...so you walk over to the bucket...and plunge your right hand in the hot water.
Picture this vividly in your mind...so that you will feel the heat.
Your hand is beginning to smart...it feels tender and painful.
Your hand is tingling...and feels warm and tender.
As soon as you feel these sensations...please signal with your left index finger again.

(Once again, the subject's finger rises.)

Right. Put your finger down again.
Now, I'm going to touch your right hand with a needle.
Your right hand is so tender and sensitive...that it feels just like a stab from a knife.
So tender and sensitive...it feels terribly painful.
See...how tender and painful it feels.
You'll notice the difference when I touch this hand...and when I touch the other hand with the needle.
I'm now going to touch the other hand...now this one, again.
See the difference!

Good subjects will actually flinch with pain when the hand is touched with the needle. It is important to get the subject to acknowledge that he felt at least some difference in the sensation between the two hands. If he feels no difference this must be repeated. He is told that this requires practice and that he will be able to detect it at his next session.

Occasionally, however, this technique does not succeed and no hypersensitivity is produced. In this case, the subject should always be questioned about his difficulties, sometimes with surprising results. A colleague discovered that his patient had no difficulty at all in picturing the bucket of hot water, but was then told 'Surely you didn't think I'd be stupid enough to plunge my hand into water that hot, without cooling it down?'

If successful, an attempt may then be made to induce analgesia. Since this is very rarely complete at the first session, it is necessary to get the subject to admit to some degree of relative insensitivity.

You'll notice that whilst your right hand is sensitive...your left hand is becoming more and more insensitive.

Now, I want you to imagine that you are consulting your doctor
because you have a boil on the forefinger of your left hand.
He is going to inject a local anaesthetic around your wrist...to
cause a wrist-block and remove the pain...like this.

(The wrist is then circled with slight needle pricks.)

Gradually your left hand is becoming more and more numb...and
soon it will become so numb and insensitive...you will be able to
feel no pain...compared with your right hand.
All the feeling will leave your hand...and it will become more
and more numb.
As you concentrate on your left hand...try to imagine that you
are wearing a thick, heavy leather glove on your left hand.
As soon as you can picture yourself wearing the glove...and feel as
if the glove is on your hand...please signal with your right index
finger.

(After some delay, during which the suggestions are repeated, the
subject's finger eventually rises.)

Put your finger down, again.
Your hand now feels as if you are wearing a thick, heavy,
leather glove...so that when I touch it with a needle...it will feel
just as if I am touching leather.
You will feel no pain at all...just a dull feeling.
Now, I'm going to show you the difference, by first touching your
right hand...the sensitive one...and then the left one.
Do you feel the difference?
And now, your hand is becoming more and more numb...more
and more insensitive...and all sensations of pain are
disappearing completely.
This dull feeling is spreading over your whole hand...over the
back of your hand...your fingers and thumb...over the front of
your hand.
This feeling is becoming duller and duller...your hand is
beginning to feel as if it were made of wood.
I can stick a needle in it...and you will feel no real pain.
It has become so numb and insensitive...that you can feel no real
pain at all.

(The hand is now pricked, and the subject questioned.)

Note how numb it feels!

(Should the subject say that he feels pain, he must be reassured.)

> Although you still feel slight pain...it is less than in the other
> hand, isn't it?

(He will usually admit to feeling a difference.)

> That's good...it shows that the hypnosis is beginning to work.
> Let yourself relax completely...and you will fall into an even
> deeper sleep.
> And next time you come...you will not only fall into deeper, deeper
> sleep...but the feeling in your hand will disappear completely.

DEMONSTRATIONS OF HYPNOTIC ANALGESIA

Experiment 1. A subject is induced into deep hypnosis, his sleeve
rolled up, and a circle of about two or three inches diameter drawn
on his fore-arm. He remains lying back in the chair, *with his eyes
closed.* He is then told: 'When I count up to five, inside that circle
your arm will become cold and numb. You will be able to feel no
pain at all...*inside the circle.* The rest of your arm will remain normal...and you will be able to feel pain everywhere else. But, inside the circle...you will not be able to feel pain.'

First, the arm is pricked *well inside the circle,* and the subject
takes no notice. Then it is firmly pricked again, *well outside the
circle,* and the subject flinches. Finally, it is firmly pricked again,
inside the circle but close to the perimeter, and the subject flinches
again. This experiment shows that because he cannot see the
circle, the subject is not quite sure where it is, and is thus unable
to produce an accurately defined area of analgesia.

Experiment 2. The same subject is then told to open his eyes
without waking up from his trance, then he will be able to see
quite clearly but will not wake up. He is then told to look at the
circle and that once again he will not be able to feel any pain inside the circle.

His arm is then firmly pricked again, *inside the circle,* but this
time it will not matter where his arm is pricked, even up to the
periphery of the circle. He will show no response whatever. When
the arm is pricked outside the circle the subject will flinch, but
when it is pricked *inside the circle, no matter how close to the per-*

imeter, he will fail to display any reaction at all. This demonstrates the fact that, with his eyes open, the subject is now able to define accurately the precise area that is to become analgesic. It thus emphasizes the fact that if the subject is to produce the desired analgesia be must be left in no doubt as to exactly where it is to take effect.

Experiment 3. The same deeply hypnotized subject is told that his arm has become normal again and that the feeling has returned. He is then told: 'When you, yourself, count up to five...your arm inside the circle will become quite numb and insensitive to pain.

You will be able to prick yourself...but you will be able to feel no pain at all...*inside the circle.*

But when you count backwards...from five to one...your arm will return to normal...and you will feel pain in the normal way everywhere in your arm.'

This demonstrates the fact that the subject can be enabled to produce and abolish analgesia for himself upon a given signal. He can also be taught how to do this, to a strictly limited extent, in the waking state as the result of post-hypnotic suggestion.

Experiment 4. Before he is finally awakened, the subject is given the following instructions: 'You will be able to produce this same numbness for yourself...after you wake up. *For the next five minutes only*...you will be able to make any part of your body that you wish, become completely numb and insensitive to pain.

When you wish to produce numbness...you will be able to do so by counting...one...two...three...four...five.

When you wish to remove the numbness and restore the part to normal...you will be able to do so by counting backwards...five...four...three...two...one.'

Experiment 5. After the induction of hypnotic analgesia, it may be useful to test the effect of transfer before proceeding. If a glove anaesthesia has already been produced in one hand it may be suggested that a tingling or burning sensation is being experienced in the other. This is confirmed by requesting the ideomotor signal (raising the index finger). The patient is then instructed to rub the numb hand over the affected area of the other and in this way to transfer the numbess to the other. Again the ideomotor signal is requested when the tingling or burning has disappeared. The loss of all abnormal sensation is emphasized and in this way the patient will appreciate that hypnosis will effectively relieve pain.

The ability on the part of a good subject to produce self-induced analgesias must always be severely restricted, either to a limited period of time, or to specific areas of his body. Hence the five-minute spell imposed above. The subject must never be allowed to leave with the carte blanche ability to relieve pain anywhere in himself for an indefinite period. He might otherwise mask some serious condition such as acute appendicitis, with the grave danger of subsequent perforation.

Additionally, the use of self-hypnosis is essential for every patient in the management of pain with instruction and practice in the achievement of 'self-analgesia' and 'transfer'.

CLINICAL APPLICATIONS IN ACUTE AND CHRONIC PAIN

In acute pain treatment should never be attempted until the diagnosis is absolutely certain.

One of the authoritarian techniques should be employed as it is important to obtain rapid eye closure and to assert the effectiveness of the method without delay. Once this has been obtained the induction may be slowed down in order to produce a maximum calming effect and as much deepening which the circumstances will allow. Continue as follows, speaking in a positive manner:

> I will now place my hand over the painful part very gently. The
> warmth of my hand feels soothing and comfortable and as I
> press very lightly this warmth and comfort passes into your
> body so that all discomfort gradually diminishes.

Organic disease and terminal illness is frequently accompanied by pain and suffering. Awareness of the cause and the often unremitting nature of the symptoms additionally result in anxiety and depression which will compound the pain. The first step therefore is to deal with the latter. If depression exists and if there are no contraindications, antidepressant medication should be prescribed without delay. The anxiety manifestations may then be dealt with through the use of hypnosis and the specific symptom of pain is treated by direct suggestion of loss of pain using one of the techniques described below. Overall, most therapists additionally utilize a holistic approach, although it must be emphasized that this method may be unrealistic to any person suffering from severe pain and certainly too altruistic for many unfortunate patients who may be well aware of the ultimate prognosis.

It must not be overlooked that chronic pain may also appear as a conversion symptom. Such patients often produce puzzling or atypical symptoms, have frequently undergone a considerable amount of investigation and will present after every other form of treatment has failed. The patient is of course saying something by this symptom and the therapist must understand its language so that he can effectively deal with the problem.

In the management of chronic organic pain or terminal pain the importance of good motivation and confidence in the therapist and the technique must once again be emphasized. Although hypnosis has something very special to offer, the placebo effect should not be minimized. In his review of studies of double blind medication for pain reduction, Evans[22,23] showed that the relative effectiveness of placebo compared to a standard dose of morphine was about 56 per cent. This emphasized the importance of expectancy—a factor which particularly applies when hypnotherapy is used.

Kroger[24] stated that 'for any kind of psychotherapy to be successful, pain cannot be treated by any one method; it is not an isolated behaviour. Rather, the therapist should try to relate the pain behaviour to the effects of prior disease processes, responses, lifestyle and current set of values; one or more of these items can reinforce or exacerbate the behaviour.' He emphasized that pain behaviour belongs to a personality and each patient must be approached as a person rather than by an attack on the pain *per se*. He stressed that, with the patient in hypnosis, how abilities to control various 'feeling' states can be utilized and each patient is given a cassette containing post-hynotic suggestions especially tailored for his own symptoms and problems utilizing many specialized hypnotic techniques such as the production of analgesia, dissociation and time distortion to make the duration of pain seem shorter.

It must be accepted that pain alleviation or even reduction cannot be achieved with every patient. Frankel[25] remarked that the masking or displacement of physical discomfort and pain by means of perceptual distortion is dependent not only upon the interaction between the patient and the therapist, but is also a function of the *capacity* of the patient to achieve such distortion and to *experience* hypnosis.

Dabney Ewin[26] sees constant pain as an idea which equates with life itself. If the patient says 'I live with it', the subconscious corollary is 'If I didn't have it, I'd be dead'. The pain gives subconscious reassurance that he is still alive and when faced with conventional treatment he will resist giving up control of that pain. Treatment involves the establishing of rapport, regressing to the origin of the pain and making the point that even though it was originally so bad 'we know now that you didn't die don't we?' He insists upon a response and attempts to show the patient that he no longer needs his pain in order to reassure himself that he is still alive! Ewin would expect however that the pain would return by the following day and even be worse and with this he would point out to the patient that if he can make the pain worse, then it must mean that he has taken control of the pain and treatment would progress accordingly. Additionally, the following problems may have to be dealt with:

Non-acceptance ('why have *I* got the pain?'), fear, negative interpretation, the threat of endless suffering, guilt and anger, negative suggestions previously made to the patient regarding the pain, identification with other pain sufferers and pessimistic comments heard during anaesthesia for surgery.

Finer and his colleagues[27] in Sweden, adopt a firm but holistic attitude to treatment of chronic pain in addition to the somatic procedures used. Patients are trained in self-hypnosis in groups, emphasizing pain reduction, increased activity, increased self-esteem, vitality, courage and endurance. They are encouraged to express their feelings related to the pain and the general life situation together with others who support and understand. Although the actual pain is hardly affected, usually most patients improve psychologically, they are better able to cope and the attitude to the pain is improved. This work continues.

The first author of this book had previously described some useful additional methods which may be employed to obtain hypnoanalgesia. These are as follows:

1. *Substitution.* The pain may be replaced by some lesser sensation which can be better tolerated or by some altered sensation, e.g. of warmth which is not painful.

2. *Displacement.* In a particularly receptive patient, the pain can be displaced from the acutal site of the lesion to a part of the body where it may do no harm, e.g. his left hand.

3. *Progressive diminution of pain.* The patient is told that if the hundred per cent of pain he is suffering could be reduced to ninety per cent he would scarcely feel the difference. These suggestions are reinforced and continued at each session.

Some Case Histories

One lady of 51 was referred to the second author by her surgeon on account of continued pain in the left breast area following radical mastectomy and chemotherapy three years previously. There had been no complication during the operation and prolonged and considerable investigations had revealed no physical cause for the pain. The extensive use of analgesics and tranquillizers was of little help and treatment with physiotherapy and with acupuncture had been to no avail. She was well clear of the menopause but there were definite biological symptoms of depression. There was nothing of relevance in the family history or childhood. She had been previously married to a wealthy but work-shy man from whom she was subsequently divorced. There was one daughter of this union, who remained with her father 'because he had the money'. She felt that she had let her down. She was then remarried to a childhood sweetheart ten years before the discovery of a lump in the breast. Unfortunately she had become almost totally involved in business with her new husband and was responsible for most of the administrative side of his affairs. On joint interview it was clear to note his successful efforts in manipulating her to continue with this work. She was highly anxious, felt degraded, diminished, a non-person, guilt-ridden but above all very angry, commenting 'I look like a lop-sided freak'.

Treatment was along the following lines.

1. Marital therapy.
2. Prescription of antidepressant medication.
3. Lowering the level of anxiety through the use of hypnosis.
4. Hallucination whilst in hypnosis, of numbness in the palm of the right hand by immersion in a bucket of ice. This was confirmed by an ideomotor signal of the index finger of the left hand and followed by removal of the right hand from the imaginary ice bucket. Transfer was then effected by placing the palm of the right hand on the left chest wall. Analgesia was confirmed once more by an ideomotor signal and by testing with a pin prick. The numbness of the right hand was then removed.
5. Instruction in self-hypnosis with repeated practice of the production of the required analgesia at every therapeutic session. Self-hypnosis to be carried out three times daily at home in order to pre-empt the occurrence of pain.
6. Ego-strengthening to enhance her self-image and to improve her feelings of herself as a woman, a wife and in all aspects of her activities.
7. Strong post-hypnotic suggestion to forget the tension feelings in her chest (the word 'pain' was not used).

After four sessions the patient was able to decrease and subsequently to relinquish all chemical analgesics. She continued with the antidepressant medication and self-hypnosis but sadly passed away two years later as a result of multiple metasteses.

Another lady of 54 presented with a 12 year history of intractable pain in the gums. Her original complaint had been treated by the extraction of a number of teeth and the fitting of a partial denture. The pain persisted however and no amount of adjustment to the denture, nor of any other dental procedure was successful in relieving her of the problem. She consulted many dental specialists of high repute but no abnormality was discovered.

There was nothing of relevance in her family history or childhood and she was happily married and had two supportive, married children. Seven years earlier she had undergone a lumpectomy which proved to be non-malignant and subsequently attended her surgeon for a biannual check-up for three years. She had initial sleep difficulties and the pain was always magnified at night. She was preoccupied by the thought that the doctors were mistaken. The lump must have been a cancer (otherwise why did her specialist see her again for so long?), the cancer had recurred in her mouth (so were her unconscious thoughts) and this, she insisted, was the cause of her continuous pain. Additionally, she had numerous other manifestations of her severe anxiety but there was no evidence of depression. Treatment was as follows:

1. Lowering the level of anxiety by regular hypnosis and emphasis on loss of all abnormal sensations in the mouth and gums.
2. Discussion whilst in the relaxed state of her cancer phobia.
3. Desensitization to her fear, by regression to the original discovery of the lump and subsequent investigations, hospitalization and operation, etc.
4. Instruction in self-hypnosis with emphasis on good health, feelings of well being and of enjoyment of her family and general life situation.

The patient made a complete recovery after six sessions and continues to be followed up for reinforcement at three monthly intervals.

A young man of 36 complained of chronic pain in the right side of the chest following an injury whilst playing football three years earlier. There had been no bone damage and neither orthopaedic surgeons nor physicians could find any pathology to account for the symptoms. He was a highly anxious person and the pain always became worse during situations of stress and would keep him awake at night. There were no biological symptoms of depression and apart from a life-long preoccupation with his health there was nothing of relevance in his personal history. All his family were described as anxious and his mother was reported as being a constant visitor to the doctor's surgery. Treatment was as follows:

1. Lowering the level of anxiety by regular sessions of hypnosis.
2. Suggestions, whilst in hypnosis of 'bringing on the pain' in the right chest by concentration on this area. Confirmation by ideomotor signal, of suggestions of displacement of the pain on taking a deep breath, to the right foot where it would be substituted by a warm and pleasant sensation. Confirmation of this was again by an ideomotor signal.
3. Instructions in self-hypnosis with strong post-hypnotic suggestion that should this particular pain occur in the normal routine of his daily life he would equally well deal with it by taking a deep breath.

The treatment was successful although the patient remains a highly anxious person. He attends for regular monthly follow-up and 'booster'.

There is no doubt that the multidisciplinary techniques available for the treatment of chronic pain afford a pool from which the physician may draw in order to apply the form of therapy most suitable for his patient. In any event the benefit of hypnotherapy for reducing the general level of anxiety which will inevitably compound the sensation of pain whatever the source, is always of considerable value.

All in all, the treatment of pain, through hypnotherapy can be one of the most challenging and rewarding of all its uses.

Milton Erickson, at the International Congress of Hypnosis and Psychosomatic Medicine held in Paris in 1965, made the following observations: 'In all such hypnotic procedures, you must speak to the patient with an utter intensity and belief. You should also realise that maybe not all these things will work in any particular patient, but surely since he is a human being, he will respond to some of them. It is consequently your duty as a clinician to be sure to present to him these ideas, some of which he may be able to accept and act upon.'

HYPNOSIS IN SURGERY AND ANAESTHESIA

The use of various hypnotic techniques for the alleviation of pain has already been discussed.

In surgery, hypnosis is usually employed for one or other of the two following purposes:

1. To produce anaesthesia or analgesia.
2. To free the patient from anxiety and to produce mental and physical relaxation prior to operation.

Hypnosis possesses practically all the prerequisites of the ideal anaesthetic agent. When complete anaesthesia can be secured it involves no dangers at all and can be induced in the operating theatre by the surgeon or his assistant. However, the necessary depth is only rarely attainable and, in so far as major surgery is concerned, hypnosis offers other important disadvantages compared with chemically induced anaesthesia:

1. Except in those cases where the patient has been previously trained and conditioned, hypnosis is certainly neither as quick nor as easy a method of inducing anaesthesia.
2. It is rarely possible to secure the deeper stages of somnambulism which are essential before major surgery can even be considered.
3. Hypnosis is necessarily more time consuming than any existing orthodox procedure.
4. The induction and deepening of hypnosis for anaesthesia is an art which has to be learned and mastered, and should consequently only be undertaken by a specialist experienced in the subject.

Even when complete hypnotic anaesthesia is possible, the best results will only occur in those operations that do *not* require a very deep state of surgical anaesthesia.

It is important to appreciate exactly what can reasonably be expected in each of the three main stages of hypnosis:

Light trance. Only seldom is it possible to produce the slightest degree of analgesia. Nevertheless fear and anxiety can be alleviated, and the psychological overlay of pain reduced.

Medium trance. At this stage, varying degrees of analgesia can be produced in some 30 to 40 per cent of patients. Hypnosis can consequently be usefully employed to reduce discomfort in painful surgical procedures that have to be repeated, such as painful dressings which normally do not justify the use of a general anaesthetic. It can facilitate lumbar punctures and similar investigations, and even certain painful manipulations necessitated in physiotherapy can be undertaken under hypnosis with a minimum of discomfort.

Deep trance. No more than 15 to 20 per cent of patients can be induced into the deepest somnambulistic trances in which considerable degrees of analgesia become possible, and of these probably even less than 15 per cent can achieve the complete surgical anaesthesia that is essential for major operations. When this does occur, however, such surgical procedures as amputations of limbs, mastectomies, Caesarean sections and appendicectomies can be performed quite painlessly. Hypnotic anaesthesia offers certain distinct advantages:

1. Pre-operative fear and anxiety can be almost completely removed.
2. There is a complete absence of toxic effects as may occur with the use of anaesthetic drugs.
3. There is no danger from inhaled anaesthetics.
4. Shock is greatly diminished.
5. The cough reflex is not interfered with.
6. Post-operative pain, discomfort and sickness can all be controlled.

Once the somnambulistic stage has been successfully achieved, direct suggestions are usually made to the effect that the patient will become completely relaxed, both mentally and physically, and will enter so deep a sleep that he will feel no pain or discomfort whatever, and will subsequently remember nothing that has taken place. More often than not, however, *anaesthesia* such as this cannot be produced and yet a complete *analgesia* may still be possible. In such cases some sensation (without pain) may be permitted, and painful stimuli allowed to reach consciousness as non-painful experiences.

Apart from its limited use in the production of surgical anaesthesia, hypnosis can prove extremely useful to the anaesthetist in his routine work. Any method that can overcome fear, conscious

378 MEDICAL AND DENTAL HYPNOSIS

or subconscious, can afford considerable assistance and hypnosis is the ideal agent for this purpose. It is a relatively easy task to secure both mental and physical relaxation under hypnosis, and once this has been achieved much less chemical anaesthetic will be required to produce and maintain the depth at which surgery becomes possible. Moreover, if it is used pre-operatively for several days, hypnosis can ensure restful sleep and can allay the fear of pain, fear of the operation itself and of untimely death. Needless to say, such reassurances as these will enable the patient to face his operation with much more confidence and in a much calmer and more relaxed frame of mind. Indeed, as an introduction to general anaesthesia, hypnosis offers all the advantages and none of the dangers or disadvantages of chemical anaesthesia.

In children hypnosis can be an invaluable asset since it can usually be induced both easily and rapidly, and fairly deep trance states secured without much difficulty.

Whenever medium or deep stages of hypnosis can be attained and a considerable amount of analgesia secured, it may be preferred to the use of general anaesthetics in minor surgical or dental operations, particularly in children. Even these minor procedures often cause a great deal of fear and anxiety, and since hypnosis is so successful in controlling and eliminating this, it offers many advantages over the use of orthodox chemical anaesthesia.

In some earlier comments Goldie[28] reported on some valuable investigation into the usefulness of hypnotic anaesthesia or analgesia in emergency work in casualty departments. He claimed that hypnosis can be advantageously used as an adjunct to the more orthodox anaesthetic facilities and he demonstrated conclusively how effective the technique can be in untrained subjects, reducing to an appreciable extent the number of general anaesthetics that would otherwise have been required.

The conclusion may fairly be drawn that whereas hypnosis can be of considerable assistance to the anaesthetist in his work, in so far as hypnotic anaesthesia itself is concerned it can in no way be considered as a serious rival to the efficiency, safety and ease of administration of modern pharmacological anaesthetics.

Minor Surgical Procedures

These can be performed quite painlessly in a large percentage of medium-depth patients. Incisions, suturing, the dressing of burns and injuries, lumbar and abdominal punctures, cystoscopy and certain otherwise painful investigations as well as manipulations of injured parts, may be undertaken without pain. There was an interesting report published in the *Lancet*[29] of hypnosis used for endoscopy in a number of cases where pain, discomfort and gagging were eliminated. Dental extractions are today frequently undertaken using hypnosis and hypnotic analgesia can offer considerable relief in obstetrics. These two latter subjects are dealt with in chapters which follow. All in all the technique lends itself to a wide area of conditions in which the problem of anxiety, aggravating pain, plays a prominent part.

An effective and simple method of preparing the patient for minor surgery is by the reduction of anxiety in hypnosis and suggestion of analgesia of the part to be operated upon. Instruction in self-hypnosis is also given. For 'cold' surgery, a behavioural method may be used. A hierarchy of anxiety-rovoking situations is prepared and the patient is 'desensitized'. The technique is as follows:

The patient is put into hypnosis and shown that he is completely calm and relaxed. He is told to maintain the feeling of calmness and relaxation whilst he thinks about the operation generally. Confirmation is obtained by the ideomotor signal (raising the right or left index finger).

He is then told, in hypnosis, that he is on his way to the hospital or doctor's surgery for the operation, still maintaining his feelings of total calmness. Confirmation is again obtained. Then meeting the doctor or surgeon and being prepared for the operation etc., then the incision, retraction of skin and so on through the entire operative procedure one step at a time—at each, confirming the feelings of complete calmness and composure. Two or three of these steps may be visualized at each session and the subject is asked to repeat them in self-hypnosis twice daily until the next session. When he is completely desensitized final suggestions of analgesia are given of the area to be operated upon. As an added advantage the patient may use self-hypnosis before the actual operation, maintaining this state throughout the whole procedure. When he is sufficiently relaxed the surgeon may commence, first testing for local analgesia by pricking the skin with a needle. The patient is told that at a verbal signal from the surgeon such as 'it's all done now' he will open his eyes and be awake and alert. Post-operative after-effects will be minimal only.

Undoubtedly however, the presence of the hypnotist to carry out the anaesthetic procedure in person is always to be preferred.

Major Surgical Procedures

Reports are still obtained from time to time of the use of hypnosis in major surgery. However these examples are far too few to suggest that hypnoanalgesia could ever be used as a routine. It would apply to the rare occasion in which the patient is discovered to be a somnambule. That is unless one would attempt the prolonged and persistent deepening of trance as practised by Esdaile[1] and others in the nineteenth century. This would have to compete with the speed with which modern chemical anaesthesia can be carried out and few surgeons would have the time or patience for this procedure today. One point which should be noted is that whilst pain results from incisions into the skin and other external tissues, most of the remaining organs of the body are insensitive to pain or incision.

Chaves and Barber[30] drew attention to six factors that play an important role in the success of hypnotic procedures and surgery. These are as follows:

1. Patient selection.
2. Interpersonal relationship.
3. Pre-operative preparation or 'education'.
4. Use of drugs (in addition to hypnosis).
5. Suggestions of analgesia or anaesthesia (regardless of the formal induction of hypnosis).
6. Distraction (under hypnosis) from the actual process of the operation).

The use of hypnotic analgesia in plastic surgery deserves special mention. David Scott[31,32], a British anaesthetist, pioneered a special technique to overcome pain and discomfort suffered by patients undergoing skin grafting and reconstructive surgery.

The effect of hypnosis in his patients was not only to help them to relax profoundly and produce a general feeling of well being but also to aid in the transfer of pedicle grafts, particularly when bizarre postures had to be maintained for a considerable period of time. The use of self-hypnosis was invariably taught in order to help the relief of general aches and cramps and as a result, analgesic medication was considerably reduced.

The technique would involve the production of very deep hypnotic trance, testing for somnambulism and the suggestion of local analgesia and of deep analgesia of the part to be operated upon. The latter is achieved by suggestion of freezing and numbness. 'Imagine you are dipping your right hand into a bucket of ice. Keep it there until it is absolutely numb with cold and when this is so bring the hand out of the bucket and raise your index finger to confirm.' When confirmation is obtained, continue as follows:

'Now I shall prick your hand with a sterile needle and you will feel no pain, only a dull pressure.' This action is now carried out and the patient is asked to confirm once more. 'I will prick the other hand for comparison.' When this is done the patient retracts the hand. The patient is now told that he can transfer the numbness and loss of all felt pain to the area to be operated upon and powerful suggestions of loss of all unpleasant sensations in that area are given.

The entire process is repeated over and over again until certain that the operation can be proceeded with.

In conclusion it must be said that although the advantages of the use of hypnosis in any operative procedure are many, the disadvantages are also considerable. In addition, since less than one in five of the population is capable of the degree of analgesia required for major surgery, the hypnotic heroics of the days of Esdaile have long been almost universally abandoned.

REFERENCES

1. Esdaile J., 1848. Dr Esdaile's practice in the Calcutta Mesmeric Hospital. *Zoist*, **22,** 115.
2. Elliotson J., 1846. *Harveian Oration.* 68, Walton and Mitchell, London.

3. Breuer J. and Freud S., 1955. Studies on hysteria. In: *Standard Edition of the Complete Psychological Works of Sigmund Freud* (ed. Strachey), Vol. 11. Hogarth, London.
4. Beecher H.K., 1959. *Measurement of Subjective Responses*. Oxford University Press, New York.
5. Beecher H.K., 1962. *Symposium on Assessment of Pain in Man and Animals*. Universities Federation for Animal Welfare, Middlesex.
6. Melzack R. and Wall P.D., 1965. Pain mechanisms: a new theory. *Science,* **150,** 971–979.
7. Wall P.D., 1978. The gate control theory of pain mechanisms. A re-examination and re-statement. *Brain,* **101,** 1–18.
8. Hughes S., 1975. Isolation of an endogenous compound from the brain with pharmacological properties similar to morphine. *Brain Res.,* **88,** 295–308.
9. Stephenson, J.B.P., 1975. Reversal of hypnosis-induced analgesia by naloxone. *Lancet,* **ii,** 991–992.
10. Goldstein A. and Hilgard E.H., 1975. Failure of the opiate antagonist naloxone to modify hypnotic analgesia. *Proc. Natn. Acad. Sci. U.S.A.,* **72,** 2041–2043.
11. Guerra G., Guantieri G. and Tagliaro F., 1985. Hypnosis and plasmatic beta-endorphines. In: *Modern Trends in Hypnosis* (eds Waxman, Misra, Gibson, Basker). Plenum, New York.
12. Frid M. and Singer G., 1979. Hypnotic analgesia in conditions of stress is particularly reversed by naloxone. *Psychopharmacology,* **63,** 211–215.
13. Finer B., 1982. Endorphins under hypnosis in chronic pain patients: some experimental findings. Paper given at 9th International Congress of Hypnosis and Psychosomatic Medicine, Glasgow.
14. Nathan P.W., 1976. The gate control theory of pain. A critical review. *Brain,* **999,** 123–158.
15. Hilgard E.R., 1973. A neodissociation interpretation of pain reduction in hypnosis. *Psychol. Rev.,* **80,** 396–411.
16. Hilgard E.R. and Hilgard J.R., 1983, *Hypnosis in the Relief of Pain.* Kaufmann, Loss Altos, CA.
17. Perry C., 1985. Neo-dissociation theory of hypnosis: some additional data. In: *Hypnosis in Psychotherapy and Psychosomatic Medicine* (ed Guantieri). I1 Egno, Verona.
18. Weitzenhoffer A.M., 1985. In search of hypnosis. In: *Modern Trends in Hypnosis* (eds Waxman, Misra, Gibson and Basker). Plenum, New York.
19. Sacerdote P., 1985. Why is hypnosis effective in pain control? In: *Modern Trends in Hypnosis* (eds Waxman, Misra, Gibson and Bas-

ker). Plenum, New York.
20. Ostenasek F.J., 1948. Prefrontal lobotomy for the relief of intractable pain. *Bull. John Hopkins Hosp.*, **83**, 229–236.
21. Wolberg L.R., 1948. *Medical Hypnosis*, Vol. 1. Grune and Stratton, New York.
22. Evans F.J., 1977. The placebo control of pain: a paradigm for investigating non-specific effects in psychotherapy. In: *Psychiatry. Areas of Promise and Advancement* (eds Brady, Mendels, Reiger and Orne). Spectrum, New York.
23. Evans F.J., 1985. Expectancy, therapeutic instructions and the placebo response. In: *Placebo. Clinical Phenomena and New Insights* (eds White, Tursky and Schwarts). Guildford Press, New York.
24. Kroger W.S., 1980. Pain. A holistic approach. In: *Clinical Hypnosis in Medicine* (ed Wain). Symposium Specialists, Chicago.
25. Frankel F.H., 1976. *Hypnosis. Trance as a Coping Mechanism.* Plenum, New York.
26. Ewin D.M., 1986. Hypnosis and pain management. In: *Hypnosis, Questions and Answers* (eds Zilbergeld, Edelstien and Araoz). Norton, New York.
27. Finer B., Lindstrom B., Melander B. *et al.*, 1980. Psychosomatic treatment of chronic pain patients. In: *Hypnosis in Psychotherapy and Psychosomatic Medicine* (eds Pajntar, Roskar and Lavric).
28. Goldie L., 1956. Hypnosis in the casualty department. *Br. Med. J.*, **2**, 1340–1342.
29. Sutherland R.J. and Knox J., 1976. Hypnosis for endoscopy. *Lancet*, **ii**, 1244.
30. Chaves J.F. and Barber T.X., 1976. Hypnotic procedures and surgery: a critical analysis with applications to 'acupuncture analgesia'. *Am. J. Clin. Hypnosis*, **18**, 217–236.
31. Scott D.L., 1976. Hypnosis in pedicle graft surgery. *Br. J. Plastic Surg.*, **29**, 8–13.
32. Scott D.L., 1980. Hypnotherapy in plastic surgery. In: *Hypnosis in Psychotherapy and Psychosomatic Medicine* (eds Pajntar, Roskar and Lavric). University Press, Ljubljana.

CHAPTER 19

Hypnotherapy in Obstetrics

Many of the ailments which human beings experience arise solely through belief, suggestion and expectation. It is generally assumed that women must suffer great pain and discomfort during childbirth. This is partly the result of folklore and gossip and thus the average woman is bound to suffer increased pain at her confinement because her mind has been so conditioned.

The earlier work of Grantley Dick-Read[1] recognized this fact, and his explanation of the *fear–tension–pain* syndrome, did much to alter the entire approach to obstetrics. The methods which he employed so successfully to deal with this, consisted of education, relaxation and suggestion. Although he described a 'trance-like' state which occurred in some of his patients during labour, he stoutly denied that hypnosis played any part in the techniques he evolved. Nevertheless suggestion formed such an integral component of the Dick-Read procedure that there is not the slightest doubt that hypnosis would have greatly enhanced the use and effectiveness of his methods.

Since the causes of pain during childbirth have a large psychological overlay, it is obvious that the most effective methods of dealing with them must also be psychological. It should be remembered, however, that the hard work and effort connected with labour cannot be avoided, but much of the pain and mental anxiety can. Training in the hypnotic state will teach the expectant mother to exercise a remarkable degree of mental control over her bodily functions.

It is remarkable that the extent to which hypnosis may be used in obstetrics is not more widely known. The reduction of the awareness of pain is not the only advantage of its use. The feeling of well being of the mother and the condition of the child after delivery are also greatly enhanced. However, it is essential that the doctor who undertakes to use hypnosis in obstetrics should *always* be present during the labour and delivery. Some practitioners delegate responsibility to the nurse or midwife who will be in attendance, but this is an unsatisfactory practice. Trust in the doctor who has cared for the patient during the weeks preceding labour is an invaluable asset to the successful conduct of the birth of the child.

Hypnotherapy may be used in obstetrics for the following purposes:

1. To create a satisfactory state of mind to the pregnancy, labour and delivery as well as to the aftercare of the child.

2. To remove associated fears.

3. To teach self-hypnosis as a relaxation technique for twice daily use in the weeks before term. Many physiotherapists teaching groups of pregnant ladies use a method of instruction which is without doubt a covert form of hypnotic induction.

4. To teach the patient to produce analgesia of the perineal area.

5. As a treatment of hyperemesis.

6. As a method of containing labour pains.

7. For use between contractions.

8. As a treatment for infertility.

The medical practitioner who uses hypnosis and suggestion will find that his efforts are amply repaid in the field of obstetrics alone. It is not nearly as time consuming as he might imagine, and whilst results vary from patient to patient there are few who fail to benefit to a considerable extent. Hypnosis is also helpful to the single-handed general practitioner obstetrician, particularly if some form of anaesthesia is required.

In obstetrics there are three essential requirements that the ideal anaesthetic agent should fulfil.

1. It should be capable of affording complete relief from pain, however severe.

2. It should not interfere with the normal mechanics of labour.

3. It should not depress either the respiration or the circulation of the child.

Whereas the most effective chemical anaesthetic agent is at the best a compromise, hypnosis fulfils all these conditions, and has been rightly called the ideal anaesthetic in midwifery.

The pregnant woman's ability to relax depends not only upon the extent of her suggestibility, but also upon her attitude to pregnancy, her emotional reaction to the event, her previous conditioning to pain, the level of her threshold of pain, and whether she is primiparous or multiparous. All the emotional factors, which play such an important part in influencing labour pains, can be controlled by hypnosis. But it also may minimize the pain 'felt' by the physical contraction of the uterus and the stretching and distension of tissues as the baby is being born.

Whereas hypnosis has a great deal to offer as an obstetric analgesic, two objections are usually put forward:

1. The time required to induce hypnosis, to produce depth and to train the patient in readiness for her confinement is considerable.

2. The degree of analgesia that can be obtained in any given case is unpredictable.

Now hypnosis itself is far from being a complicated or difficult procedure; moreover, since no apparatus or expense is involved, it is ideal for use in either home or hospital. Considerable depth is, of course, necessary to ensure complete anaesthesia and freedom from pain, but even if this is aimed at, since pregnancy affects mainly the younger age groups, in which hypnotizability is at its greatest, and the motivation for it is usually very strong, a sufficiently deep state can fairly easily be obtained, and even somnambulism is likely to occur in 20 to 25 per cent of cases.

As far as the training and preparation of the patient for her confinement is concerned, initially weekly, then fortnightly sessions of 20 to 30 minutes' duration are all that are required in the early stages, and even these may be extended to longer intervals, if necessary, provided she regularly uses self-hypnosis, until shortly before term. To ensure the best results, the patient should be seen weekly for about the last 6 weeks. At this stage, each individual treatment can be completed in approximately 15 minutes, and whilst it is true that the patient will have to be seen rather more frequently than under ordinary conditions, there is no doubt whatever that the extra trouble involved will be found to be well worth-while.

The objection regarding the unpredictability of the degree of analgesia that can be secured is certainly not valid since that is far from being the main objective of hypnotic treatment. Heron and Abramson[2] consider that the greatest value of hypnotic training lies in its ability to achieve the following:

1. The eradication of erroneous ideas by use of counter-suggestion.
2. The teaching of relaxation.
3. The teaching of self-hypnosis to the patient and the ability to produce such relaxation whenever required.

In their view, the induction of hypnotic analgesia is of secondary importance since relaxation itself will always automatically raise the threshold of pain. When the patient receives proper psychological preparation for labour, it is questionable whether induced anaesthesia is necessary since labour will tend to proceed with a minimum of discomfort except for that associated with hard work.

It is certainly true that if the expectant mother can be taught to relax, to feel confident, and to look forward to her confinement with pleasure as a most rewarding and satisfying experience, her labour is likely to be shortened in duration, much easier and far less distressing. Fortunately this can be achieved without deep hypnosis or somnambulism. Early training in both mental and physical relaxation can be achieved even in the lighter or medium stages of hypnosis, and can prevent a great deal of anxiety, apprehension and tension. Moreover, the increased confidence acquired will minimize the amount of anaesthesia required, should this have to be reinforced in the later expulsive stage. Heron and

Abramson[2] reported an average reduction of 20 per cent in the length of the first stage of labour in women who had received pre-natal hypnotic training, and some 20 per cent of their patients were able to achieve the deepest hypnotic states with spectacular results in the complete elimination of pain. In a study of 70 preg-nant women treated by hypnosis, Davidson[3] was able to show that the duration of labour was considerably reduced and nearly 60 per cent required no chemical analgesia.

In a more recent paper presented at the Second European Con-gress of Hypnosis held in Dubrovnik in 1980, Tiba *et al.*[4] showed that hypnotherapeutic preparation in obstetrics was highly effec-tive in the following:

1.   Decreasing fear of labour and delivery, independently of hyp-notic susceptibility.

2.   Increasing painlessness and co-operation during labour and delivery.

3.   Decreasing the amount of anaesthetic required.

They additionally found that hypnotherapeutic preparation seemed not only highly beneficial in the gestational period but that it may also help to develop an appropriate attitude in the mother towards the child.

Probably 90 per cent of all pregnant women can achieve some degree of hypnosis, depending largely upon the skill of the oper-ator and the personality of the individual patient. This always has to be taken into account, for the woman who has responded to menstruation, marriage or motherhood with fear and ap-prehension, will more likely tend to feel over-anxious, tense and apprehensive during pregnancy and labour. The great value of hypnosis is amply confirmed by the patient's subjective reactions to the experience when questioned post-natally. Almost invari-ably the reply will be that future confinements will hold no ter-rors whatever, and that the patient will even look forward to having another baby under similar circumstances.

Summary of the Advantages of Hypnosis in Obstetrics

1. *It can greatly increase the patient's ability to relax, both men-tally and physically.*   Under hypnosis, the patient will readily ac-

cept the fact that there is nothing to fear, and that since she will be able to relax completely, the tension and pain will disappear, and her labour will become very much easier. She is easily taught to gain much more control over her bodily functions.

2. *It produces no depression of the respiratory or circulatory functions, in either mother or child.* In using chemical anaesthetic agents or other medication the potential risk to the foetus must always be considered. This is particularly a problem when powerful analgesics are employed. Not only is this danger avoided in hypnosis, but there is much less need for the use of any drugs at all, and consequently much less risk to mother and child. Fuchs *et al.*[5], evaluating the influence of maternal hypnosis, noted a significant increase in foetal activity as a result. This, they believed, was due to a reduction of maternal anxiety and improvement in placental blood perfusion.

3. *Hypnosis usually effects some shortening of the first stage of labour.* Evidence has shown that this reduction will generally amount to at least 2 hours in the case of multiparae, and possibly to between 3 and 4 hours in primiparae.

4. *Hypnosis increases the patient's resistance to obstetric shock.* The risk of shock is greatly diminished since the mother becomes much less exhausted during the first stage. Under hypnosis, she can eat, drink, sleep and attend to her natural functions. She is able to co-operate fully with both doctor and midwife, even when the contractions are strong and frequent. The mother is also enabled to relax her muscles so completely that the danger of foetal injury is much reduced.

5. *Hypnosis does not interfere in any way with the normal mechanics of labour.* Both general anaesthetics and analgesic or sedative drugs have the disadvantage of exercising a depressing action upon uterine contractions. They consequently tend to delay and to prolong labour. Under hypnosis drugs may often be dispensed with altogether, and even when some supplementary medication is required the effective dosage will be much reduced.

6. *In the lighter and medium stages hypnosis greatly reduces the liability to pain by relieving the fear–pain–tension syndrome, and*

substituting the ability to relax, both mentally and physically. Even in the second stage, when the contractions become stronger and more frequent, the patient who has been taught in hypnosis to couple suggestions of increasing relaxation with deep, rhythmic breathing, can greatly relieve, and sometimes even remove all feelings of pain. It is only as the head descends and the perineum becomes distended that pain is likely to be felt, and supplementary measures are needed to keep it under control. In the course of her prenatal training, the patient should always be told that inhalation anaesthesia and analgesic drugs will be readily available should she require them. Whether they are actually used or not should be left to the mother herself. Some women resent a general anaesthetic as they feel they have missed the delight of hearing the baby's first cry; for this reason alone the mother's wish should always be respected.

7. *In the somnambulistic stages of hypnosis partial or complete analgesia and anaesthesia may be produced in any part of the body by direct suggestion.* The patient's ability to produce complete muscular relaxation is tremendously increased and the perineum can often be rendered completely insensitive during the second stage. Acute pain is most likely to be felt as the head crowns, but direct suggestion can greatly lessen its intensity and may sometimes succeed in removing it altogether.

In complete somnambulism, particularly if amnesia has been obtained during prenatal training, labour can usually be rendered completely painless. Kroger[6] pointed out that the subjective pain element need not be completely lost. In his view, the pain of childbirth is a necessary psychological experience, and he therefore considers it important that the patient can be awakened at any time to feel the contractions and to see the birth of her baby.

Somnambulistic patients always enter deep hypnosis immediately upon a prearranged signal. They can be told that whenever the contractions occur, no matter how heavy or frequent they may be, no pain will be felt. The only sensations experienced will be those of a certain amount of discomfort and pressure, and even this will be rendered much less uncomfortable by bearing down when instructed to do so. The behaviour of somnambulistic patients is remarkable as they remain calm, quiet and relaxed throughout their labour.

8. *In these stages, hypnosis affords almost complete control over the rate of expulsion of the head and shoulders.* As the head is about to emerge, the uterine contractions become so powerful, frequent and urgent that the mother feels it impossible to stop pushing, even when told not to do so. The perineum is consequently given no opportunity to stretch and will often tear. However, the moment that the hypnotized patient is told to stop pushing she will obey implicitly and so allow her abdominal muscles to relax completely leaving the contractions to do their own work, and when she is told to push, she will do so more effectively. The obstetrician therefore has control over the rate of delivery, and perineal tears are much more likely to be avoided.

9. *An episiotomy can be performed quite painlessly, under hypnosis alone.* If perineal repair is required, it can easily be done without pain and without anaesthesia. The third stage and the expulsion of the placenta usually proceeds quite normally under hypnosis, and the average blood loss seems to be appreciably diminished.

10. *Post-operative recovery is usually both smooth and uneventful.* Most women feel remarkably fit and well after hypnotic delivery and show much less physical and mental exhaustion. The fact that they can move their legs freely and exercise their muscles immediately following the birth greatly diminishes the risk of any subsequent venous thrombosis. Other complications also seem much less likely to occur, and there is also less danger to the child.

11. *Lactation can be stimulated, and breast feeding facilitated by direct suggestion under hypnosis.* This is hardly surprising, for it is well known that the physiological process of lactation can often be seriously influenced by conscious and unconscious emotional disturbances.

In brief, the greatest value of hypnosis in the field of obstetrics lies in its ability to produce complete mental and physical relaxation, together with the relief of fear and anxiety. Once the element of fear is removed the patient will approach her confinement with confidence, and consequently only a minimum of analgesia is likely to be required. It is important that the general practitioner should remember that even when the depth of hypnosis is insufficient to remove all pain, repeated suggestion, with or without supplementary medication, can still render labour a great deal easier by abolishing the *fear–tension–pain* syndrome.

The Disadvantages of Hypnosis in Obstetrics

1. *Prejudice against the idea of hypnosis itself.*

2. *The time and effort required to produce and deepen the trance and to give adequate prenatal training.*

3. *The variability of degrees of susceptibility to hypnosis.* These three objections have already been fully discussed.

4. *Lack of co-operation and understanding on the part of trained personnel.* The patient may lose whatever composure she has acquired during her prenatal training if she is admitted to a ward where other women, in various stages of labour, are causing disturbances. In domiciliary midwifery, this difficulty will not arise, but the practitioner may have to work with a midwife who fails to understand or is totally unsympathetic to the idea of hypnosis. Even during the early stages of labour, it is essential that the patient should remain quiet, and be allowed to relax and sleep. She should be aroused only when necessary. In too many instances, the midwife fails to grasp this fact, and often disturbs and worries the patient by rousing her and talking to her unnecessarily.

THE TECHNICAL APPLICATION OF HYPNOSIS IN OBSTETRICS

If delivery is to take place in hospital it is essential that ward staff be fully advised as to the procedure.

The most successful results will always be obtained when the obstetrician undertakes the induction of hypnosis and the prenatal training of the patient, and is subsequently present to conduct the confinement. In the case of home confinement, the general practitioner is in a much better position to use it successfully than anyone else. Hypnosis can be undertaken by a professional colleague, and provided that both are present at the confinement and working as a team, excellent results will be obtained.

Hypnosis is not necessarily contraindicated when the patient is to be delivered by a midwife alone. Provided that the mother has been adequately prepared, she will still be able to relax completely and greatly diminish her discomfort, particularly if she has been taught how to put herself into a trance whenever she wishes to do so. She can then be put 'en rapport' with the midwife, whose instructions she will be told to follow exactly as if they were given by the obstetrician himself. The midwife must naturally be fully instructed as to the conduct of the labour, and *must co-operate fully* in complying with any special conditions that need to be observed. For instance, no matter how successful the patient may have been throughout the earlier stages of labour, she is quite likely to break down and lose control as the actual delivery becomes imminent. At this point, she should certainly be given some form of supplementary analgesia should she desire it.

It is essential that the patient should receive adequate preparation for her confinement during the prenatal period. It is unlikely that hypnosis will achieve any degree of success if the first induction has to take place whilst labour is in progress. It is necessary to see the patient for the first time as soon as possible after the pregnancy has been confirmed, although some authorities defer this until just before the seventh month of gestation. The sooner misconceptions, fears, anxieties and tensions are removed, the more quickly the patient can be trained to look forward to her confinement rather than to dread it. Moreover, the necessary contact can be made with the midwife, and early discomforts such as morning sickness, heartburn or flatulence can be dealt with.

The patient should initially be seen weekly in the course of which she is trained to achieve as deep a state of hypnosis as possible, any existing problems are dealt with, and further training and conditioning of the patient's mind is commenced. Very often, depending upon the personality of the individual, these preliminary sessions may be extended to fortnightly intervals. As soon as sufficient progress has been made, the sessions may be spaced out, and then the patient is told to return between the seventh and eighth month or, should she so desire, is seen at monthly or six weekly periods in the interim. It is essential to see the patient once a week for the last six weeks of her pregnancy.

Prenatal Training

This is by far the most important part of the patient's preparation for her confinement, and has two main objects:

1. To teach the patient to relax, both mentally and physically, to the greatest possible extent in order to ensure as easy a labour as possible.
2. To teach the patient to gain increased control over her body functions by achieving a positive and healthy attitude of mind.

There can be no doubt that by far the best and easiest way of securing a satisfactory delivery lies in the proper antenatal preparation for the event.

The first interview. Contact should be made with the patient, and every possible step taken to put her completely at ease. As in every other kind of hypnotic work, this is of vital importance, for if you have failed to gain the patient's complete confidence by the end of the first session, it is most unlikely that you will ever be able to achieve really satisfying results. In the course of general conversation, directed towards the discovery of her ideas and attitudes concerning pregnancy and childbirth, try to assess her potentialities, both as a possible hypnotic subject, and with regard to motherhood. If it is felt that she may be a suitable subject, try to introduce the possibilities of hypnosis, and explain its many advantages. At the same time, be equally frank concerning its limitations.

Begin by telling the patient that since childbirth is a perfectly natural process, there is no reason why it should be either painful or unpleasant. That pain largely occurs because the patient expects it, and is afraid of it, and because she is unable to prevent all her muscles from becoming rigid and tense. Since hypnosis will teach her to be able to get rid of all this tension by relaxing her muscles during her confinement, there will be no reason why she should expect to have pain, and that she should consequently have a much easier time. Tell her that if she wishes hypnosis to be used it can help her greatly, but that she must not expect magical results. What can be achieved will depend firstly upon her own desire and ability to co-operate, and secondly upon the depth of hypnosis she can achieve with training.

Never make any over-enthusiastic promises. Try to discover her own ideas, fears and reservations concerning hypnosis, and deal with these by explaining, as simply as possible what hypnosis is really like, and how it works. In this connection, emphasize the fact that there is not the slightest question of giving up control but that it is purely a matter of team work.

Tell her that it will probably take two or three sessions to discover that greatest depth of hypnosis that she is capable of achieving. If she is a deep subject then it should be possible to render her confinement almost painless. This, however, must not be relied upon since only about 20 per cent of women are capable of this depth. She can, however, be sure of one thing. Even as a result of the lighter stages, she will be able to relax, both mentally and physically, so much more successfully during her labour that she will certainly have a much easier time than she would otherwise have done.

Never, under any circumstances, make any attempt to induce hypnosis in the course of this first interview. This should be limited to eliciting the facts, to the removal of doubts and fears, and to the encouragement of the patient's motivation. Invite her to think over carefully, during the forthcoming week, all that she has been told, and to ask any questions that may occur to her next time.

The second interview. Begin by asking the patient whether she has been thinking about last week's discussion, and whether there are any questions she would like to ask. Deal with these first in order to dispel as far as possible any remaining doubts and uncertainties. Then explain, in the simplest possible terms, the method of inducing hypnosis, and tell the patient exactly what she has to do and what she may expect to happen. Follow by inducing hypnosis for the first time but make no attempt to gain real depth. Awaken the patient and discuss with her in some detail her own subjective sensations and reactions. Explain to her that learning hypnosis is just like learning to ride a bicycle for the first time. On the first occasion, somebody has to give support by holding the saddle all the time. On the next occasion, this support can be withdrawn for brief periods, during which the patient would be able to proceed on her course, wobbly and uncertain though this progress might be, to be supported only if there was any danger of falling off. On subsequent occasions the rider would do more and more on her own, until eventually riding would become just as natural an act as walking.

Tell the patient that, as soon as she has achieved the necessary depth, she will be taught how to use hypnosis herself, during her confinement. It is always important to obtain the husband's consent before hypnosis is induced for the first time.

Subsequent interviews. The hypnosis should be deepened until the patient has achieved the greatest depth of which she is capable. Should this prove insufficient for any marked degree of analgesia, instill into the patient's mind, under hypnosis, the following idea:

> During your confinement...*you will feel so very relaxed...so very, very sleepy and drowsy...that you will feel much less discomfort than if you were wide awake.*

In all future discussions with the patient, it is wise to avoid the words 'pain' or 'labour pains', when referring to uterine contractions, which should be simply described as such, even in connection with the actual confinement. The word pressure or contraction is infinitely preferable to the word 'pain'.

When it is possible to induce localized analgesia to a painful stimulus such as pin prick, test for somnambulism (by getting the patient to open her eyes without awakening from the trance) and for amnesia. If these are successful the labour can be rendered entirely painless throughout, but you, the doctor, *must* be present. This can still occur in your absence, but there is a risk of the patient's control breaking down at the worst moment just as the head is about to emerge. This will be the only point at which some form of supplementary anaesthesia may be needed.

If localized analgesia can be produced by suggestion, it is useful to demonstrate to the patient how it can be transferred to any region of the body. Deep subjects can be taught how to produce it for themselves, at will, under certain restricted circumstances which must also be clearly defined when the appropriate post-hypnotic suggestion is given. Such patients as these, however, will unfortunately always be in the minority. Nevertheless, the majority will still be able to attain a calmness of mind, and a satisfactory relaxation during light- or medium-depth hypnosis to serve them well at their confinement.

The fact that it may prove impossible to produce any marked degree of analgesia to pin prick does not mean that the patient will be unable to exercise a considerable amount of control over physiological pain in her confinement. But it will naturally be necessary for the patient to attend more frequently for antenatal training than if complete somnambulism were achieved. In the latter case, not only need the prenatal training be less prolonged, but much greater use may be made of direct suggestion and post-hypnotic suggestion in the conduct of the labour itself. Moreover, it is possible for analgesia to be produced very rapidly indeed, either upon word of command or as the result of a predetermined signal. The question has been raised as to whether hypnotic analgesia is, in effect, nothing but amnesia. This seems to be disproved by the fact that analgesia can often be obtained in waking hypnosis, when no amnesia at all has been secured.

The Use of Self-hypnosis in Labour

The teaching of self-hypnosis can prove to be an invaluable asset in all cases in which sufficient depth has been obtained. In medium depth, the patient can usually be taught to produce a trance state herself at will, and to produce complete mental and physical relaxation by self-suggestion. Whilst the average depth of such auto-hypnosis is not great, it is quite sufficient to be of material assistance, particularly in the first stage of labour. The resulting analgesia is due to relaxation, and the relief of tension, fear and anxiety rather than to direct suggestion. The technique should be taught as early as possible and the patient encouraged to use it daily in her own home throughout her antenatal period. In this way she gradually gains confidence, not only in her own power of control, but also in her ability to secure complete relaxation and diminution of pain and discomfort during her confinement.

During her labour, the patient can make use of self-hypnosis in one of two ways:

1. She can induce it shortly after the onset of labour, and maintain the trance state undisturbed for considerable periods of time.

2. She can induce it each time she feels a contraction, and maintain it solely for the duration of each contraction.

She may elect to use either method or both alternately according to circumstances. The medium-depth patient usually appears to derive most benefit from the first procedure, and it is only the somnambule who is likely to achieve complete success and relief from the second.

The patient using self-hypnosis will generally 'sleep' or relax continuously throughout the earlier stages. She will often lie quite motionless and will require no attention other than routine care and observation. She will be able to converse, to empty her bladder or attend to her bowels, or to be fed at her own request. The midwife should be instructed not to talk to her or disturb her unnecessarily at this stage. An understanding and sympathetic midwife can greatly enhance the effectiveness of self-hypnosis, indeed it may even be said that her attitude may well determine the difference between success and failure.

Somnambulistic patients, however, can be taught to induce a deep trance state, a complete analgesia and often, amnesia, within a matter of 5 to 10 seconds. This speed is essential if the patient is to retain full control during the height of delivery, when there is little intermission between the strong and frequent uterine contractions. In these cases self-hypnosis can be taught through post-hypnotic suggestion.

> In a few moments...when I count up to *seven...you will open your eyes and be wide awake, again.*
> After I have wakened you, I shall talk to you for a minute or two. *You will then put yourself straight off to sleep again...into a sleep, just as deep as this one.*
> You will lie back, comfortably...fix your eyes on a spot upon the ceiling...and count slowly up to five.
> As you count...your eyes will become more and more tired...you will feel drowsier and drowsier...and, the moment you have reached

> five...your eyes will close immediately...and you will fall
> immediately into a sleep, just as deep as this one.

Then wake the patient, chat to her briefly, and tell her to put herself to sleep again. This she does without difficulty. Continue by telling her that, whenever she needs to put herself to sleep, particularly during her confinement, she will always be able to do so immediately by counting up to five. Subsequently teach her how to produce complete mental and physical relaxation through appropriate self-suggestions, and how to induce localized analgesia whenever she needs to do so, by simply suggesting to herself that all pain will completely disappear the moment she counts up to three. For obvious reasons, however, she must *not* be left with the ability to do this with regard to each and every kind of pain. Strictly limited conditions must be clearly defined, and she must be told that she will be able to remove pain in this way only during her confinement: no other type of pain will respond and on no other occasion will this method achieve the slightest success.

Instruct the patient to practise this self-hypnosis regularly in her own home to produce complete mental and physical relaxation, and renew the post-hypnotic suggestions that she will be able to exercise complete control over pain *during her confinement* at each subsequent prenatal training session.

Brief hypnosis may also be taught for use when required during early labour.

THE MANAGEMENT OF ANTENATAL HYPNOTIC TRAINING

Once satisfactory trance depth has been obtained and the technique of self-hypnosis mastered, whenever this is possible, the next most important step is to give the patient as simple an explanation as possible of the three stages of labour, and what she may expect to feel or to happen in each of these stages. Explain it to the patient in the following manner:

> In every confinement, there are three separate and distinct stages.
> The first and longest of these is concerned with the necessary
> preparation for the birth of the child. This could not occur unless
> time were given for all the muscles to relax, and the passages to

widen and dilate sufficiently to permit the passage of the baby. Once these are wide open, the second and more active stage occurs. During this, the child descends through the passages, and eventually emerges and is born. When this has happened, there is still the final stage, which is not completed until the afterbirth has come away.

Now, probably the first sign that you will have that labour has started is a slight show of blood, almost as if a monthly period were beginning. With this you will feel some weak contractions of the womb, with long intervals between them. Sometimes, the show does not occur, and the only sign of commencing labour is the presence of these weak, infrequent, but regular uterine contractions. When you first feel these, look at the clock and time them. No matter how long elapses between them, if they are occurring at regular intervals, you have probably started in labour, so either send for the midwife, or go straight into hospital according to your previous arrangements.

You must not induce any hypnotic trance until this has been done.

During this first stage, you will find that the contractions will be weak, and will not occur very often. They will gradually cause the passages to open up, but this is a slow process and takes time. They will cause so little discomfort to begin with, that the only thing you will need to do is to sleep as much as possible, and to relax. You will be able to do this by putting yourself to sleep and relaxing in hypnosis as you have been taught. Because of this, you will feel the contractions merely as pressure in your stomach, and they will not distress you at all. If anything, or anyone disturbs you, you will immediately put yourself straight off to sleep again, as a result of which your labour will progress more steadily and easily. You will remain perfectly calm and unworried, and not in the least bit afraid.

Later, as the passages open up, the contractions will become stronger, heavier and more frequent. You will not become frightened or try to resist this, because this is perfectly normal and helps the baby to be born. This is a sign that your labour is progressing well. You will be able to stay in your trance and remain relaxed by taking a series of deep, rapid, rhythmic breaths. With each of these, you will relax more and more completely. All tension will disappear and you will feel only the discomfort of heavier pressure from each contraction. You will not lose control, and will remain perfectly passive, allowing the contractions to do their own work, without trying to assist in any way.

A short pause may occur, after which the contractions will recommence with increased strength. About this time, the membranes will rupture and the waters escape. There is no need to become worried or alarmed about this. It merely means that you have entered into the second stage of your labour, and the actual birth and expulsion of your child is about to begin. Although the contractions become much heavier and more frequent, they will not frighten you, because soon it will be necessary for you to co-operate and help in getting your baby born. As the contractions continue, you will begin to feel an almost irresistible desire to assist by bearing down. No matter when this occurs, *you must not give way to it, until you are told to do so.*

If you do, you will delay the birth of your child, render it more difficult, and wear yourself out unnecessarily, without doing a scrap of good. As soon as you feel this urge, tell the midwife or nurse, but do not give way to it until she tells you to. When she does, take a deep breath, hold it as long as you can, and push down as hard as you can as long as each contraction lasts. If you have to breathe out before the contraction is over, take another deep breath as quickly as possible and continue to hold it and push down, since it is usually the last part of the contraction that produces most progress. You will find that this will greatly reduce the discomfort. Remember, as you bear down and push, how much you are helping to bring your baby into the world, because this could not be done without some hard work and physical exertion. It will be well worth while. In each interval, between the contractions, you will be able to relax completely, and sleep.

As the baby's head descends, and appears at the outlet, the final process of delivery is about to begin. At this point, you will be able to obey all instructions implicitly. Whenever you are told to stop pushing, you will stop pushing immediately, and indulge in rapid deep breathing instead. As a result of this you will relax more and more completely, and as the head presses down harder and harder on the outlet, the whole area will become quite numb and insensitive. You will experience a feeling of stretching, and the sensation of something passing through the outlet.

Although you will probably require no extra help, suitable drugs

or anaesthetics will be available if you feel the need of them.
They will not be given to you unless you request them. You have
only to ask. If, on the other hand, you wish to remain awake as
your baby is born, you have only to say so. When you have seen
the baby, and the afterbirth has come away, you will fall into a
deep refreshing sleep. You will wake up from this feeling really
fit and well, and remembering very little of what has occurred.
Throughout the whole of your labour, you will be able to talk, or
answer questions if necessary, without waking up from your deep,
relaxed, hynotic sleep. You will be able to co-operate in every way,
but you will feel far too sleepy and drowsy to become disturbed.
You will carry out faithfully every instruction that you are given,
just as effectively as if I had given them, myself.

The main object of subsequent antenatal hypnotic training sessions is to condition the patient to become completely relaxed,
both mentally and physically, whenever she enters the trance
state; to remove fear and apprehension, and to instil suggestions
of confidence and general and physical well being. This conditioning is more effective if the patient is taught self-hypnosis and
practises it regularly at home, thereby gaining much more confidence in her own power to control her reactions during the confinement.

When teaching self-hypnosis and in the course of each ordinary
hypnotic induction, it is always advisable to couple suggestions
of increased relaxation with deep, rhythmic breathing. Once this
technique has been mastered by the patient, it will prove invaluable in the alleviation of pain and distress during her actual labour.

The suggestions to be impressed upon the patient's mind at each
training session can easily be constructed from the detailed description of labour under hypnosis which has already been given
to her. These should be selected and phrased to suit each individual case, in accordance with certain general principles:

1. Suggestions that the patient will continue to keep fit and
well throughout her pregnancy.
2. That she will look forward to her confinement with pleasure
and happiness, and not with dread and apprehension.
3. That everything is perfectly normal (provided, of course, that

this fact has been clinically established).

4. That, during her labour, she will fall into a deep hypnotic sleep whenever she is told to do so, or upon a pre-arranged signal she gives herself to induce self-hypnosis, and all subsequent suggestions will be both accepted and acted upon.

5. That each contraction of the womb will be felt as a not altogether unpleasant sensation. Even during the second stage, the feelings experienced will be simply those of increasing pressure, comparable in every way to ordinary physical exertion.

Care must be taken not to abolish *all* her sensations, otherwise labour might well commence without the patient becoming aware of the fact.

6. That every time she puts herself into a deep hypnotic sleep, she will be able to relax her muscles and relieve tension so completely that she will feel much less discomfort. The contractions will bother her very much less, and the delivery of the baby will become much easier.

7. That subsequently her breasts will more likely produce plenty of milk, so that she will be able to breast feed her child should she so wish, without difficulty.

This last suggestion is likely to be successful since the commonest causes of deficient lactation are worry and fear. Hypnosis seems to abolish these by inducing an attitude of positive expectancy.

8. That once the confinement is over, and she has slept, she will wake up feeling perfectly fit and well, and may, if she so desires, remember little or nothing about it.

These specialized suggestions should be preceded by the usual ego-strengthening routine on every occasion. During the last six weeks of pregnancy, special emphasis is placed upon those suggestions relating to the patient's reactions and behaviour, and the instructions she is to follow during her confinement.

If the practitioner by any chance, will be unable to be present at the confinement, the patient must be placed post-hypnotically 'en rapport' with some other individual—doctor, nurse or midwife—with whose instructions she will comply as if they had been issued by the hypnotist. For this procedure to succeed, the deeper stages of hypnosis will have to be attained, and the individual to whom rapport is transferred fully informed as to the correct method of conducting a labour under hypnosis.

Hyperemesis Gravidarum

This is a very common problem which may be considered to be psychogenic in origin and to represent an expression of disgust and rejection and a conscious or unconscious wish to get rid of the pregnancy. It has also been suggested that the customary disappearance of the symptom between the third and the fourth month occurs because foetal movements compel the mother to accept it as a separate individual. Other psychological factors may lie behind this symptom: disturbed marital relations, a craving for or even lack of affection, and fears concerning the birth and subsequent rearing of the child may all play a part. Sometimes vomiting is regular and really severe, in other instances there is nothing more than nausea. No matter how severe the case, hypnosis can always prove extremely useful, even when it is combined with other therapeutic measures. Direct suggestion under hypnosis, constantly repeated and re-inforced, is capable of curing over 50 per cent of cases. In resistant cases treatment should also be directed towards the patient's emotional attitudes and not aimed at the symptom alone.

A modified version of the routine 'ego-strengthening' suggestions, followed by direct symptom removal has been found effective:

> As you focus your attention on your stomach...*you will begin to experience a feeling of warmth, spreading into your stomach.*
> That feeling of warmth is increasing...with every word that I utter, warm and comfortable...warm and comfortable...As soon as you feel that warmth...please raise your index finger.
> That's right.
> Now, put it down again.
> *And as your stomach feels warmer...it is beginning to feel more normal...more and more comfortable.*
> All feelings of sickness are passing away completely...you no longer feel at all sick.
> Your stomach feels perfectly normal...and comfortable, in every way.
> And in a few moments...when I count up to *seven*...you will open

your eyes, and be wide awake, again.
You will wake up...with your stomach completely
comfortable...without the slightest feeling of sickness or
*discomfort...*and you will find that...*when you wake up, each*
morning...you will not feel the slightest trace of sickness
whatever...your stomach will remain perfectly normal...without
the slightest discomfort of any kind.
And, with every one of these treatments...this trouble is going to
disappear...more and more quickly...more and more completely.

In a further interesting paper, Fuchs *et al.*[7] published a report
on 138 women suffering from extremely severe vomiting in the
first trimester of pregnancy who were treated by medical hypnosis. Eighty seven of the patients were treated in groups and 51
were treated individually. In the former, no patients were hospi-
talized and treatment was easier and more efficient. Sixty one patients were cured of vomiting and nausea, 24 patients were cured
of vomiting but some nausea remained and two patients only
failed to improve. Suggestions given under hypnosis were of calmness and composure, of happiness and the good general progress
of the pregnancy.

Heartburn and Flatulence

Causation is most frequently psychogenic, and a great deal can
be achieved simply by the alleviation of anxiety and tension. The
condition usually subsides quickly under direct hypnotic suggestion, if this is combined with a full discussion and explanation of
the harmlessness of the symptom.

Many other prenatal symptoms such as backache, pruritus and
insomnia can be greatly relieved by hypnosis.

HYPNOSIS IN COMPLICATED OR OBSTRUCTED LABOUR

Much has been written to advocate the use of hypnosis in obstetrics, but there are few authenticated reports of its possible dangers and disadvantages in any particular case. Attention should
be drawn to certain practical difficulties that may arise in complicated cases if relations between hypnotist and obstetrician are
not sufficiently close. The following case history should conse-

quently prove of interest:

Case history.   Mrs Blank, 25 years old, was referred on January 7th. She was expecting her first child in April and was anxious to gain any relief that hypnosis might offer her in the course of her confinement. Since there seemed to be some degree of pelvic contraction she was sent to a consultant obstetric and gynaecological surgeon, who arranged for her to be confined in the local maternity hospital. She subsequently attended for hypnosis once a week for the first six weeks, and from then on once a fortnight until her confinement on April 15th.

There was no difficulty in inducing hypnosis, and by the end of several sessions she was trained to achieve reasonable depth and to enter the hypnotic state on a selected cue word. She never became completely somnambulistic, and she developed only a partial amnesia. At this depth her sensitivity to painful stimuli could be blunted but never completely abolished, so that absolute analgesia was never actually achieved.

She learned the technique of self-hypnosis without difficulty and she was able, during antenatal training, to achieve complete relaxation and to gain some control over pain such as backache. But considering her repeated failure to produce satisfactory analgesia to painful stimuli artificially induced, it was not expected that her confinement would be completely painless, and it was doubtful as to how far she would be able to exercise her power of control over pain during labour.

At each antenatal session, during hypnosis, it was impressed upon her that she would be able during her confinement to put herself into a trance, to relax all her muscles and thus to remove her pains. She would *not,* however, be able to free herself entirely from sensations of discomfort, and she would always remain fully conscious of the pressure of her uterine contractions.

On one occasion she arrived with her arm in a sling. It appeared that she and her husband had been involved in a motor accident in which she had sustained injuries to her right arm and shoulder. When her husband extracted her from the car she was in great pain, and he went off to the nearest farmhouse to seek assistance. On his return he found that she had put herself into a hypnotic trance and was completely free from pain.

The onset of labour occurred on April 14th. The patient was seen by her own doctor and admitted to hospital. When visited that evening she was fast asleep. She was quite comfortable, but little progress had been made because her contractions were very poor. The following afternoon it was evident that a Caesarean section would almost certainly be necessary. The operation was performed successfully under ordinary anaesthesia and both mother and child subsequently did well.

In view of the difficulties in deciding upon surgical intervention in this case, the obstetrician involved has kindly supplied his own detailed account of the case:

Obstetrician's case history. I saw Mrs Blank on three occasions during the second half of pregnancy and she impressed me very much with her calm composure and happy anticipation of natural childbirth. She seemed entirely free from the physical and emotional strains that often complicate the antenatal period, and this may well have been partly due to the powers of inducing self-hypnosis. It became apparent from physical and X-ray examination that she was suffering from pelvic contraction which would undoubtedly lead to some degree of disproportion, but although she realized the implication of this it seemed to cause little, if any, anxiety.

Early labour. The onset of labour was marked by rupture of the membranes and regular uterine contractions which produced sensations of pressure, but no pain. It was thus difficult for her family doctor to advise that labour had started, and the same difficulty was encountered by the medical and nursing staff when she was admitted to the maternity hospital. It was unfortunate in view of the disproportion, that she should suffer from primary uterine inertia with rather poor contractions, but it was confirmed by examination that labour had commenced although little progress was made during the first 24 hours.

Advanced labour. In order to ensure that a full trial of labour had been carried out, she was treated by an intravenous infusion of oxytocin, using 2 units in 500 ml dextrose solution. This soon produced very strong uterine contractions which could be felt by observers, but there was still some doubt regarding their nature as Mrs Blank appeared to experience very little pain and repeatedly asked that they should be made more powerful to give her every chance of producing the baby naturally. It was only when a decision was reached some hours later that a Caesarean section would almost certainly be necessary that she lost her composure for the first time, indulging in a short fit of weeping and complaining of backache. There was still some doubt in the mind of at least one observer regarding the degree of uterine action that had in fact been achieved.

Delivery. When the uterus was explored and the baby delivered by lower segment Caesarean section, it was a surprise to find that the lower segment was very thin and that the retraction ring had risen almost to a dangerous height. It was clear that labour had advanced to a greater extent than had been apparent, due to the extreme composure of the patient and her failure to show any sign of systemic reaction to the strong contractions. There was in fact no danger to mother or child, but it is conceivable that in a multiparous patient labour might become dangerously advanced, possibly leading to some serious complications in similar circumstances.

Discussion. One difficulty of this case lay in arriving at an accurate decision as to when surgical intervention should be undertaken in the interest of both mother and child. This difficulty could have been minimized, and others eliminated, if conditions had permitted a closer co-operation between us as hypnotist and obstetrician, and if it had been possible for the hospital staff to have been fully instructed regarding the changed conditions imposed by hypnosis on the course of labour.

The ideal situation would be for the obstetrician himself to undertake the induction of hypnosis, the prenatal training of the patient and to conduct the confinement. In practice one must often be content with the closest co-operation between the obstetrician and the medical hypnotist concerned. The fact that such a difficulty can arise as that in the case described above leads us to underline the positive dangers that may occur when expectant mothers are trained to produce self-hypnosis and analgesia by unqualified hypnotists. We agree in drawing the following conclusions:

1. Where the medical hypnotist undertaking obstetric work is not himself conducting the confinement he should at all times be readily available for consultation during the labour, *but it is desirable that he should be present at the actual delivery.*

2. In complicated obstetric cases hypnotic analgesia should only be employed after full investigations have been undertaken and when the closest co-operation between medical hypnotist and obstetrician can be ensured.

3. In multiparous or complicated obstetric cases it is unwise and possibly dangerous to instruct the patient in the technique of self-hypnosis unless the above safeguards can be guaranteed.

4. Whenever the technique of self-hypnosis is taught, it is essential that both the attending obstetrician and midwife should be warned that the signs and symptoms of maternal distress or impending catastrophe may be dangerously masked, or even absent.

5. Ideally, any physician wishing to utilize the benefits of hypnosis for patients in his special field of training should properly be the one to induce the hypnosis in the patient.

HYPNOTHERAPY AND INFERTILITY

The problem of infertility is one which brings a great deal of distress to many married couples. Just as sexual potency in the male is the essential expression of manhood, so the ability to conceive is an affirmation of the woman's femininity.

Extensive investigations are invariably carried out in such cases but little attention is given to the individual personalities of the partners or to the relationship between them. Of the utmost importance is an assessment of the psychological status of the infertile female, in particular of her status before the infertility was known and of her level of anxiety both at that time and subsequently. The discovery of the infertility and the failure of investigatory procedures to reveal abnormality in either partner can result in considerable marital disharmony and thus the amount of stress is compounded.

In a recent paper, Mackett and Maden[8] point out that stress, acting via the hypothalamus, can modify pituitary function, upsetting the fine endocrine balance and thus interfere with the development and release of the ovum.

Acting upon this hypothesis and assuming that investigations have revealed no abnormality in either partner some consideration may be given to attempt to reduce the stress in order to achieve conception.

They further postulate that hypnotherapy seems the ideal method of reducing stress whilst avoiding any additional factor such as the interaction between the endocrine system and anxiolytic drugs. They describe the treatment of four patients who had failed to conceive over a period ranging from two to six years. The technique used involved relaxation, ego-strengthening and the teaching of self-hypnosis. All four patients managed to conceive, the duration of treatment being five days (three sessions) to two months (six sessions). Mackett and Maden conclude that where no physical bar to conception has been demonstrated, where hormone treatment has failed and where excessive anxiety is present, then hypnotherapy is a worthwhile adjunct to the management of certain cases of infertility.

REFERENCES

1. Dick-Read G., 1944. *Childbirth Without Fear*. Harper, New York.
2. Heron W.T. and Abramson M., 1952, Hypnosis in obstetrics (a psychological preparation for childbirth). In: *Experimental Hypnosis* (ed. Le Cron). MacMillan, New York.
3. Davidson J.A., 1962. An assessment of the value of hypnosis in pregnancy and labour. *Br. Med. J.*, **ii,** 951–953.
4. Tiba J., Balogh I., Meszaros I. *et al.*, 1980. Hypnotherapy during pregnancy, delivery and child-bed; first steps in Hungary. In: *Hypnosis in Psychotherapy and Psychosomatic Medicine* (eds Pajntar, Rŏskar, Lavrič), University Press, Ljubljana.
5. Fuchs K., Zimmer E.Z., Eyal A. *et al.*, 1987. Is there any influence of maternal hypnosis on foetal well-being in uterus. Paper read at 4th European Congress of Hypnosis in Psychotherapy and Psychosomatic Medicine, Oxford.
6. Kroger W.S., 1962. *Psychosomatic Obstetrics, Gynaecology and Endrocrinology*. Thomas, Springfield, Ill.

7. Fuchs K., Paldi E., Abramovici H. *et al.*, 1980. Treatment of hyper-emesis gravidarum by hypnosis. *Int. J. Clin. Exp. Hypnosis,* **XXVIII,** 313–323.

8. Mackett J. and Maden W., 1987. Simple hypnotherapy for infertility. Paper read at 4th European Congress of Hypnosis in Psychotherapy and Psychosomatic Medicine, Oxford.

CHAPTER 20

Paediatric Hypnotherapy

The use of hypnotherapy with children can produce some remarkable and effective results which are extremely rewarding, not only to the patient but to parents and all who are involved with his or her care.

It is essential that the therapist is experienced in the treatment of children, is kindly, non-authoritarian and entirely non-threatening in his approach. It is usually suggested that hypnosis should not be used with any child below the age of seven years. This age is entirely empirical however. What must be the deciding factor is that the patient should have an understanding of what will be happening, with due regard to his age, intelligence and environmental background. Obviously, no child should be treated by hypnosis without permission of parent or guardian and it might be a wise precaution to have the practice nurse in the room or within earshot at all times. Another essential prerequisite is to interview parents or guardian and possibly other members of the family both together with the child and separately. Indeed, one may often find that the cause of the trouble lies with the attitude or behaviour of one or more persons other than with the patient. If this is the case, it may also be that direct counselling of the offending person or persons will be all that will be required.

Children are generally good subjects, responding well where a trusting relationship is established and often quite obviously enjoy the deepening process where fairy stories or the appropriate fantasy is used.

THE INDUCTION OF HYPNOSIS

Most children are readily hypnotized. The use of the word 'hypnosis' should be avoided as this may have certain fictitional connotations and could arouse undue anxiety.

The induction technique should be consistent with the child's level of intelligence and understanding of language, as well as with his interests and abilities. Emphasis should be placed on the fact that he is being taught to achieve this particular state of relaxation *by himself*, just as if he was learning to ride a bicycle or some other activity requiring personal control.

The child is first seated comfortably in a chair. He should not be asked to lie down except perhaps when treating nocturnal enuresis as this could possibly evoke feelings of insecurity. Normal lighting is essential, that is, daylight if sufficient or electric light if at night. Full reassurance must be given that he is being taught to achieve a very special kind of sleep by himself. That in that sleep he will hear everything that is being said and will be able to talk and move and yet remain asleep. One of the following methods of induction may be used.

1. *Eye Fixation with Progressive Relaxation*
The child is asked to fix his eyes on some point of his own choosing and told:

> I will count from one to ten and as I count your eyes become more and more tired and will want to close...One, two, three...More and more tired...Four, five, six...Wanting to close, more and more...Seven, eight, nine,
> Heavier and heavier...Blinking and wanting to close...Ten...Let them close.

He is then told that he will increase his feelings of comfort and relaxation by concentrating on each part of his body in turn from his head to his toes, as you speak about it. This is then done. Further deepening may be obtained by further counting. Subsequent to this the child is told to think of a situation that he had actually experienced at some time, during which he had felt totally happy and relaxed. This information had earlier been elicited during routine history taking and may for example be a memory such as playing on the beach whilst on holiday by the sea. Then he is asked to see himself, in that situation as you describe it to him. Or he may be asked to visualize his favourite television programme (provided of course, that it does not involve violence). The child himself may play the part of the hero as you elaborate upon it.

Further deepening can be obtained by balloon levitation as follows:

> Now just imagine yourself sitting on the grass in the park and
> resting back against a tree. The sun is shining and it's a lovely day.
> You are holding a large balloon in your hands. It is blown up
> and tied with string.
> What colour is the balloon?

The child answers. Successful visualization is thus confirmed by the identification of a specific colour of balloon and the depth of hypnosis is increased by the subsequent response to suggestions of arm levitation.

> Good...now just loop the end of the string around one finger of
> your right hand. Have you done that?

Wait for the answer, repeating the instruction if necessary.

> Good...now the balloon is filled with air and a gentle breeze is
> blowing...so just watch that balloon floating up in the air. Up, up
> and up, higher and higher...your finger goes up with it, so does
> your hand and your arm, higher and higher, higher and higher.

The limb is gently coaxed into the air by verbal suggestion, with the balloon at the end of the string tugging at the child's arm.

> Now suddenly the breeze has stopped, the balloon comes
> tumbling down...and so does your arm and hand and as your
> hand lands on your tummy (or your thigh or the chair) you drop
> into a very deep sleep instead.

The subject is now ready for treatment.

However, it must be noted that not all subjects can successfully visualize colour. The balloon may be some hazy object floating in the air. In addition, although the arm may not actually rise in the air, the patient will often have the *subjective* impression that it is so doing. This is not an infrequent occurrence and no reference should be made to this after the hypnotic session as the patient may feel that he has failed in some way.

2. *Erickson's Hand Levitation method*
This is an excellent technique for hypnotic induction in children.

> Now you are sitting comfortably in the chair. Just rest back and place your hands on your knees. Keep your eyes fixed on your hands and don't look away for one moment. Try to keep your hands as still as you can...but as hard as you try to keep your hands still, there will be some movement somewhere, in one of your hands...Keep watching your hands...
> Don't let your eyes wander away for one moment...
> There...did you see that...there was a tiny twitch of your left thumb.

The therapist has assiduously been observing the hands and picks up the smallest movement which will inevitably occur.

> Now watch for another twitch...
> There it goes...even more than before...And as you watch your hand, which has twitched, watch now how slowly the fingers begin to separate...ever so slowly...and as this happens the hand is lifting slowly up from your knee...the hand and the arm...there is goes...Keep watching...higher and higher...towards your face...and now your eyes feel heavier and heavier...heavier and heavier as your hand and your arm go higher and higher...towards your face...Now...your finger touches your eyelid...your eyes close...and sleep...deeply, deeply asleep.

Further suggestions of relaxation and deepening may then be given and the patient is ready for treatment.

3. *Raised Hand Technique*
The child is asked to hold his hand above his head and to look at his thumb nail. Alternatively he may be asked to hold a small picture or other interesting object above his head.

> Now fix your eyes on your thumb nail (or the picture or object)...don't look at anything else...watch it closely...As you watch it closely...note how your eyes become blurred...more and more

blurred...more hazy and blurred...so you can hardly see
clearly...and at the same time your eyes are becoming more and
more tired...more and more tired...and your arm and hand as well,
more and more tired all the time...Your eyes are so tired, they
want to close...Your arm and hand so tired, they want to drop onto
your lap...Let it happen...Your arm and hand drop to your lap and
your eyes close...There!
And deeply, deeply, deeply asleep.

Relaxation and deepening is reinforced as with previous methods.

It is useful to know that young children can also be hypnotized
with the eyes open if considered desirable. This might be an advantage where it is evident that fear might prevent the child from
entering the hypnotic state.

SOME PROBLEMS ARISING IN CHILDREN AND THEIR TREATMENT

Many of the problems from which adults suffer may also be
found in children.

Ambrose[1] maintained that tension is often the kernel of the
child's difficulties. The corollary would be therefore that by relief
of that tension the symptoms should disappear. To commence
with, the child, in spite of his age, should be given a simple and
rational explanation of his problem so that some understanding
may be obtained.

Coping abilities are just as relevant in childhood as they are in
adult life. Any situation of stress which raises anxiety to a level
which is above that with which the child can cope may be internalized. As a result, one or more of a wide range of neurotic disorders may follow, as they do under similar circumstances in
adults. Acting-out behaviour may occur, the child responding by
some action which is considered quite out of character.

Personality difficulties may arise or the child may become depressed. The latter is a problem which is certainly seen in children but because it is generally unexpected or not properly
explored, often fails to be recognized. More commonly a young person will present with many of the neuroses or problems earlier
described.

1. Generalized Anxiety

Certainly generalized and non-specific anxiety is a common problem. The inability to find adequate expression to these anxieties may compound the situation so that the label 'very nervous' is easily acquired by the child, whose inner fears are often totally misunderstood by his loving parents.

After induction and when the child is sufficiently relaxed, he may be gently encouraged to discuss his difficulties. Adequate explanation must be given so as not to arouse further anxiety and the child is shown that he can tolerate those problems which cause the symptoms or the individual behaviour of whoever the offending party may be. Ego-strengthening plays an important part in treatment. This may be related to modelling on the child's favourite hero or heroine of film, television or magazine. Self-hypnosis also has a role in treatment but the usefulness of this depends entirely upon the age and understanding of the child.

2. Psychosomatic Symptoms

These may be apparent in any system of the body but commonly occur in children in the respiratory, gastro-intestinal or urinary systems or in the skin.

Moreover, as the symptoms are repeated they become a conditioned response. As such they may be treated by de-conditioning or desensitization under hypnosis.

Respiratory System

The common problem is 'nervous asthma'. This may often be noted to occur on Monday mornings—the beginning of the school week, or perhaps at weekends, with daddy home from work and all the family gathered and the many problems which may arise therefrom.

The use of hypnosis has brought very considerable benefit to many sufferers from this condition. Instruction in self-hypnosis is given for regular twice daily use in order to reduce the general level of anxiety. It should also be used whenever this patient feels that an attack may be imminent. However, *hypnosis should never be used in any attempt to treat an acute asthma attack*.

Much of the credit for the development of the use of hypnosis in the treatment of nervous asthma must go to a London chest physician, Dr Gilbert Maher-Loughnan[2] who stated that 'General experience has shown that children who have had asthma for many years acquire habits of response which resemble psychogenic asthma but which when analysed, prove to be a form of conditioning. The frequent recurrences of asthma when excitement mounts—at the start of a holiday, for instance, or at weekends, or before examinations—are examples of this.' Any family physician or paediatrician will be familiar with this and the problem lends itself ideally to deconditioning under hypnosis.

Gastro-intestinal System

'Tummy ache' is a very common reason for missing school, where the real cause may be fear. Fear of the teacher or the child's peers or of the general ambience of the school situation. 'Nervy tummy', 'coliwobbles', although unscientific terms, are common and very adequate descriptions.

Such problems may be a precursor to the irritable bowel syndrome in adults.

Another and not uncommon symptom affecting the bowel is encopresis. Although ideas of an excessive preoccupation with potty training on the part of the mother, or of excessive purging or of repeated punishment for soiling may apply, or perhaps the therapist has theories relating to sensuous pleasure or childhood erotic fantasies, these should not be discussed with the child. Certainly where a parent is obviously at fault, that parent should be appropriately advised. The child however will usually respond to hypnotherapy, with ego-strengthening and emphasis upon the great disadvantages associated with the problem and upon the fact that he alone, a strong and intelligent person, can control the workings of his body.

Urinary system

Most children have attained control of the sphincter of the bladder by the age of three but enuresis may occasionally persist. When it occurs at night it may be associated with deep sleep and every doctor will be aware of the considerable frustration and anger which arises in the parent when the symptom persists.

The use of drugs, including stimulants such as ephedrine and amphetamine and antidepressants such as imipramine have already been tried. Equally, the alarm system (buzzer and pad) has usually failed to have any lasting effect. Unfortunately every failed attempt at treatment only serves to reinforce the problem.

It is essential to interview the parents and to assess their attitude to the child. To explain to them that the problem is not due to laziness or disobedience, but to fear. Frequently the parents will have little insight into, or understanding of the child's needs and at least as much sympathy and understanding must be reserved for them if the child is to benefit. The child should be treated as an equal and a warm and friendly attitude must be adopted towards him. He should never be punished for waking with a wet bed. A simple explanation of bladder function and control is given as well as an explanation of the use of hypnotherapy. Treatment commences with the induction of hypnosis and wherever possible instruction in self-hypnosis, which is to be used nightly, is also given. Powerful suggestions of ego-strengthening and adult development, with control over body functions, are given and incorporated into the self-hypnosis. Positive suggestions are added that if his bladder becomes full during the night he will awaken and go to the toilet. This too, is incorporated into the self-hypnosis. It is useful to suggest to the child, whilst he is under hypnosis, that he can be aware of his bladder filling and of the need to empty it. Then, and whilst he remains in hypnosis, he may be told that he will awaken, walk to your toilet, empty his bladder and return to the consulting room chair (or couch, i.e. his bed) and immediately relax into hypnosis once more.

> Now I will count to three. When I say three you will be aware of a feeling of fullness low down in your stomach, you will awaken, go to the toilet, empty your bladder and return to your bed. Immediately you lie on it again your eyes will close and you will be in a deep sleep once more.

Further complicated dynamic exploration or the involvement of some Freudian interpretation of unconscious erotic thoughts as the patient emerges through the oedipal phase are quite unnecessary and will only serve to confuse. Every dry night should be acknowledged by praise and reward in order to reinforce the confidence of the child.

The Skin

Dermatological problems, particularly eczema can cause considerable difficulties both to the child and family. The relationship between eczema and 'nervous' asthma in childhood must not go unnoted.

The considerable difficulties involved with any skin condition which other parents may consider to be contagious, are well known and the child at least must be totally reassured that the condition is not 'catching'.

A child suffering from eczema was brought to one of us (D.W.) and had been told by the teacher that she was dirty. She had to sit in class and eat her meals separately from the other children. One can well imagine what a devastating effect this must have had upon her.

Treatment involves a thorough understanding of the child's early and present environment. An interview with the parents is essential as is knowledge of any family history of skin conditions. Instruction in self-hypnosis and ego-strengthening are again a *sine qua non* as far as hypnotherapy is concerned. At the very least, with the reduction of anxiety and the increase in self-confidence which results, irritation and scratching will be reduced. At the best the rash will subside and will be kept under control by the persistent use of self-hypnosis until it eventually disappears.

3. Phobic Symptoms

Irrational fears are not uncommon in childhood and a family history of phobic anxiety is often found.

Perhaps the most famous case in the history of childhood phobias is that of little Hans who had 'a fear that a horse would bite him in the street'. This young Viennese child aged five years, was treated by Freud[3], although not with hypnosis. He used instead his newly developing analytic technique (with the aid of a history and interpretations supplied by the boy's father!).

The outcome was Freud's deduction of the boy's erotic feelings for his mother. As a result he feared the jealousy of his father. The horse represented the wrath of the father and by avoiding horses, Hans avoided the wrath of his father. In addition, 'Hans's phobia of horses was an obstacle to his going into the street and could serve as a means of allowing him to stay at home with his beloved mother'.

There is a great deal more in the discussion of this fascinating case history but perhaps the most interesting comment was that made by the Professor himself when he said 'analysis does not undo the *effects* of repression'.

Nevertheless there are few of us who could emulate the successes of the father of psychoanalysis. We may better therefore satisfy ourselves with the use of hypnotherapy for the relief of phobic symptoms using the methods described.

In the realities of the paediatric neuroses seen today, school phobia often presents a considerable problem. This should be distinguished from truanting and simple refusal on the part of the immature child to leave the mother or parent, which is in effect a separation anxiety. The school phobic child will complain of a variety of fears and psychosomatic symptoms and may develop a panic attack. The problem is often associated with a disturbed parent–child relationship and this possibility must be thoroughly explored. Lawlor[4] enumerated some of the problems and fears which a child may be unable to bring into consciousness and talk about and which may be responsible for the symptoms. These include the following:

1. A fear of abandonment by the parents.

2. A fear of some disaster befalling the parents, particularly the mother.

3. Fears based on destructive wishes towards siblings due to sibling rivalry.

4. Fears that exhibiting angry feelings will be punished by the parents.

5. Fears of annihilation and starvation.

Treatment consists of full discussion and counselling of the parents followed by a full discussion with the child, both separately and together with the parents. Hypnotherapy should be used for reduction in the level of anxiety and desensitization. The results are usually good but one must watch carefully for symptoms of depression. The problem of school phobia is also discussed in Chapter 15.

4. Obsessions and Compulsions

These are faily common in children and usually disappear as the child matures. Unless severely incapacitating no treatment is indicated but if the concomitant anxiety is high this may be treated with hypnotherapy.

5. Hysterical or Conversion Symptoms

These may certainly occur in children. Treatment is by relaxation in hypnosis, exploration of possible aetiology of the conversion and desensitization as with adults. Symptom removal by direct suggestion should never be attempted. Ego-strengthening should also be included.

6. Personality Difficulties

Stammering, tics and other nervous habits frequently originate in childhood. The earlier that treatment is commenced, the better is the prognosis. Hypnotherapy may be used in the same way as for adults but with particular emphasis upon ego-strengthening especially tailored to suit the child's difficulties.

7. The Problem of Pain

Perhaps the greatest contribution to the treatment of children has been made by E.R. and J.R. Hilgard[5]. They particularly focussed on the pain and anxiety experienced by children and adolescents before and during treatment for leukaemia, for example during bone marrow aspiration. It was found that hypnosis helped considerably to abolish fear. Seventy-nine per cent of highly hypnotizable subjects showed a good response to suggestions of pain reduction. Since children are generally highly hypnotizable, then hypnotherapy is a very worthwhile procedure in such cases.

Hypnosis is also extremely useful in abolishing nausea and vomiting occurring during the administration of cytotoxic drugs. It is also most useful in anticipatory vomiting which may occur in patients who become conditioned to this response (Kaszab[6]).

It may additionally be used to allay anxiety and to reduce pain in other surgical interventions such as venesection and lumbar puncture. Zeltzer *et al.*[7] demonstrated that hypnosis was significantly more effective than non-hypnotic techniques during all such assaults upon the sick child.

These results alone indicate the value of hypnotherapy for the relief of suffering in paediatric practice.

REFERENCES

1. Ambrose G., 1961. *Hypnotherapy with Children*. Staples, London.
2. Maher-Loughnan G.P., 1970. Hypnosis and auto-hypnosis for the treatment of asthma. *Int. J. Clin. Exp. Hypnosis*, **XVIII**, 1–14.
3. Freud S., 1955. Analysis of a phobia in a five-year old boy. In: *Standard Edition of the Complete Psychological Works of Sigmund Freud* (ed. Strachey), Vol. X. Hogarth, London.
4. Lawler E.D., 1976. Hypnotic intervention with 'school phobic' children. *Int. J. Clin. Exp. Hypnosis*, **XXIV**, 74–86.
5. Hilgard E.R. and Hilgard J.R., 1975. *Hypnosis in the Relief of Pain*. Kaufmann, Los Altos, CA.
6. Kaszab Z., 1987. Supportive hypnotherapy for children with malignant diseases. Paper read at 4th European Congress of Hypnosis in Psychotherapy and Psychosomatic Medicine, Oxford.
7. Zeltzer L., LeBarron S. and Zeltzer P.M., 1982. Hypnotic and non-hypnotic techniques for reduction of distress in children with cancer. Paper read at the 9th International Congress of Hypnosis and Psychosomatic Medicine, Glasgow.

CHAPTER 21

Hypnotherapy in the Treatment of Depression

As has already been mentioned repeatedly the taking of a full and accurate medical and psychiatric history is an essential prerequisite of any treatment in which hypnosis is likely to be used. This is never more true than where symptoms of depression are identified. Indeed, if the use of hypnotherapy fails, then the therapist should look again at the history, for where the patient is depressed and if the depression has been missed, that problem may well be compounded and the case could end in disaster.

At the outset then, it must be clearly understood that *hypnosis alone is not a routine treatment for depression.*

If the patient is depressed or if depression is suspected then it is essential to prescribe adequate antidepressant medication and not to commence hypnotherapy until a positive response to the drugs is shown.

West and Deckert[1] warned that 'depressed patients can become worse, even suicidal...when the somatic expression of depression is removed by hypnosis.' This fact was supported by a publication in the British Medical Journal (Waxman[2]).

Having said this, it must be added that there are experts in hypnotherapy and with specialist psychiatric training who do use hypnosis by itself to treat certain depressed patients. Nevertheless, one should never lose sight of the fact that the choice which should always be made is that which would be the safest and most beneficial for the patient.

With the best intentions in the world, the condition may be difficult to identify. Feeling low and gloomy and dispirited does not signify pathological depression. When referring to the latter, we are talking of a host of biological and physical symptoms in addition to the change in affect with which the word is usually associated.

Depression may appear in many guises. It is ubiquitous and all-pervading and reaches into areas which the commonly accepted teachings and clinical assessments may not anticipate. It is a problem which has been said to fall only a short way behind disorders of the cardiovascular system and chronic bronchitis as one of the major causes of serious morbidity. Perhaps the most important comment which can be made regarding the importance of accurate diagnosis and correct treatment is that one of the major complications of depression is suicide or parasuicide.

In the search for the symptoms of depression, listed below are some of the more common features which may be elicited either singly or in any permutation or combination and often *in addition* to the presenting symptoms or the problem for which the patient has been referred.

1. Depressed mood often on waking and with diurnal mood swing.
2. Sleep difficulties. Classically the complaint is of early morning waking but certainly initial and intermediate sleep problems may predominate.
3. Loss of appetite.
4. Loss of weight.
5. Loss of energy.
6. Loss of interest.
7. Constipation.
8. Loss of libido.
9. Inability to concentrate.
10. Morbid thoughts and ideas.

Having listed these symptoms it must be understood that much of that which is so important may be masked by that which appears to the patient to be the main problem. In the event it is the experience and judgement of the doctor which is the overriding factor in making the correct diagnosis.

The search for some positive criteria upon which to base a diagnosis of depression has existed for many years.

The Hippocratic idea was that melancholia was a disorder of mood associated with an excess of black bile. In the nineteenth century it was thought that depressive disorders were the consequence of some biological defect of genetic origin. Then under the influence of the new schools of psychoanalysis, there developed the psychodynamic idea of aetiology. Depressive disorders were perceived as the result of serious object loss, either real or symbolic, or frustrated hostility turned inwards against the self.

More recent ideas of a biological and biochemical cause of depression have been developed and continue to be researched and there is no doubt that there is considerable evidence of endocrine, serum electrolyte and biogenic amine changes which may take place in any depressive illness.

Be that as it may, most authorities additionally subscribe to genetic and psychodynamic ideas and it is with the latter in mind that we can find a place for the use of hypnosis in addition to other therapies.

Having established that the patient is depressed, the next essential, before instigating treatment is to elicit exactly what type of depression we are dealing with. The illness may fall into any of the following categories:

1. *Reactive Depression*

This may be associated with any of the neuroses. It may be secondary to a situation which is worrying or disturbing in some way so as to produce this particular change in affect. It is transitory and will often resolve when the precipitating cause is resolved. It will be helped by the appropriate antidepressant medication and when the latter is seen to be taking effect then hypnotherapy may be applied to explore possible causes and to treat any associated neurosis.

2. *Endogenous Depression*

This is a primary depression where there is no obvious triggering cause. It may be chronic or recurring and it is the sort of mood which is built-in to the personality of the patient.

At this stage, let us consider the following possibilities. A patient is referred to the doctor with a diagnosis of agoraphobia. A history is taken and the presenting symptoms are confirmed. Some biological symptoms of depression are also revealed and the conclusion is that this highly anxious patient has become agoraphobic and as a consequence additionally suffers from a reactive depression. It is perfectly safe to desensitize this patient to the phobic symptoms using hypnosis and it is strongly advised to prescribe an antidepressant before commencing hypnodesensitization. This will certainly facilitate treatment and be far safer. However, it is possible that the diagnosis is not quite correct. It is possible that a depressive illness preceded the onset of phobic symptoms and that this was missed in the assessment. It is possible that the primary illness is depression and that the anxiety symptoms and agoraphobia are secondary to the depression.

Removal of the protective facade of anxiety by the use of hypnosis or by any other method would mean that the patient, with his mood unclouded by anxiety, could well see some intolerable reasons for his depression and as a result he may then take the only solution that he considers will end his suffering. This example is given to emphasize the absolute need for a correct diagnosis before considering hypnotherapy.

3. *Mixed Depression*

As the name implies, this is a reactive depression superimposed upon a chronic or endogenous depression perhaps in temporary remission, or aggravating already existing symptoms. From the practical point of view of treatment, it should be considered as endogenous.

4. *Bipolar Depression (Manic Depressive Psychosis)*

No attempt should be made to treat manic symptoms with the

use of hypnosis. Hypomanic patients may temporarily respond but only for a brief period. In any case, lithium, major tranquillizers and antidepressants would certainly be the appropriate medication to be considered, with hypnotherapy at a later stage to help work through the patient's problems.

5. *Psychotic Depression*

In this we are referring to the more severe phase of the illness where psychotic symptoms begin to appear and the subject loses touch with reality. It is most important to recognize that hypnosis has no place in the treatment of this condition.

6. *Puerperal, Pre-menstrual or Involutional Depression*

Here again, it is better to tackle the problem through the use of the appropriate psychotropic medication or hormone therapy although hypnosis may additionally reduce any associated anxiety symptoms.

7. *Depression Following Bereavement or Loss*

In exploring the history of any patient suffering from depression, it is not uncommon to discover recurring attacks over many years and this may be found to date from the loss of a loved one. In such cases it may further be found that the patient had not successfully negotiated the stages of mourning and is suffering from an unresolved grief reaction.

Hypnotherapy lends itself ideally to treatment in such cases. Nevertheless once again antidepressant cover is strongly advised. Hypnoanalysis will allow the patient to ventilate his feelings of denial, guilt and anger, etc. Discussion and explanation of the symptoms will allow the patient to come to terms, albeit even years later, with that particular loss and to reintegrate into society.

Symptoms of loss may also occur as a result of loss of some loved object, loss of a job or loss of prestige and may be similarly treated.

Any therapist wishing to treat this very difficult problem is advised to study the classic paper, 'Mourning and Melancholia' by Freud[3] and the more recent work of Parkes.[4]

8. *Depression and its Relationship with Aggression*

Many clinicians from Freud until the present day have commented upon the psychodynamic idea of the co-existence of hostility and depression. This was also investigated by Kendall[5] amongst others, who found that suicide and homicide were inversely related. Suicide was found to be less common in cultures in which expressions of aggression are permitted and more common where aggression is discouraged. This does seem to indicate that if such aggression can be expressed outwardly then the depressed mood could be alleviated.

Once more therefore a possibility of the use of hypnosis is revealed. Exploration of the problem under hypnosis should allow the patient to ventilate his anger and by ridding himself of the repressed emotions, to rid himself also of his symptoms.

9. *Depression Associated with Other Illness*

This is not unusual in older people, where the presenting symptom may well be that of a depressive illness. However, the patient could, for example, have a carcinoma of the bowel. This possibility should always be considered in depression of recent origin in the elderly. Also, of course, the depression may follow an illness such as influenza or may result from a prolonged or severe illness. In addition, the therapist may fall into a trap if the patient has already been prescribed some medication which could cause him to be depressed. Commonly, antibiotics effect some people in this way as do certain hypotensive drugs. In all such cases hypnosis is unsuitable and the appropriate medical treatment should be commenced.

10. *Other Manifestations of Depression*

Alcoholism, gambling and migraine are amongst some of the conditions which may be associated with depression. Where symptoms of the latter are elicited, successful treatment of the presenting complaint may well depend upon successful treatment of the depression. Hypnotherapy may prove invaluable in reducing the level of alcoholism or gambling or in treating the migraine, if the depression is concurrently treated. Hypnoanalysis may then be used in order to elicit, if possible, the cause of the original complaint.

A more recent addition to the armamentarium for the treatment of depression is that known as cognitive therapy. This is a form of brief psychotherapy which was developed by Aaron T. Beck[6]. It considers that a person's conceptualization of things will determine his feelings and behaviour. For example, thinking and seeing negatively will result in depression and therefore by changing the cognition, the depression will also change.

It is also claimed that more acceptable social adjustment is obtained with cognitive therapy than with the drugs in patients suffering from unipolar depression. Beck et al.[7] characterized thought content in depression in terms of a cognitive triad of negative feelings about oneself, the world and the future. This would point to the possible value of hypnosis as an adjunct to cognitive therapy. It is interesting to consider that the first author[8], discussing the value of his ego-strengthening technique, might well have been using hypnosis with cognitive therapy in order to effect change.

In a more recent paper Alladin[9] described the use of 'cognitive therapy' in reactive, unipolar depression. In outlining the advantages of clear goals, the many and long-lasting distinct gains and the reduction of suicide ideation in a limited number of cases, he also discussed the value of hypnosis in his treatment approach (cognitive–hypnotherapy) and demonstrated the need for further development of this technique.

However, it is not a method for the amateur hypnotherapist. It should be reserved for use by highly qualified psychologists, well versed in this form of treatment and experienced in the clinical use of hypnosis.

In summarizing the treatment of depression, if hypnosis is to be used, the following procedure may be adopted *bearing in mind all the precautions that have already been indicated*.

1. Hypnoanalysis.
2. Ventilation of problems leading to depressed mood (with possible abreaction).

3. Discussion, with insight-directed psychotherapy if applicable.

4. Reduction of associated anxiety.

5. Cognitive–hypnotherapy with ego-strengthening.

We must conclude however as we began, namely with a warning.

'The risk of employing hypnosis to focus on the emotionally laden areas of a patient's life is that such an intense concentration might exacerbate the severity of the depression' (Terman[10]).

REFERENCES

1. West L.J. and Deckert C.H., 1965. Dangers of hypnosis. *J. Am. Med. Assoc.*, **192,** 9–12.
2. Waxman D., 1978. Misuse of hypnosis. *Br. Med. J.*, **2,** 571.
3. Freud S., 1957. Mourning and melancholia. In: *Standard Edition of the Complete Psychological Works of Sigmund Freud* (ed. Strachey), Vol. XIV. Hogarth, London.
4. Parkes C.M., 1972. *Bereavement*. Penguin, Harmondsworth.
5. Kendall R.E., 1970. Relationship between aggression and depression. *Archs. Gen Psychiat.*, **22,** 308–318.
6. Beck A.T., 1976. *Depression: Clinical, Experimental and Theoretical Aspects*. Harper and Row, New York.
7. Beck A., Rush A., Shaw B. *et al.*, 1979. *Cognitive Therapy of Depression*. Wiley, Chichester.
8. Hartland J., 1971. Further observations on the use of 'ego-strengthening' techniques. *Am. J. Clin. Hypnosis*, **14,** 1–8.
9. Alladin A., 1987. Cognitive hypnotherapy for depression. Paper read at 4th European Congress of Hypnosis in Psychotherapy and Psychosomatic Medicine, Oxford.
10. Terman S.A., 1980. Hypnosis in depression. In: *Clinical Hypnosis in Medicine* (ed. Wain). Symposia Specialists, Chicago.

CHAPTER 22

Hypnotherapy in Chronic and Terminal Illness

Hilgard and Hilgard[1] have identified two major components of pain. These are sensory pain and suffering. The relevance of this is that pain and suffering are so often associated with terminal illness.

To the patient, pain and suffering is one. It is the threat and expression of approaching death and inevitably anxiety will increase. Hypnotherapy can do much to lower the level of anxiety but must also be directed towards the reduction of the awareness of any associated pain. It is a mistake to assume that the reduction of anxiety *per se* is the same as the reduction of felt pain. Particular attention must be given to both aspects of the experience.

It may be that the level of pain and fear of the inevitable outcome will be denied by the patient. Close observation must be kept on the situation and no attempt may be made to reduce the patient's defences.

In addition, in any approach to therapy we may be met with anger, hostility and resistance. Perhaps because of the failures of other modalities already attempted, a negative attitude will be maintained to any further intervention. The feelings of the patient must be respected. There must be no suggestion of an intrusion into his very personal inner world. A slow and gentle approach is essential so that in a sense, the patient gives the doctor permission to enter.

Now over and above all these problems it would be surprising indeed if the patient was not additionally depressed. Depression will compound the pain which will increase the anxiety. The possible prescription of some antidepressant medication must be seriously considered and probably one of the non-activating tricyclic drugs would be indicated.

The use of hypnosis for the treatment of pain has been fully discussed in an earlier chapter. In chronic pain however, which is associated with terminal illness, apart from direct and various indirect suggestions of analgesia which may be given, many other aspects of the patient's situation must be taken into account. Additional procedures may therefore be indicated. The doctor is not only involved with the patient as a person who is in pain, not only is a very special relationship established through the particular use of hypnosis, but the doctor must also have the understanding to guide the patient and all who are involved, into a peaceful acceptance of the inevitable.

Whenever a patient becomes physically ill, without doubt many powerful emotional factors as have been mentioned, will enter into the picture. These will tend both to influence his symptoms and, in many instances, to retard his recovery. The extent to which they do this will depend largely upon the way in which the patient regards his illness, and if such factors are also taken into account and treated adequately, a great deal can be achieved in increasing the patient's incentives and accelerating the process of healing.

Hypnosis can be extremely useful in chronic, incapacitating diseases in helping the patient to accept both his illness and his limitations philosophically. He can be encouraged to accept the fact that whilst there are certain things that he may not be able to do again, there are others that he will be able to achieve successfully despite the handicap imposed by his illness. Even when little more than this can be accomplished, the resulting improvement in his morale and general outlook will frequently prove most gratifying.

In incurable, painful and ultimately fatal conditions, hypnosis may often be used advantageously to alleviate pain and suffering in addition to helping the patient to accept his illness. When employed in this way the greatest success is likely to be achieved when the depth of hypnosis is sufficient to secure complete analgesia. Unfortunately this is not easily obtained; even so, a considerable degree of relief from pain can often be secured, as a result of which the amount of analgesic and sedative drugs administered can frequently be substantially reduced. Even in cases of inoperable cancer, hypnosis can sometimes augment and prolong the action of the milder pain relieving drugs and thus delay considerably the need to resort to more powerful analgesia.

In our approach to this type of case we often tend to adopt too perfectionistic an outlook, and the fact that the pain seems so intense and the possibility of securing any significant degree of analgesia so remote only too frequently discourages us even from considering the use of hypnosis. Such an attitude is entirely wrong, for we should always remember that even when hypnosis can only be used to minimize the distress suffered by the patient, the pain itself tends to become rather less severe and more easily tolerated. Relaxation and the reduction of tension, worry and anxiety, all of which can be achieved in the light or medium stages of hypnosis, can afford some relief to the sufferer. In many cases, this alone will reduce the amount of medication necessary, without resort to additional techniques required for the production of analgesia.

In addition to the reduction of anxiety and the production of analgesia, there are a number of other methods which may be usefully attempted in order to help the patient. *'Distraction'* will sometimes succeed for we all know that it is possible to forget pain, just as we can forget a headache for example, whilst watching an exciting film. We should also be more willing to settle for things that *can* be endured, rather than to fail to change things that cannot otherwise be changed. Indeed, one of the things we can sometimes do is to *substitute or replace pain by a lesser or altered sensation*. It may be possible to transform a distressing pain into a feeling of unpleasant, but not painful, warmth which is much more easily tolerated and infinitely preferable to the original pain. Indeed in a receptive patient in a reasonably deep trance, pain can be *'displaced'* for it need not necessarily be experienced at the site of the lesion or disease. After all, a gall bladder pain is felt between the shoulders, and a cardiac pain in the upper arm. Under these circumstances, whilst in hypnosis, a patient can be told that the pain he is feeling in his stomach, would be tolerated better if it were in his left hand, and proceed to induce it in the latter as a replacement of the former. In certain instances, *'time distortion'* can afford relief from pain. When friends visit, time passes quickly, but when unwelcome visitors arrive one wonders whether the day will ever end. This is a common example of 'time distortion' or subjective time. Using this principle, the patient can be taught how to experience 20 minutes of pain in only 10 seconds of actual time, thus decreasing its duration to such an extent that the painful periods appear very short in comparison with the time he is pain free.

It may also be suggested to the patient that he can achieve a *slowly progressive diminution of his pain.* In this case, tell him that if the 100 per cent of pain he is suffering were reduced to 90 per cent he would hardly be able to notice any difference. That the level might even drop to 85 per cent...or 80 per cent...75 per cent...or even 70 per cent...and so on, and the patient will often go along with this idea because he has not been asked to perform a major task. In deeper hypnosis of course *'dissociative'* procedures may be most effective.

In a masterly review of the subject, Sacerdote[2], drawing attention to the distinction between pain and suffering, pointed out that patients with advanced illness often function at two levels of awareness. At one level, every kind of rationalization and reassurance is used to sustain faith in an optimistic outcome and at another level there is the awareness of the inevitability of further suffering and of ultimate death. The danger may therefore be, he suggests, that hypnosis will help a patient to have a clearer perception of the inevitable end and as a result will refuse further hypnotherapy.

Ewin[3] attaches a special psychological meaning to the complaint of constant pain and utilizes this in his treatment. When a patient gives a history of pain that is constant, continuous, always there and never goes away and when he says 'I live with it', he is often expressing a subconscious corollary, 'If I did not have it, I would be dead'. 'Obviously', Ewin says, 'if the pain proves he is alive, it cannot be relinquished completely for even five minutes...even when he is asleep'. From this interesting hypothesis, it follows that any person that attempts to take the pain away from the patient is his enemy. Treatment would consist of regressing the patient to some precipitating incident, perhaps one in which he actually experienced some life-threatening event which was associated with pain and then showing him, whilst in hypnosis, that he can be free from pain and yet alive.

O'Connell[4] pointed to the rapport which develops between the doctor using hypnosis and the dying patient. Not only does this provide the necessary emotional support but also can reduce the need for analgesic drugs and ameliorate other symptoms such as nausea, insomnia, dyspnoea and itching.

It is preferable to avoid the use of the word 'pain', if possible choosing some word which has less significant connotations. Perhaps substituting the word 'colic', if it is abdominal or 'tension' or 'sensitivity' if it is elsewhere.

In conclusion let us summarize the objectives of any treatment of chronic or terminal illness associated with intractable pain and as agreed by the many experts in this field of hypnotherapy. These are as follows:

1. To reduce anxiety.
2. To diminish the awareness of pain.
3. To decrease the dependence on analgesics and thus increase their effectiveness when required.
4. To improve the patient's attitude to his illness and his general outlook.
5. To encourage and enhance any available and remaining capabilities.
6. To counsel family and friends.
7. To prepare the patient for the inevitable.

Hypnosis may be used to achieve these ends in the following way:

1. The reduction of anxiety by suggestion under hypnosis, instruction in self-hypnosis and the production of a tape recording if necessary to assist with and reinforce the latter.

2. The direct suggestion of pain relief coupled with progressive relaxation and decrease in sensitivity.

3. The production of analgesia by suggestions, if appropriate, of glove anaesthesia. For example immersing the hand in an imaginary bucket of ice until it is numb with cold and transferring the numbness to the affected area.

4. Suggestions that the hand of the doctor, placed on the painful part of the body, will remove, absorb or diminish the pain. If the technique is effective, the patient may be taught to accept the hand of the nurse, or of some loved member of the family. By practice in self-hypnosis, he may be taught that his own hand will be equally effective.

5. By substitution of the feeling of pain for something more tolerable such as pressure.

6. By displacement of the symptoms to another part of the body, for example from the abdomen to the arm or leg where it would be more easily tolerated.

7. By dissociation. In deep trance the 'hidden observer' technique may be used (see Chapter 18). The patient will 'observe' what is happening to his body without the actual perception of painful subjective sensations.

8. By the use of the phenomenon of time distortion in hypnosis so that the patient perceives the period of pain as much shorter than it really is. This may be coupled with suggestions of progressive diminution of the pain.

9. By hallucination. That is the patient seeing himself in some pleasurable setting of his own choice or by guided age-regression into one which he has previously experienced and enjoyed.

10. By guided age-progression. This may be used to suggest some future time where discomfort and illness will have been left behind. This is a very sensitive area however. The patient may perceive no future at all and extra care must be used if this particular technique is applied.

If these techniques are carefully studied, there is no doubt that the doctor can provide what is certainly the most valuable service of his profession, namely the relief of pain and suffering.

For further understanding of this highly emotive subject the reader is advised to consult the classic work of John Hinton entitled 'Dying'[5].

REFERENCES

1. Hilgard E.R. and Hilgard J.R., 1975. *Hypnosis in the Relief of Pain.* Kaufmann, Los Altos, CA.
2. Sacerdote P., 1985. Why is hypnosis effective in pain control? In: *Modern Trends in Hypnosis* (eds Waxman, Misra, Gibson and Basker). Plenum, New York.
3. Ewin D.M., 1980. Constant pain syndrome: its psychological meaning and cure using hypnosis. In: *Clinical Hypnosis in Medicine* (ed. Wain). Symposium Specialists, Chicago.
4. O'Connell S., 1985. Hypnosis in terminal care: discussion paper. *J.R.S.M.*, **78**, 122–125.
5. Hinton J., 1967. *Dying*, Penguin. Harmondsworth.

CHAPTER 23

The Use of Hypnosis in Dental Surgery

Every dental surgeon is bound to encounter a limited number of patients who could successfully undergo all their dental operations, painful or otherwise, under hypnosis alone. Often, however, it is felt that many of the hypnotic procedures recommended for dentistry in the past are too time consuming and laborious for the ordinary practitioner, working in his own surgery. But in view of what is known today about the number of patients who can be hypnotized into light, medium or every deep trances, it is now realized that the employment of these various trance states can afford the dentist considerable assistance in selected cases. Furthermore, in the Hospital Service, where the time factor is not so pressing and the condition of many patients is so serious that it requires more time to be spent upon them, hypnosis could well be used more widely than it is at the present time.

Light Trance Hypnosis

By far the largest number of patients will achieve light or medium trance only unless the hypnotist is prepared to go to a great deal of time and trouble. Even under these circumstances, hypnosis can still prove to be a valuable supportive measure towards the completion of the treatment envisaged. We all know the type of patient who finds it difficult to pluck up his courage sufficiently to visit the dentist. We all know the type of patient who is overcome with anxiety and apprehension when he finally arrives in our consulting rooms. We are also familiar with the patient who, whilst making strenuous efforts to control himself, is obviously finding it so difficult that he remains highly excitable and tense for as long as we are operating upon him. In all these patients induction into the hypnotic state will alleviate their fears, reduce their anxiety and apprehension, and produce sensations of relaxation, comfort and well being to a greater or lesser degree. Under hypnosis, the dentist can suggest directly to the patient that he will be able to relax, that there is no need for him to worry, that he will become less tense, less apprehensive, and that he will be able to try to assist the dentist in whatever procedure he is carrying out. Even this level of trance, at which suggestions can be quite potent and effective, constitutes one of the most valuable and widely applicable uses of hypnosis in dentistry.

Medium Trance Hypnosis

A considerable number of patients can attain an intermediate stage of analgesia. Whilst they undoubtedly feel some pain, they feel much less under hypnosis than they would in the waking state. Although they are by no means completely analgesic, these patients can be considerably helped by hypnosis. The prick of the needle when giving a hypodermic injection can be greatly mitigated by the direct suggestion under hypnosis that analgesia of the muco-periosteum in the area of the injection has been obtained.

Deep Trance Hypnosis

Obviously with those patients who can achieve the deep trance state on the first or second attempt, dentistry will present no problems. Most of these will succeed in producing complete analgesia, and many will develop a total amnesia for such operations as are performed. In these circumstances there is no quicker or easier way of carrying out any dental operation. The patient can be seated in the chair and put into the trance state instantaneously by a conditioned signal, or within 10 seconds by a normal induction procedure. Anaesthesia of the intended area of operation can be obtained in a further 10 seconds, and the dentist can be proceeding about his business within 30 seconds of the patient entering the surgery. Unfortunately, this is only possible in a very small percentage of the total population and is consequently quite unattainable as a routine measure.

The would-be dental hypnotist should be warned against the blandishments of patients who wish to undergo hypnosis unnecessarily, or request it for the relief of conditions that do not fit into the dental picture. It cannot be emphasized too strongly that the dentist who ventures outside the sphere of dentistry, in order to enhance his image or to oblige his patients, is doing so at considerable risk to himself.

Most medical and dental practitioners who use hypnosis regularly consider that any attempt by a practitioner lacking psychiatric experience, to go outside his normal field of activity, is fraught with danger. The dentist should, therefore, confine his activities entirely to the dental field, and even at the risk of upsetting people he should decline to treat them for other conditions. For instance, dentists who practise hypnosis are constantly being asked to cure people of the habit of smoking. Whilst it is true that hypnotherapy can help to achieve this, it should still only be undertaken under competent medical guidance since there is always the danger that the addiction may become transferred from nicotine to something more dangerous.

THE MAIN USES OF HYPNOSIS IN DENTISTRY

1. Obtaining relaxation.
2. Ensuring co-operation from the otherwise uncooperative.
3. The reduction of anxiety and fear.
4. The preparation of the patient for local or general anaesthesia.
5. The production of analgesia.
6. The production of amnesia.
7. The control of fainting.
8. The control of bleeding.
9. The control of salivation.
10. The induction of muscular rigidity of the jaw and neck.

11. The extension of the period of analgesia.

12. The toleration of impression taking without gagging or sickness.

13. Improvement of the effort necessary to learn the wearing of prosthetic or orthodontic appliances.

This list constitutes a fairly complete catalogue of most of the uses to which dentists put hypnosis in the course of their normal practice.

1. *Obtaining relaxation.* It is well known that the highly nervous patient invariably has a lower threshold of pain, and will consequently be under increasing tension as the operation proceeds. It is also recognized that if this state of tension in the patient can be reduced either by drugs or, in the case of dental hypnosis, by suggestion, the patient's pain threshold will be elevated to such an extent that simple operations not involving too much pain will become tolerable to that patient.

2. *Ensuring co-operation.* Even without the induction of hypnosis, it has been found that many patients who are reassured and talked to quietly in the waking state as their treatment progresses will become much more relaxed and co-operative, thus rendering the whole procedure very much easier. In the light and medium trance states, this effect can be tremendously enhanced.

3. *The reduction of anxiety and fear.* Most normal patients who visit their dentist are in some condition of fear. Those who have been coming for a long time probably willbe less frightened. But newer patients whose confidence we have not fully gained through lack of opportunity, and those who have experienced somewhat unsuccessful sessions in the past will exhibit a very active fear. If suitable steps can be taken to eliminate this, a state of mind will be produced in which treatment will become much more acceptable, and the pain threshold will once again be elevated. This can sometimes be achieved by a straightforward talk in the waking state, in the course of which the confidence of the patient is obtained. On other occasions, hypnosis can be used to great advantage since it can be directly suggested to the patient that his fears of a dental appointment will cease to exist; that he

will be able to allow the necessary treatment to be carried out; and that he will experience no fear whatever during the whole of the time he spends with the dentist. In a similar manner, direct suggestion under hypnosis can be employed to reduce the fear of any particular operation that is contemplated. Fortunately, suggestions of this kind can prove very effective in the lightest stages of hypnosis, so that the vast majority of our patients can actually be helped in this way. Indeed, in so far as the reduction of anxiety and fear, and the attaining of relaxation are concerned, at least nine out of ten patients can be assisted by the use of hypnosis.

4. *Preparation for local or general anaesthesia.* Most specialist anaesthetists are in the habit of using a relaxing technique in talking to their patients before inducing anaesthesia. In the dental surgery this method can usefully be adopted before giving nitrous oxide and oxygen, and possibly some of the intravenous anaesthetic agents. Appropriate suggestions are made in a quiet, drowsy voice, and the monotony is maintained throughout the actual induction of anaesthesia. Hypnosis often supervenes well before anaesthetization is complete. Should local anaesthesia only be required, an extremely relaxed, sleepy state of mind can be induced by using a similar hypnotic technique, and it is interesting to note that under these circumstances the quantity of local anaesthetic necessary to obtain adequate anaesthesia for the operation contemplated can often be substantially reduced.

5. *The production of analgesia.* Some degree of analgesia, partial or complete, is obtainable in no more than 30 per cent of patients, but complete analgesia will only be obtainable in some 10 per cent, and even then will often require several visits to achieve. Thus complete analgesia, whilst being delightful to work with when it can be secured, must be regarded as the exception rather than the rule, whereas varying degrees of partial analgesia can often be attained.

6. *The production of amnesia.* A complete loss of memory for a dental procedure can often be induced in those deep-trance subjects who are capable of high degrees of analgesia. This can be utilized with great benefit to the patient whenever an operation has been protracted or particularly unpleasant. Under such cir-

cumstances, one can try to increase the patient's susceptibility to amnesia by various suggestions such as that the mind is going blank.

7. *The control of fainting.* This is readily susceptible to treatment by hypnotic methods. We are all only too familiar with the type of patient who, during a hypodermic injection or immediately following it, breaks out in beads of perspiration, blanches or goes grey, and in next to no time passes out in the chair. If, at the onset of the attack, he is told with confidence and authority to place his head between his knees, thereby compressing the abdominal viscera, his colour will return in a matter of seconds and the whole episode will be over within a minute or two. Any recurrence of this can be guarded against and avoided by hypnotizing such patients and making strong, positive and authoritative suggestions that fainting will *not* occur on any future occasion. This is particularly effective if it is also explained to the patient that fainting is directly due to fear, and that next time he will no longer be afraid.

8. *The control of bleeding.* Bleeding from a post-extraction wound or immediately following an extraction can be controlled if a strong suggestion is given to the deeply hypnotized patient that the blood flow in the particular area will be reduced for some hours. Under these circumstances, the bleeding will often cease completely. An extraction can frequently be performed without the loss of more than two or three drops of blood if the blood flow is reduced by hypnotic suggestion before the extraction is made.

9. *The control of salivation.* In a similar manner, direct suggestions that the patient's saliva will dry up for a limited period will result in a definite lessening of the flow of saliva. This can be of great assistance in the type of patient who has a profuse or ropey saliva which constitutes an increasing hazard during the preparation of a cavity in a lower tooth.

10. *Induction of muscular rigidity of the jaw and neck.* This can be produced most efficiently in the hypnotic trance by simple, direct suggestion. This is usually done to a count of five, and it is suggested to the patient that the muscles of the jaw, head and

neck will become completely stiff and rigid with the jaw locked widely open until the operation is completed. The rigidity *must* subsequently be removed by a reverse count.

11. *Extension of the period of analgesia.* When it is anticipated that an operation will produce a certain amount of after-pain, it is quite reasonable to suggest to the patient that the area of operation will remain analgesic for the next 12 to 24 hours, thereby affording the patient a degree of post-operative comfort which would not exist nearly so long if an ordinary local anaesthetic had been used. Such instructions, however, must be strictly limited in application since severe pain following an operation may indicate the onset of a spreading infection, or that something else has gone wrong. In this case, it is essential that the patient should receive adequate warning of the necessity of revisiting the dentist.

12. *Impression tolerance and control of gagging.* The control of gagging and of sickness can undoubtedly be effected by hypnotic suggestion. The patient is told that the palate and upper portion of the pharynx is becoming anaesthetized, and that he will consequently have no need to retch. This renders the taking of impressions which have to stay in the mouth for 3 minutes or more much easier in patients who are susceptible to this type of complaint.

13. *Tolerance of prosthetic and orthodontic appliances.* The co-operation of patients in the wearing of new dentures can be actively enlisted under hypnosis, and this is equally applicable to children in the wearing of fixed or removable orthodontic appliances. When suggestions to this effect are made, it is always wise to stress the reasons for the patient's co-operation and the benefits that are going to accrue from the wearing of the appliances. A further use of hypnosis in the field of orthodontics can be found in dealing with the normal thumb-sucking or tongue-thrusting type of child, whose dental abnormality is due to some extent to these two factors. A child can be instructed under hypnosis that if it must suck something, it will suck a finger rather than a thumb. This has the advantage of reducing considerably the size of the object that is sucked. The matter can be taken further and the patient can be told that any part of either hand which is placed in

the mouth will taste so unpleasant that it will have to be removed. This has been known to occur after only one session of hypnosis.

TECHNIQUES FOR THE INDUCTION OF HYPNOSIS

The problems of hypnotic induction for dental purposes are rather different from those confronting the doctor or psychotherapist. In one sense, the dentist has a distinct advantage because the patient knows that hypnosis is only being used for a limited purpose, and consequently has the assurance that no exploration of his mind will be attempted. On the other hand, most dental patients suffer from the disadvantage that the fear and dread evoked by the prospect of dental treatment makes it more difficult for them to co-operate and relax. This can usually be overcome, however, provided that sufficient time and care are devoted to the preparation of the patient's mind before any attempt at induction is made. This step may well determine the difference between success and failure.

The Induction of Hypnosis in Adults

Any of the usual methods of induction are applicable to dental purposes. The choice should always be made with due regard to its suitability for the individual patient and the personality of the operator himself.

In the dental chair, the eye fixation–distraction method will usually be found to be both rapid and efficient.

The patient is seated comfortably in the dental chair and his eyes are fixed either on a point on the ceiling or on the tip of a pen or pencil (the intra-oral lamp is a very suitable object upon which the patient can be asked to fix). The object is held above and slightly to the rear of the patient's eyes, so that a pronounced effort has to be made to keep it in view, and is sufficiently near for the eyes to focus convergently upon it (i.e. not more than a foot or 18 inches away).

The patient is asked to relax his muscles completely...to get really comfortable in the chair...and to fix his eyes upon the point. He is then told to count quietly to himself, backwards from 300. As he does this, suggestions are made of increasing heaviness of his eyes...of heaviness of the eyelids...and of a general feeling of lassitude.

These suggestions are given in a monotonous tone of voice, and in a very short time, the eyes will appear to focus away in the distance and will become rather more moist than they normally are. Then the eyelids will begin to flicker a little, at which point the suggestions of heaviness are pressed with more emphasis and the patient told that his eyelids are wanting to close...that they are heavier and heavier...and are wanting to close, more and more. Eye closure usually follows rapidly, and can be accelerated at the right moment by the instruction to go to sleep. The patient is then told that he will not want to open his eyes until instructed to do so.

Both the eye fixation progressive relaxation method and the thumb nail technique (see Chapter 5) are equally suitable, the latter being the speedier.

The 'Dropped Coin' Technique

Another simple and quick method of induction favoured by many dental surgeons is the *'dropped coin technique'*. This is another 'eye fixation' procedure, using the patient's thumb as a fixation point. Ideomotor activity in the actual opening of the fingers is also involved:

I want you to relax as much as possible...don't try to make
anything happen...don't try to stop anything happening...just let
everything happen...as it wants to happen.
All you have to do is to follow my instructions...and you will find
it very easy to drift into a sleep-like state...but although your
eyes will close...and will remain closed...you will not actually be
asleep.
You will know everything that is going on...but you will not have
the slightest desire to open your eyes...until I tell you to do so.
You could open them at any moment...if you wanted to...but you
won't...simply because you have no desire to do so.
Let us use this coin.
I am going to place this coin in your right hand...and I want you
to close your fingers gently...so that when I turn your hand
over...the coin does not fall.
Now...hold your right arm straight out...at shoulder level...and

stretch out your thumb.

Keep your eyes fixed on it...because I want you to follow these instructions carefully.

Fix your eyes upon your thumb nail...and don't let them wander from it for a single moment.

Whilst your eyes are fixed upon your thumb nail...I want you to pay close attention to your fingers...and to the coin...which is loosely held in the palm of your hand.

Notice the position of your fingers with regard to the coin...the position of your fingers with regard to each other...and to the palm of your hand. You can actually feel the coin...in the palm of your hand...and as you do so...you will become aware of a number of different sensations.

Now...I am going to start counting slowly upwards from *One*. With each count...you will feel your fingers becoming more and more relaxed...more and more relaxed.

And as they do so...they will gradually straighten out to a point when the coin will drop out of your hand...and will fall on the floor.

When the coin drops...that will be a signal for three things to happen.

Your eyes will close...your whole body will sink back into the chair...and you will fall into a deep, deep sleep.

Your eyes may become so tired...through gazing at your thumb nail...that they may even close before the coin drops.

If they do...that's fine.

Just keep them closed...and when the coin drops...let your whole body sink back comfortably into the chair...without bothering about your eyes which are already closed.

It may be...that as I count...your eyes will begin to blink.

If so...just let them blink as much as they want...and they will begin to feel so heavy...that it will be more comfortable to let them close on their own.

ONE...Your fingers are beginning to relax...more...and more...and more. They are no longer touching the palm of your hand...and they are beginning to open...just a little bit.

TWO...Relaxing more...and more...and more.

Your fingers are beginning to straighten out...they are opening more and more...so that the coin is now resting mainly on your fingers.

THREE...You can notice quite a bit of movement now...in your fingers...and soon...that coin is going to drop to the floor...even

sooner than you think.
FOUR...You're making excellent progress...just continue to
relax...and let yourself go, completely.
FIVE...Your fingers are straightening out now...more...and
more...and more. Soon...that coin will drop...and as it strikes the
floor...let yourself slump limply down into the chair...let your
eyes close...and enjoy that feeling of complete and utter
relaxation.
SIX...You're doing splendidly...just let those fingers
relax...more...and more...and more.
SEVEN...With each count...your fingers are relaxing...more and
more...straightening out...more and more...so that your hand is
slowly opening...and, very soon now...that coin will drop.

(Suppose at this point, the coin drops).

Deeply relaxed...deeply relaxed...go very, very deeply asleep.

The subject can then be told to take several very deep
breaths...and that with each breath that he takes...he will become
more and more deeply relaxed...deeper and deeper asleep. The
hypnosis can be deepened by whatever method seems appropriate.

The Induction of Hypnosis in Children

Once a child's confidence has been gained, the induction of hypnosis becomes relatively easy since most children are readily susceptible unless they are exceptionally timid and nervous. The
dentist's prestige will assist him in establishing satisfactory rapport, and in many cases, the deeper stages will be established
without difficulty. The precise age of the child is not the most important factor. What does matter is whether the child's interest
and attention can be held long enough for the suggestions to take
effect. Consequently, the method may have to be varied from time
to time in order to achieve this object. Provided that the child is
able to count at all, a modified version of the eye fixation–distraction method is usually most successful.

Tell the child to keep looking at the light, and to count slowly as
far as it can. When it has reached this point, it is to start at the
beginning again and repeat the count. In younger children it is
often advisable to allow them to count out aloud, for this often

seems to help considerably. During the count, the usual
suggestions are made, suitably reworded and simplified, until the
eyes close. This usually happens very quickly indeed.

If the very young child can be cajoled into keeping its eyes fixed
upon the light, or dental mirror, the count can often be omitted
for hypnosis will frequently supervene as a result of verbal suggestion alone.

The 'Picture Visualization' Technique

Some dentists favour the picture visualization technique described by Moss[1], an effective version of which is as follows:

> Now it's time for us to play a game together...you'd like that,
> wouldn't you?
> I'll teach you what to do...and it's going to be a lot of
> fun...because all you have to do is to close your eyes...and
> pretend that you're asleep. You won't be really asleep, of
> course...but it will be most exciting...because during this
> 'pretend' sleep, you can watch films...television...circuses...or
> anything else you enjoy.
> So...make yourself as comfortable as possible...and start
> pretending, as soon as you're ready.
> Close your eyes...and don't open them again until I ask you.
> Now, I'd like you to pretend that you are back at home watching
> your favourite television programme.
> I'm just going to lift up your hand...and as I lift it...the picture
> becomes sharper and clearer.
> The better the picture...the higher your hand will rise...and the
> higher your hand rises...the better the picture will become.
> And presently...you'll find that your elbow will begin to
> bend...and your hand will move towards your face.
> And when your hand touches your face...that picture will be
> perfect.
> But don't let your hand touch your face...until you are satisfied
> with the picture. That's fine. Keep on watching the picture...and
> don't lose it...and you'll find that your hand will drop down to
> your lap...and as it does...you can pretend to be really asleep.
> And notice how limp and slack your muscles have become.
> Now, with television pictures...there is usually some music.
> Just listen to that music...and as soon as you can hear it...start
> marking time to the music with your hand or finger.

Keep on watching the picture...and don't lose it.
As long as you have the picture...lift up the finger of your other
hand...and keep it up.
Then I'll know that this is the 'picture' finger...and the other is
the 'music' finger.
What sort of picture are you looking at?
Are there people or animals in it...or both?
It really doesn't matter...because if you want to change the
picture...you can do so quite easily.
Don't lose the picture...or the music.
And I'd like you to know...that when you watch television like
this...you can feel things...but they won't bother you.
I can even pinch you...like this...and although you can feel the
pinch...it doesn't bother you at all. That's right...isn't it?
Now I'm going to be working on your teeth...and although you
can feel something going on...as long as you go on watching the
picture...and listening to the music...it won't bother you...and
really won't matter.
Is the picture still there? Is the music still there?
Just keep on watching...and listening.

Children have such vivid imaginations that one might almost
say that they spend a considerable part of their time in 'a world
of pretence'. Consequently, a technique of this kind is quite natural to them. You will notice that whilst watching the picture and
listening to the music, they become completely relaxed and 'miles
away', so that it is quite easy to work on them. They can still feel
things, but it no longer matters or bothers them.
To awaken the child, you can say that someone has turned the
television off, so it really isn't much use going on pretending. So
tell it that it can stop pretending now, open its eyes, and be wide
awake again.

Trance-deepening Procedures

A similar trance-deepening routine to that which has already
been described may be followed. Begin by eliciting arm heaviness
followed by arm catalepsy (raising the arm and telling the patient
it will remain in the air without any conscious effort on his part,
until he is told to lower it). Deepening is then continued by the
induction of automatic movement, either through the continuous

rotation of the patient's hands, one around the other, or through a to and fro movement of the forearm, the patient being instructed to visualize a piece of cord pulling the hand backwards and forwards. Should these tests prove successful, the final deepening technique may consist of dream induction. The patient is asked to visualize in his mind some simple action such as combing the hair, washing the face or undoing a tie. He is then instructed to dream that he is performing this simple action, and as he does so, to act it out as he sits in the chair.

Tests for somnambulism can subsequently be applied. The patient can be told to open his eyes without awakening from the trance, and to rinse out his mouth, and that when he sits back in the chair again and his head touches the head-rest his eyes will close and he will remain in a very deep sleep. If he accomplishes this successfully, he has achieved the stage of somnambulism.

The breathing technique is another useful deepening agent which seems to work extremely well with many patients. The patient is instructed to breathe in deeply...to hold his breath for two seconds...and as he breathes out, he will go into a deeper trance. This is repeated five times, and it is often quite dramatic to watch the patient deepening and relaxing, and his muscles becoming completely limp and flaccid as he breathes deeply in and out.

Dental Procedures at the Various Levels of Hypnosis

Even when the patient only succeeds in achieving light hypnosis, it should still be possible to enlist greater co-operation on his part and a considerable degree of relaxation. One can also expect to reduce his anxiety and fear, and to induce a certain amount of drowsiness and sleepiness in preparation for anaesthesia, either general or local. Moreover, the efforts made by the patient to tolerate the wearing of dentures or orthodontic appliances can often be improved.

In medium-depth hypnosis, all the above can be obtained even more easily and completely. Varying degrees of analgesia can also be produced, together with some control of fainting, bleeding and saliva flow. Gagging, during the taking of impressions, can be reduced, and muscular rigidity of the jaw and neck can be secured.

In deep hypnosis, in addition to the above, complete analgesia and possibly some amnesia can be obtained. In our experience, however, analgesia and amnesia are not necessarily both obtainable in every deep-trance subject. There may be complete analgesia without amnesia or the reverse. Unfortunately, the phenomena that can be elicited at different levels of hypnosis vary considerably from patient to patient, and it is fair to say that no general rules can be laid down as to what one can expect in any one individual.

The Time Factor in Dental Hypnosis

No more than three sessions should ordinarily be devoted to attempting to induce hypnosis. If satisfactory progress is not made within three to five minutes on each of these separate occasions, then the patient is not a suitable subject for hypnosis in a busy practice, since treatment will necessarily be both protracted and unremunerative.

It will be realized that nearly all dental patients could be assisted to some extent by hypnosis—at least 90 per cent—so that the use that any individual dentist makes of hypnosis in his own practice is bound to depend upon the amount of time he is prepared to devote to it, and whether the patient is strongly in favour of it. When dentists first begin to use hypnosis they could spend many hours in attempting all the various phases of its application in dentistry, but most who have worked in this field for a number of years find it no longer necessary to employ hypnosis regularly, since many of the patients who were hypnotized in the first place have gained so much confidence that they do not require it any more.

Some patients are interested to have hypnotic treatment merely for the experience, and unless the dentist can see a real need for it, such requests should be firmly discouraged. On the other hand, there are a limited number of patients whom we should never be able to treat without the aid of hypnosis, used in one of the ways already mentioned. It is in such instances as these that the greatest benefit is to be found, since these patients can be rendered quite amenable to treatment if a little time and care is taken in their preparation.

REFERENCES

1. Moss A.A., 1952. *Hypnodontics.* Kimpton, London

PART FOUR

OTHER USES AND SOME ABUSES OF HYPNOSIS

CHAPTER 24

Hypnotherapy and Competitive Sports

With the increase in the numbers and variations of national and international competitions, especially where sponsorship is involved, sport has become a major industry. Considerable sums are offered as rewards and untold wealth, fame and glory, annually await the new champions.

As competitions have grown in importance so the physical and psychological demands upon the participants has resulted in the standard of medical care assuming a major role. Thus sports medicine has now reached specialist status, the doctors themselves being examined as to their proficiency in treatment.

Many disciplines are involved and where psychological problems exist, a range of techniques can be offered. These include training in relaxation, in assertiveness and in mental attitudes, desensitization, autogenic training and biofeedback. Although numerous experts exist in these fields however, hypnotherapy, which can often be the treatment of choice, has so far received only limited recognition. This is probably as a result of ignorance of the nature of the hypnotic state as well as of its applications.

Specific problems can be identified in which hypnosis may be used in competitive sports and these are as follows:

1. *Trait Anxiety*
This is the situation in which a high level of anxiety exists as a particular quality of the individual. That is, it is always present.

Thus although it will sometimes be of advantage in that performance will commence at a higher level of arousal, yet the ceiling to that arousal will be reached sooner and responses will begin to deteriorate.

Treatment is as for anxiety in general. Hypnosis and instruction in self-hypnosis to be performed as a minimum twice daily and additionally before any sporting event, in order to reduce the level of anxiety. This is followed by exploration of any other possible related worries. Then, desensitization to as extensive a hierarchy of anxiety-producing situations as can be devised. 'Self-desensitization' or mental rehearsal in self-hypnosis is a useful addition.

2. *State Anxiety.*

In any individual there may be a response of severe anxiety to a specific situation, for example the approach and the challenge of the actual game, competition or performance. In the acute state it is equivalent to stage fright or 'freezing' and this is discussed separately. Prolonged training, exhortations to win, reports of unbeatable challengers and so on, all add to the stressful demands. Stress has been generally too loosely defined. It should be confined specifically to the effects of 'pressure of some adverse force or influence' (O.E.D.), that is external pressures. Such pressures are only tolerable to a certain level above which the cracks begin to appear. This is the state of the *person,* in which psychic and somatic symptoms of anxiety are noted. In other words increase in stress will result in increased levels of state anxiety. Therefore, performance will initially improve but will then reach a point beyond which it will begin to deteriorate.

Maximum performance must depend on maximum *tolerable* arousal. That there is a direct interrelationship between anxiety and arousal was effectively demonstrated at the beginning of the century by Yerkes and Dodson[1]. The inverted 'U' hypothesis which demonstrates this relationship of performance to stimulus is well known. As arousal is increased so performance is enhanced. But when the stimulus reaches a certain limit that level of performance can no longer be sustained and begins to diminish. This conclusion subsequently led to many studies which have largely validated the idea. However, Jackson[2] has shown that the issue regarding the relationship between performance efficiency and arousal still remains a contentious one. At some point nevertheless, a delicate balance between arousal and performance is reached and this must not be exceeded. The question that arises is where does arousal end and where do anxiety symptoms begin? The answer to this may be found by very gentle exploration under hypnosis. In addition, hypnosis must be used to help the subject to tolerate maximum arousal without the production of symptoms. Krenz *et al.*[3] presented an excellent paper in a study of athletes and the use of post-hypnotic suggestion in the reduction of state anxiety. Their findings also could be interpreted to confirm that state anxiety and stress are independent phenomena.

Other problems that need to be researched are the mental attitude of the competitor during the actual performance and the level of 'need' for achievement.

Desensitization for state anxiety will differ from that of trait anxiety in that more specific fears can be identified and particular emphasis may be given to these fears. A typical hierarchy would be as follows:

1. The status of the event (local, national or international).
2. The environment of the event (hall, theatre, stadium).
3. High expectations.
4. Media coverage.
5. Status of major opponents (publicity, bragging, etc.).
6. At the event itself (changing or dressing rooms).
7. In front of spectators (focus of attention, noise and cheers).
8. Ready to start...start.
9. Actual performance...to win.
10. Attitude at completion.

One competitive golfer complained that every time he reached the green and addressed the ball with his putter his arm would stiffen so that he was unable to play his stroke efficiently. He believed that the condition originated six months earlier when playing an important club match. At that time he was suddenly distracted at the twelfth hole by an aeroplane which appeared to be diving from the sky directly at him. 'Reminded me of those days in the desert when we were repeatedly strafed from the air and had to dive for cover', he said. 'Were you afraid?' he was asked 'Scared stiff' was the prompt reply. He at once understood the slip of the tongue and had inadvertently provided the route of his cure. Treatment was as has been described.

Relaxation under hypnosis and discussion of some of his traumatic wartime experiences as an infantryman in the Middle East helped him to obtain a rational explanation of the common fear response of increased muscular tension. Desensitization by visualization of himself on the green, looking at his golf ball and then the hole and experiencing a feeling of total relaxation before taking his shot in the best professional manner, relieved him of his acute anxiety in five sessions. Instruction in self-hypnosis was an integral part of the treatment.

3. Acute Performance Anxiety

This is the equivalent of stage fright. The difference between this and state anxiety again is often confused and should be looked upon as one of degree only.

Naruse[4] treated such patients by direct hypnotic suggestion and self-hypnosis in conjunction with other modalities. He also used a technique which he called an 'escape from reality into happy trance'. Whilst in hypnosis it was suggested to the subject that he was living far away from his usual everyday life, that he was indifferent to the opinion of other persons or society and that critical evaluation of him by others did not matter to him, that he would remain calm until the coming game, recall only his successful games and not recall the unsuccessful ones. He repeated the treatment several times until the actual day of the event.

4. Injury and Pain

These are problems which have taken on a very important dimension in competitive sports. In a leading article in the British Medical Journal[5] it was stated that between 2.5 and 10 per cent of attendances at accident and emergency clinics follow acute sports injuries. This certainly indicates the need for the establishment of specialized sports injury units in major hospitals in the sports centres of the world.

The results of injury not only mean that there is physical damage which will inhibit or prohibit performance, or that pain will be an inevitable result, but the damage may also affect the person's attitude to future competitive events.

It is possible to alleviate pain through the use of hypnosis, by the production of an area of analgesia over the affective part. This could be, however, a dangerous and ill-advised procedure. The nature of the injury must be clearly identified before any hypnotic intervention is attempted. Minor injuries which have been positively diagnosed and in which any use of the affected part would not aggravate the condition, may be treated by hypnosis. Since most injuries however, involve strain or damage which may necessitate immobilization and rest, the use of hypnosis must be very selective indeed.

Its most valuable application is to reduce the inevitable overlay of anxiety which compounds any pain, particularly that which will occur when there is a great deal at stake.

Many athletes have difficulty in adjusting to injury. Career prospects could be jeopardized and repeated injury to a particular part may inhibit performance even when the person is otherwise perfectly well. Anxiety may be readily aggravated by fear of yet further damage. Repeated injury however, may also have a different meaning. Does the injury serve a purpose? Is the competitor unconsciously avoiding the competiton? Perhaps a minor injury will even avoid the possibility of a major injury. Perhaps withdrawal from the competition will mean the avoidance of the need to win.

Some athletes may acquire a reputation for being accident prone. This problem may be one merely of coincidence. It may be due to the mood of the person at the time. It may be expression of some emotion deeply hidden in the unconscious, of anger or of guilt. It may be due to lack of confidence or some other manifestation of anxiety which can be explored within the relaxed state of hypnosis. The possibility of unconscious motives behind repeated injury should always be considered. After discussion and the necessary insight-directed psychotherapy, then ego-strengthening and ego-assertive retraining to meet the next competitive event can be of considerable benefit.

5. *Failure to Achieve Potential and Repeated Mistakes.*

This problem requires very thorough investigation as no single factor may be responsible. Performers who have ability and fail to function to the level of that ability may not only be anxious but may also be depressed and this is a possibility which should be seriously addressed. Repetition of poor performance may result in a learned response which could be extremely difficult to rectify. Yaffé[6] conducted a study amongst English competitors at a prestigious international sporting event, asking which was the most important psychological factor upon which good performance depended. The results are reproduced below.

The most important psychological factors for doing well
(responses represented as percentages)

Factors	Competitors		Coaches
	Male	Female	
Concentration	30.9	26.3	45.0
Selective attention	4.4	2.8	5.0
Control of anxiety	6.4	5.4	21.1
Relaxation	13.8	21.1	15.8
Assertiveness	2.2	2.6	5.3
Self-confidence	40.8	39.5	26.3
Other	36.4	20.0	66.7

As can be seen self-confidence was of supreme importance for doing well and concentration was also highly rated. The scores for coaches may also be seen. This is particularly relevant in any psychological approach to treatment as increasing self-confidence and improvement in concentration can be repeatedly emphasized when using hypnotherapy by the techniques already described.

If early symptoms are neglected and the competitor continues to lose confidence so he will begin to make mistakes which only increase his loss of confidence. He becomes anxious and angry and will make more mistakes and thus if depression was not one of the precipitating causes of his problem in the first place, it will certainly be present by now and other symptoms will appear. Early and accurate diagnosis and treatment is therefore essential.

6. *Depression*

Persistent failure to achieve expected results may be due to a variety of reasons and the possibility of depression as a cause or result of that failure is one which requires immediate attention. This is a problem which can result in failure in many activities, not least of all in sports.

All sporting activities involve a physical and a mental component and although anxiety and perhaps other mental disturbances may readily be revealed, the possibility of depression should be deliberately explored and identified if any biological symptoms are present. Amongst the features are the following:

1. Sleep difficulties, initial and intermediate difficulties and particularly but not necessarily, early morning waking.
2. Depressed mood on waking with possible diurnal mood swing.
3. Loss of appetite.
4. Loss of weight.
5. Loss of energy.
6. Loss of interest.
7. Constipation.
8. Loss of libido.
9. Pre-menstrual depression or menstrual irregularity in females.
10. Loss of concentration.
11. Loss of drive and of the mood to win.

If a diagnosis of depression is made, what sort of depression is it and what is the possible cause? Look into the following:

1. Fear of failure.
2. Repeated failures.
3. Injury.
4. Repeated injury.
5. Other illness.
6. Life events (e.g. financial or domestic difficulties).

7. Side-effects or drugs (e.g. antibiotics).

8. A recurrence of a chronic endogenous depression.

9. The depressed phase of a hitherto undetected bipolar depression.

10. Pre-menstrual depression in a female competitor.

Any depressive illness must be treated as a serious illness. It should not be ignored for the sake of the sport and it is ethical and proper to withdraw the candidate if the nature of the depression is sufficiently serious and if the treatment would normally demand this. Drug treatment may be essential and side-effects such as weight increase or the sedation which occurs with certain antidepressants, should be watched for. On the other hand, complete withdrawal from the sport may be counter-productive and running, for example may even be therapeutic.

Hypnosis may be used in any type of depression provided that antidepressant medication has been prescribed and when it is evident (say after two to four weeks) that the drug is exerting its effect.

Hypnosis will reduce any accompanying anxiety but it is emphasized again, should *not* be used in an attempt to remove the symptoms of depression. It *may* be used to explore the precipitating causes of a reactive depression and to restore to the patient his positive feelings, self-confidence, drive and goals. Cognitive-hypnotherapy would be a great advantage (see Chapter 21).

Finally, in the use of hypnosis for problems arising in competiting sports any or all of the following techniques may be employed:

1. The reduction of anxiety to the upper limits of arousal.

2. The restoration and maintenance of confidence, drive and goals.

3. Hypnoanalysis to enable the competitor to ventilate his feelings, followed by insight-directed psychotherapy.

4. Desensitization along a hierarchy of anxiety-producing situations.

5. Self-hypnosis to help reduce anxiety with self-desensitization, that is the mental rehearsal for training and for the event.

6. Practical retraining where possible, through competitive events graduated in importance.

7. Ego-strengthening for self-confidence and self-image.

8. Ego-assertive retraining.
9. Specific treatment for pain if required.
10. Post-hypnotic suggestion to win.

It must be emphasized that hypnosis cannot produce a performance beyond the physical capability of the athlete. It is not a substitute for training, skill and experience. Competitors under *stress* are more likely to make errors. However, performance will improve if the upper level of arousal can be tempered with feelings of calmness and complete control. Hypnosis can certainly help to bring a healthier attitude to any sport or competition.

REFERENCES

1. Yerkes R.M. and Dodson, J.D., 1908. The relation of strength of stimulus to rapidity of habit-formation. *J. Comp. Neurol. Psychol.*, **18,** 459–482.
2. Jackson J.A., 1982. The hypnotic management of sports anxiety. Paper read at 9th International Congress of Hypnosis and Psychosomatic Medicine, Glasgow.
3. Krenz E.W., Gordin R. and Edwards S.W., 1985. In: *Modern Trends in Hypnosis* (eds Waxman, Misra, Gibson and Basker). Plenum, New York.
4. Naruse G., 1965. The hypnotic treatment of stage fright in champion athletes. *Int. J. Clin. Exp. Hypnosis,* **XIII,** 63–70.
5. Stableforth P.G., 1987. Why sports injury clinics? *Br. Med. J.,* **295,** 799.
6. Yaffé M., 1979. The contribution of psychology to sport: an overview. *Medisport,* **1,** 18.

CHAPTER 25

The Use of Hypnosis in Criminal Investigation

Forensic medicine is a speciality which has made considerable advances over recent years so that the investigator is often enabled to identify various signs or clues with indisputable accuracy.

Unfortunately the same does not apply to forensic hypnosis. It is certainly a specialized subject. However modern research has more clearly defined not only its uses but also its weaknesses.

It has generally been employed as a means of 'reviving' and exploring the memory of a victim or witness of some serious crime. However, not only may that memory be lacking or at fault, but often the technique used can be somewhat wanting.

A popular misconception is that hypnosis is an infallible means of making a person confess to or deny, some crime or misdemeanour of which he may have been accused. It certainly cannot do that. Nor is it in any way guaranteed to provide any information which could not ordinarily be obtained in the waking state.

Hypnosis has no facility for revealing the incontrovertible truth. No disclosure made under hypnosis can have the validity of a fingerprint.

Hypnosis, however, is a useful tool which is employed by many police forces in the world in order to attempt to obtain information that could *lead* to certain clues which would otherwise not have been revealed.

Such information is not evidence.

It is a fallacy to believe that every event or experience, however trivial, is somehow registered in the mind, never to be forgotten. Many events of course, are recorded and can easily be recalled. Others may fade with the passage of time and be completely lost, whilst others perhaps which are frightening or humiliating, or which are associated with an experience too traumatic to tolerate, may be repressed below the level of conscious awareness and there retained.

In an effort to recover earlier memories some investigators prefer the euphemistic phrase 'memory enhancement'. Perhaps this is rather an attempt to describe what happens with the use of hypnosis, whilst ensuring that not too much should be expected. For example we know that some 'forgotten' memories may be recaptured simply by concentration in the waking state. As we have all experienced, sitting quietly with the eyes closed and excluding all external sounds and other stimuli will aid concentration and a particular memory may come to the surface. Additionally, in any situation of stress, anxiety may cloud the memory of that incident. Hypnosis can be of great help in such cases. By reducing the level of anxiety and with the subject's mind 'locked' to the words of the therapist all external stimuli can be ignored and concentration and memory will then be enhanced.

Repressed memories may sometimes be recalled under hypnosis. This depends upon the hypnotizability of the subject and the skill of the hypnotist. The release of repressed memories however could be accompanied by a highly traumatic display of emotions and should only be attempted by a specialist experienced in the handling of an abreaction. One must remember also the possible post-hypnotic effects that the release of repressed emotions may have upon the hypnotized person so that suitable arrangements may be made for careful observation, follow-up and counselling if necessary.

Any 'information' obtained by age-regression is certainly not infallible. It should be noted that subjects are also able to age-progress under hypnosis[1]!

Nevertheless, we may recall, from the work of Breuer and Freud that an abreaction may also bring considerable benefit to the subject. This they demonstrated whilst working with their patient Anna O[2].

Freud also noted that a patient's 'recall' under hypnosis may not necessarily be a true record of events as they actually happened. It is of the utmost importance to understand this when hypnosis is used for forensic purposes.

In the clinical situation the therapist is able to discuss with the patient whatever he may be saying. He may be expected to give him insight and understanding into any reported experiences and to his responses. In forensic investigation under hypnosis however, it is important that no guiding remarks or suggestions are given in any circumstances. Any chance comment, any sound or movement by the hypnotist, may be picked up by the subject and may influence his thoughts and words. There must be no non-verbal communication whatsoever so that there is no possibility of the subject being 'contaminated' by external cueing.

Memory is not necessarily more accurate in the hypnotic state than it is in the normal waking state. Moreover, if any information given by the subject has been the result of fantasy or confabulation it may be perceived by him on waking as a true 'memory' of the events under investigation and that person would then be an unreliable witness.

Both hypnotist and police must be aware of some basic problems which have emerged as a result of the work of Orne[3] and many others. They may be summarized as follows:

1. Subjects may simulate hypnosis.
2. They may wilfully lie, even in deep hypnosis.
3. They may confabulate or fantasize[1].
4. Such confabulation or fantasy or some subtle or unwitting suggestion made by the hypnotist may result in the development of 'pseudo-memories' which may come to be accepted by the subject as his actual recall of original events.
5. The veracity of 'recall' under hypnosis must always be in doubt. It must be regarded as information only and further corroborative evidence is *always* essential.

One of the first known cases of an application to the courts for the use of hypnosis to be admissible as evidence occurred in Cali-

THE USE OF HYPNOSIS IN CRIMINAL INVESTIGATION

fornia in 1897[4]. An accused man was questioned under hypnosis and denied his guilt. The court held that 'the law in the United States does not recognize hypnotism'.

Nevertheless in more recent times many people including witnesses, victims and persons accused of crime have appeared before the courts both in the USA and other countries in order to give 'evidence' obtained whilst that person was under hypnosis.

Fortunately, research into the subject has been considerable and the debate continues.

Summary of Relevant Literature

In discussing the problem of recall where emotional factors are involved Kroger[5] found hypnosis to be an effectual tool to achieve hyperamnesia. Similarly, Goldstein and Sipprelle[6] found that if emotional trauma had resulted in the production of amnesia for the precipitating event then hypnosis seemed to facilitate the recall of that event. Field and Dworkin[7], however, introduced a note of caution. They reported that people who have something to hide, can successfully hide that material even if deeply hypnotized. Kleinhauz et al.[8], researching the literature found that improvement of recall increased with the significance of the memory and also depended upon the amount of anxiety evoked by the event itself. Schafer and Rubio[9] made the very important point that the ideal case for hypnosis of a witness as an aid for justice is where the information obtained is additional to that obtained by ordinary interrogative processes and leads to the investigation of a suspect who can be convicted or exonerated only by material evidence additional to that obtained by hypnosis. As a result of their laboratory investigations, Hilgard and Loftus[10] drew attention to the need for extreme care in the wording of questions put to a subject as these can not only affect the answers given but may also distort the memory of the witness for the actual reported experience. The manner in which questions are put can also lead the witness, and this was emphasized in a paper by Zelig and Beidleman[11]. Wagstaff[12,13] recognized two very important points regarding the difference between laboratory investigaton and any actual case of forensic examination of a witness under hypnosis. These were that:

1. The greater value of hypnosis may lie in its ability to create a social situation in which witnesses may feel able to divulge distressing or embarrassing information.

2. In many eyewitness situations the witness is under a great deal of stress, whereas in most laboratory situations the subjects are not.

Perry and Laurence[14], reviewing the enhancement of memory by hypnosis, found that the two main problems are confabulation and the creation of pseudo-memories. They stressed the need for stringent safeguards.

In the summary to a Council Report on the subject, the American Medical Association[15] suggested yet a further need. They advised that the subject's response to the termination of hypnosis and the post-hypnotic discussion concerning the experience of hypnosis are of major importance in assessing the subject's response to hypnosis.

The views of an English court were unequivocal. In a judgment given in 1986, Mr Justice Tucker stated 'As a matter of principle, evidence produced by the administration of a mechanically or chemically or hypnotically induced test on a witness so as to show the veracity or otherwise of that witness is not admissible in an English court of law'[16]. This statement ensures that in England at least any information obtained under hypnosis is not *evidence* and confirms the need for corroboration.

Nevertheless, Le Page and Goldney[17] reported a case in Australia, where hypnosis was used to retrieve memory loss due to post-traumatic retrograde amnesia resulting from a severe head injury sustained in a road-traffic accident. The information obtained was subsequently accepted as admissible in court proceedings. This provided a precedent for the acceptance by courts of law of previously amnesic information retrieved by means of hypnosis, where the amnesia was due to trauma.

There is no doubt therefore that considerable differences of opinion still exist in courts of law throughout the world.

Haward[18] deplored the attempt to discourage the use of investigative hypnosis on the grounds that it has no validity when considerable positive (if anecdotal) evidence exists to the contrary. He asked 'How much relevant anecdotal evidence is required to outweigh irrelevant experimental evidence?' But if certain strict safeguards are utilized with hypnosis, suggested Perry and Nogrady[19], and provided the hypnotized witness is not permitted to testify in court, there is little danger of abuse and miscarriage of justice.

Summary of Safeguards Required

1. The subject must be entirely willing to undergo hypnosis. The process should be fully explained and signed and witnessed consent must be obtained.

2. The perpetrator or suspected perpetrator of the crime should never be hypnotized.

3. Immunity from prosecution should never be offered to the person being hypnotized.

4. Hypnosis should only be carried out by a physician or psychologist with experience in the clinical use and with special training in the forensic use, of hypnosis.

5. He must be an independent consultant with no responsibility to either side in the case.

6. He should be given only some basic known facts of the case with no information which could possibly bias his opinion. He must be given no knowledge of any suspect and must remain completely impartial.

7. The specialist undertaking the hypnosis must make a full medical and psychiatric evaluation of the subject before commencing. He must be satisfied that the subject is a fit person to undergo hypnosis.

8. Tape recordings and videotape recordings covering the total area of the room in which the interview is to take place should be made of the *entire* proceedings from the moment the subject enters the room.

He must be told that the interview is being recorded. The sealed tapes should be opened and subsequently resealed by the police officer in charge of the case.

9. Only the specialist and the subject should be in the interview room during the period of the examination in order to avoid inadvertent cueing of the subject by other persons.

10. Full discussion should take place after the termination of

hypnosis. The specialist should allow the subject to make his comments but must make no suggestion of enhanced memory. This discussion should be included in the taped recordings. Arrangements for follow-up must be made. This could be with the subject's general practitioner.

11. Any information obtained under hypnosis should be regarded as hearsay.

It must never be admissible as evidence in any court of law. Corroborative evidence should always be obtained by the police. The corollary is that information at the interview cannot be used to corroborate other information for which there is no evidence.

12. The person undergoing hypnosis should not be called upon to give evidence in court thus avoiding the danger of the introduction of 'pseudo-memories'.

Summary of Technique

The investigation of any subject for forensic purposes must conform to these safeguards. Failure to do so may prejudice the case and all involved. It may mean the loss of vital evidence or even a miscarriage of justice. It is a discrete and time consuming exercise but one which can often be of considerable assistance in the pursuance of the perpetrators of crime.

Of great importance is the initial assessment of the subject and the establishment of rapport. This all serves to reinforce hypnotizability and very rarely would further testing be required. Before hypnosis commences, the subject is asked simply 'What happened to you regarding the event under investigation?' No further questions are put. We have thus a base line for the patient's conscious recall. The technique of induction should be explained and must always be totally non-authoritarian.

Hypnosis and deepening is then carried out and the subject is taken back to the morning of the day in question, well before any known or suspected time of the relevant event and he should be simply asked 'Tell me what is happening.'

There must be no prompting, no suggestions, no further questions and no advice put to him. The specialist takes on a silent and purely passive role whilst observing the subject continuously.

The officer in charge of the case has been instructed to pass a note under the door should he require some further information and the subject is warned that this may occur so as not to cause alarm. The relevant questions may be put to the subject during the hypnosis but in a manner in which no cueing could be interpreted. Otherwise the only remarks permitted are an occasional 'uh-huh' or 'what then?'

The subject may commence by saying 'I remember...' This is recall and he should be allowed to continue. On the other hand he may regress and relive the day and the event. He speaks in the present tense and there is no doubt by his expression and attitude that he is 'reliving' those events, albeit possibly fantasizing.

Should a severe abreaction occur then appropriate calming words are necessary. If the subject awakens during the abreaction he should be allowed to calm himself for a few minutes and then when he is ready, he is re-hypnotized and the session is continued.

At the end of the investigation, the subject is awakened with the usual suggestions of well being. No post-hypnotic suggestion should be given that he will recall further material as a result of the hypnosis. If, in the subsequent discussion, further information is forthcoming, this should be entirely unprompted.

It should be remembered that in true regression not only may there be visual and auditory recall. Any sensation previously experienced may be once again perceived.

One young victim of rape had become extremely depressed after the event. She had however extensive recall but insufficient to give the police any worthwhile information. At one point under hypnosis she looked puzzled and remained silent for a while. When she spoke again she said 'There's that funny smell again...it's a sort of farmyard smell...'

A few days later a tramp, who had been sleeping rough, was arrested for some petty theft. A bracelet which he had taken from the victim's wrist was found in his pocket...

He eventually confessed to the crime.

However, an additional dividend in this case was that the victim's depression lifted and she was able to reintegrate once again into her normal life.

There is no doubt that the use of hypnosis in criminology has in the past been applied in a manner leaving much to be desired, particularly in the United States of America.

Those who have utilized this method have been exposed to a great deal of criticism and laboratory research has revealed many of the weaknesses.

If we are to recognize the true value of this technique, stringent safeguards as outlined must be applied and the guidelines strictly observed.

If under such conditions hypnosis is used, there is no doubt that it may offer a valuable additional modality in the investigation of serious crime.

REFERENCES

1. Rubenstein R, and Newman R., 1954. The living out of 'future' experiences under hypnosis. *Science*, **119,**472–473.
2. Breuer J. and Freud S., 1955. Studies on hysteria. In: *Standard Edition of the Complete Psychological Works of Sigmund Freud* (ed. Strachey), Vol. 11. Hogarth, London.
3. Orne M.T., 1979. The use and misuse of hypnosis in court. *Int. J. Clin. Exp. Hypnosis*, **XXVII,** 311–341.
4. Warner K.E., 1979. The use of hypnosis in the defense of criminal cases. *Int. J. Clin. Exp. Hypnosis*, **XXVII,** 417–436.
5. Kroger W.S., 1963. *Clinical and Experimental Hypnosis.* Lippincott, Philadelphia.
6. Goldstein M.S. and Sipprelle C.N., 1970. Hypnotically induced amnesia versus ablation of memory. *Int. J. Clin. Exp. Hypnosis*, **18,** 211–216.
7. Field P.B. and Dworkin S.F., 1967. Strategies of hypnotic interrogation. *J. Psychol.*, **67,** 47–58.
8. Kleinhauz M., Horowitz I. and Tobin Y., 1977. The use of hypnosis in police investigation. A preliminary communication. *J. Forensic Sci. Soc.*, **17,** 77–80.
9. Schafer D.W. and Rubio R., 1978. Hypnosis to aid the recall of witnesses. *Int. J. Clin. Exp. Hypnosis*, **XXVI,** 81–91.
10. Hilgard E.R. and Loftus E.F., 1979. Effective interrogation of the eyewitness. *Int. J. Clin. Exp. Hypnosis*, **XXVII,** 342–357.
11. Zelig M. and Beidleman W.B., 1981. The investigative use of hypnosis: a word of caution. *Int. J. Clin. Exp. Hypnosis*, **XXIX,** 401–412.

12. Wagstaff G.F., 1985. Hypnosis and the law: the role of induction in witness recall. In: *Modern Trends in Hypnosis* (eds Waxman, Misra, Gibson and Basker). Plenum, New York.
13. Wagstaff G.F., 1982. Hypnosis and witness recall: discussion paper. *J.R.S.M.,* **75,** 793–798
14. Perry C. and Laurence J-R, 1983. The enhancement of memory by hypnosis in the legal investigation situation. *Can. Psychol.,* **24,** 3.
15. American Medical Association, 1986. Scientific status of refreshing recollection by the use of hypnosis. Council report, *Int. J. Clin. Exp. Hypnosis,* **XXXIV,** 1–12.
16. Tucker Mr. Justice, 1986. Fennel v Jerome Property Maintenance Ltd., Judgement November 21.
17. Le Page K.E. and Goldney R.D., 1987. The use of hypnosis in the retrieval of memory loss due to post-traumatic retrograde amnesia. *Aust. J. Forensic Sci.,* **19,** 85–90.
18. Haward R.C., 1984. Comments on the BSECH Report on the Home Office draft circular on the use of hypnosis by the police in the investigation of crime. *Br. J. Exp. Clin. Hypnosis,* **1,** 68.
19. Perry C. and Nogrady H., 1985. Use of hypnosis by the police in the investigation of crime: is guided imagery a safe substitute? *Br. J. Exp. Clin. Hypnosis,* **3,** 25–31.

CHAPTER 26

Some Dangers of Hypnosis: Stage Hypnotism, Lay Therapy and the Law

The use of hypnosis from antiquity to the days of Mesmer, from the magnetizers and the great thinkers and theorists of the nineteenth century, from magic, mystery and misunderstanding has struggled hard to reach its present high ethical standards in the many disciplines of medicine, dentistry and psychology. Sadly, when Freud abandoned hypnosis to chart the course of psychoanalysis, the field was left wide open for its exploitation by charlatans and stage performers. Hypnotherapy, having reached a new status and new pinnacles of achievement in symptom relief, sank into oblivion. Then when the dust had settled, the real value of hypnotherapy was reassessed. It was realized that when properly used it could be of considerable benefit in the alleviation of a broad range of problems. Consequently, because of the persistent interest and curiosity of a number of research workers, the study of hypnosis has today found its rightful place in the laboratories of the experimental psychologists. Simultaneously, the development of effective techniques has emerged for its clincical use.

Unfortunately, however, what has become an important form of treatment continues to be abused, devalued and degraded. The spirit of Svengali still looms large in the folklore which has hindered the progress of hypnotherapy and which lingers in certain quarters, as a result of the persistent exploitation of hypnotism for purposes of entertainment. A great deal of investigation has been carried out through the years, of the ill effects of such misuse.

The possible complications of hypnosis were investigated by Schultz in the early 1920s. He cited 50 cases of hysteria, 30 cases of schizoid psychoses and 26 with various other harmful effects. Kleinsorge[1], in a later article, reported various cases of sexual misuse and of improper suggestions made under hypnosis as well as cases of sudden death. He concluded 'There is no doubt that the use of hypnosis should be reserved by law for therapeutic purposes by doctors and clinical psychologists.'

In a paper published in *The Journal of Nervous and Mental Disease*, Hilgard *et al.*[2] stated that 'symptom removal in patients on the verge of psychosis can deprive such patients of a major area of ego-defense and is ill-advised'. They believe that many psychosomatic or related complications would not have occurred had careful histories been taken. They also make the point that 'unexpected behaviour may occur in the induction phase, in the established state (either spontaneously or following some specific kind of suggestion) or after leaving hypnosis (spontaneously, or in relation to post-hypnotic suggestions)'. All this emphasizes the dangers of the improper use of hypnosis.

Numerous other adverse effects due to symptom removal by suggestion under hypnosis are also reported. These include many substitution symptoms, acute schizophrenia, depression, murderous impulses, suicide and suicidal risk, paranoid and other psychoses and other mental disturbances.

Erickson[3] reported 'about a score' of back injuries possibly due to stage demonstrations of hypnotism.

Some of the most frequently mentioned dangers of hypnosis have been summarized by Nesbitt[4]. These include the following:

1. Treating symptoms of unrecognized organic disease.
2. Uncovering traumatic emotional situations in the patient's past.
3. Presuming to know the patient's source of trouble.
4. The development of dependence by the patient on the therapist.

5. Precipitating a pre-psychotic into a frank psychosis by disturbing the balance of repressive safeguards.

6. Possible activation of latent homosexuality.

7. The danger of a claim of sexual assault by unstable patients.

8. Release of antisocial behaviour in psychotics.

9. Panic reactions in certain patients.

10. The giving of inappropriate post-hypnotic suggestions.

11. The failure to remove post-hypnotic suggestions.

12. The operator using hypnosis to fulfil his own neurotic or psychotic needs to the detriment of himself or his patient.

West and Deckert[5] also summarized the dangers of the use of hypnosis many years ago. These are just as relevant today and equally apply if hypnosis is being used for entertainment, or improperly in medical practice. The following problems are included:

1. The danger of precipitating a psychiatric illness. The authors quote the case of severe anxiety hysteria in a young female student following the suggestions under hypnosis that she was cutting off her hair.

2. The danger of making an existing disorder worse. For example using hypnosis in schizophrenic, depressed or even anxious persons can be 'profoundly disrupting'.

3. The danger of causing recurrence of symptoms in persons whose illness is in remission. This applies particularly to a person suffering from schizophrenia.

4. The danger of prolonging an illness particularly if attempting to cut short treatment using hypnosis.

5. The danger of masking effect. The subject behaving as healthy if he feels that this is what the therapist desires.

6. The danger of superficial relief. This could apply to a person complaining of suffering say from 'migraine' when the underlying cause, possibly a cerebral tumour, has not been investigated, or diagnosed.

7. The danger of excessive dependency. Here we are back to Breuer and Freud again and the problems arising from a powerful positive transference.

8. The danger of sexual seduction. Although this may appear remote and indeed was one of the charges levelled against the

'magnetizers' of the eighteenth century, it remains a distinct possibility and there are many recent reports of problems arising in this area.

9. The danger of criminal activity. Again, this is a remote possibility and Campbell Perry has shown[6] that the subject must have some predisposition towards criminal behaviour prior to compliance. Nevertheless, such acts have been reported following hypnotic suggestion.

10. The danger to the operator. A rarely considered possibility, but the sense of power and grandiosity has been noted to be potentially dangerous.

'Virtually every serious hypnotherapist has a built-in aversion to hypnosis for entertainment purposes' stated Clagett Harding[7]. This exhibition 'involves exploitation and exposure to substantial risks without reasonable gain for the subject or the audience'. Nelson[8] in remarks made in his book of instruction for stage hypnotists indicated that what is required is rapid and sensational routines, comedy relief, and of course audience participation! Thus a valuable therapeutic weapon is effectively exploited.

Harding reported the case of a normal healthy female who went into a hypnotic state whilst she was *a member of the audience* watching a performance of hypnotism. She was ordered to the stage and rigidity was produced. She was then suspended on her head and ankles between two chairs, subsequent to which the hypnotist stood on her abdomen (the 'human bridge' effect). This was not only an assault but the result for this unwitting subject was an orthopaedic, neurological and psychiatric disaster. Moreover, Harding showed that the offer frequently made by stage performers of help with problems of smoking, obesity or other habits has a high potential for undesirable side-effects. In addition he indicated that witnesses to stage performance of hypnosis may develop a 'block' to possible future therapy which could be difficult to overcome.

Kleinhauz *et al.*[9] pointed out that since hypnosis is a procedure which 'enables intervention into the function and emotional process in man...it carries a potential hazard'. In a case report they described a middle aged lady who was regressed to her childhood for the purposes of entertainment. Since no history had been taken, the hypnotist was unaware that this was a highly traumatic period of her life during the second world war when she had been in hiding. Unfortunately her repressed emotions relating to that time were reactivated and a neurosis developed which remained untreated for 11 years. The authors considered that hypnosis is a precipitating factor which may trigger psychopathological manifestations not only during trance but also after the trance has been terminated. These include anything from mild symptoms such as vertigo, nausea and drowsiness to anxiety, depression or obsessive preoccupation and the exacerbation of a full-blown psychosis.

There is no doubt that these possibilities have a marked potentiation of their expression in stage hypnosis and the authors had encountered a number of such problems.

Since interest in the use of 'complementary' medicine has increased in the UK dozens of so-called 'qualified hypnotherapists' have advertised their wares through the post, in magazines and in the popular press, purporting to cure stress-related illnesses (including depression) as well as a multitude of unrelated problems. Quasi-'psychotherapy' clinics have been established in dozens of cities and an assortment of new 'degrees' or 'diplomas' have been issued by self-appointed 'specialists'. First of all it must be understood that there is no authentic degree or diploma in hypnosis issued either in Great Britain nor in any other country in the world. There is no such person as a 'qualified' hypnotherapist and the only recognized courses of instruction in the UK are those held by the British Society of Medical and Dental Hypnosis (BSMDH) for registered medical and dental practitioners and by the British Society for Experimental and Clinical Hypnosis (BSECH) for properly qualified psychologists as well as for doctors and dentists.

The BSMDH issues a Certificate of Accreditation to those doctors or dentists who have studied with the Society and whose knowledge and work satisfies certain very rigid criteria. The members of the BSECH are responsible for much of the experimental work on hypnosis which has recently been forthcoming. These studies relate to a large range of subjects concerning both hypnotherapy and the hypnotic state. Additionally, both societies have contributed considerably to the clinical use of hypnosis and maintain the highest ethical standards.

As the study of hypnosis in the experimental field together with its clincial use, began to develop renewed interest worldwide, so the phenomena of hypnosis were increasingly exploited from the stage. The first half of the twentieth century culminated in the now historic case of Rains-Bath v Slater[10].

Ralph Slater was a stage hypnotist who in December 1948 was appearing in Brighton. During the performance he hypnotized a young lady who subsequently alleged assault and professional negligence. As a result the plaintiff was awarded damages. Later, an appeal on the issue of negligence was allowed, but dismissed on the issue of assault. Nevertheless, although a minor event in itself, it was sufficient to draw attention to the need for some legal control over the performances of hypnotism.

The cause of establishing the ethical status of hypnosis in the UK was championed by a well-known member of the British Parliament, Mr Leo Abse. This was in the form of a Private Member's Bill, as 'An Act to regulate the demonstration of hypnotic phenomena for the purposes of public entertainment' and was placed on the statute book on 1 August 1952[11]. In short, the new Act conferred power to any local authority which granted licences for the regulation of places used for various forms of public entertainment, to attach conditions to that licence, regulating or prohibiting the giving of an exhibition, demonstration or performance of hypnotism in those places.

In addition amongst other safeguards it was forbidden to give an exhibition, demonstration or performance of hypnotism upon any person who had not attained the age of 21 years.

Although this new enactment was a step forward, its weaknesses were soon to become obvious. Many local authorities, being unaware of the problems inherent in the performances of hypnotism, readily granted licences and the difficulties in policing such places of entertainment rendered the Bill virtually ineffective.

It fell to the lot of the British Medical Association to take the next step.

The Psychological Medicine Group Committee appointed a Subcommittee with the following brief: 'To consider the use of hypnotism, its relation to medical practice in the present day, the advisability of giving encouragement to research into the nature and application and the lines upon which such research might be organized'[12].

The Subcommittee noted the remarkable and striking nature of the phenomena induced in hypnotism and the ease with which they may be induced which has led to exploitation in the hands of charlatans. In spite of the many therapeutic uses which were listed it issued a warning that persons predisposed to severe psychoneurotic reactions or antisocial behaviour could be in danger when hypnotism was used without proper consideration to such conditions. They emphasized the possible source of danger resulting from the transference which developed, as well as any harm which could arise from the use of hypnosis by persons ignorant of the morbid complications which could ensue. In its concluding paragraph 'strong disapprobation' was expressed of public exhibitions of hypnotic phenomena with the hope that some legal restriction would be placed upon them.

Unfortunately, in spite of these restraints, stage performances of hypnotism continued and the numbers of lay therapists advertising their wares as 'qualified hypnotherapists' proliferated. Simultaneously, reports of the resulting ill effects of stage hypnosis multiplied. Many of these were hearsay but very many were reported to various interested parties and in view of his particular interest, reached the second author of this book. These included many types of physical injury from simple back strain to damage to the spinal column. Additionally, gastro-intestinal symptoms resulting from the ingestion, for example, of an onion (having been told it was a juicy apple), as well as vertigo, fainting and other nervous symptoms. Other subjects have become overtly anxious or depressed and another report is of a man admitted to hospital suffering from schizophrenia after offering himself to the 'entertainer' as a volunteer. Other cases of death and suicide have been recorded and in a personal communication, a young man who had been hypnotized, on driving home after the performance, was reported to have lost control of his vehicle which struck a tree. One passenger was killed. It was considered that the actions of the driver were quite out of keeping with his normal behaviour and care whilst at the wheel.

Apart from all these unfortunate reports, the persistent failure of so-called entertainers to remove post-hypnotic suggestions before subjects *or audience* left the theatre, resulted in innumerable embarrassing situations. The general public becoming more aware of frequent, unexpected, unpleasant and often damaging side-effects, continued to report complaints.

From the ongoing discussion and the numerous learned papers on the general subject of the improper use of hypnosis we can see that the problems that have emerged are threefold. These are:

1. Ethical and moral issues. As a result of the increasing use of hypnosis for entertainment many patients who would benefit from hypnotherapy are frightened and suspicious of the process and possible outcome.

2. Physical problems, especially related to the 'human bridge'.

3. The psychological problems.

These points were elaborated in a letter published in the *British Medical Journal* (Waxman[13]). This included the following details concerning the use of hypnosis for entertainment and by lay 'therapists' without any form of medical or psychological qualifications.

1. No medical history is taken and existing medical or psychiatric conditions could be aggravated.

2. Anxious patients could become more anxious or even depressed.

3. Depressed patients could become more depressed with the removal of the overlay of anxiety and the possibility of suicide should not be disregarded.

4. The psychotic person, perhaps in remission or giving no indication of his condition when on stage or even in therapy, could relapse or become more psychotic, particularly if sensory imagery is involved.

5. Conditions such as cerebral tumours and various neurological disorders, hypoglycaemia, thyroid dysfunction and drug dependence can only be recognized by the medically trained. All these illnesses may present psychological problems which the unwary and lay hypnotist may meet.

6. Well-known phenomena such as limb rigidity or catalepsy may be produced under hypnosis. Demonstration of the 'human bridge' could result in serious injury.

7. The use of hypnosis can be easily abused. For example, certain susceptible subjects could be made to perform immoral or improper acts.

8. The practice of hypnosis is a psychotherapy and as such should only be used by those properly trained and when adequate psychiatric safeguards are available.

9. Doctors and dentists are bound by a code of ethics which safeguards both public and patients against any abuses. As such they assume full clinical responsibility for their patients. Unqualified persons are not so bound.

10. The ability to recognize mental illness is essential so that drug treatment may be prescribed if necessary. Non-qualified persons can do neither.

Finally, it was added that the use of hypnosis by unqualified persons and for amusement debases and devalues a valuable therapeutic aid. Those who have watched a stage performance of hypnosis will agree that it is degrading to human dignity.

The dangers and opinions enumerated above apply not only to the use of hypnosis by entertainers and lay therapists but to the improper use of hypnosis in any situation.

So many bizarre incidents involving the misuse of hypnosis were received that one of us (D.W.) decided to launch a campaign for an amendment to the Hypnotism Bill. The intention was to make further provisions for regulating the demonstration of hypnotic phenomena and for controlling the demonstration of hypnosis at clubs, etc. in addition to theatres, for prohibiting advertisements of performances of stage hypnotism, prohibiting recordings of treatment by hypnosis and increasing the penalties for infringement.

Members of Parliament and all possible interested parties were lobbied. Support was obtained from the British Medical Association, the British Dental Association, The Royal Colleges of General Practitioners, Physicians and Psychiatrists as well as from The Law Society[14] and from many eminent persons interested in the proper use of hypnosis and its therapeutic value. A new Private Member's Bill was drawn up and passed through the House of Lords with the support of the Earl of Kinnoull[15]. It was read in the Commons by David Crouch MP[16] but as a result of last minute lack of support by the government reached only the second reading. Unfortunately it appeared that other powerful influences blocked its passage.

Nevertheless, realizing the need for restrictions, the British Home Secretary was directly instrumental in setting up a committee of stage hypnotists and representatives of the British Society of Medical and Dental Hypnosis in order to formulate a Code of Conduct for the performances of stage hypnosis[17]. This was duly established following a number of meetings at the Home Office and reads as follows:

1. No treatment of any condition should be attempted from the stage.
2. No suggestion of rigidity or catalepsy should ever be given.
3. No age-regression should ever be attempted.
4. No noxious substance should ever be given to the subject.
5. All post-hypnotic suggestion to be removed from all subjects as well as from all members of the audience before leaving the theatre.

The Federation of Ethical Stage Hypnotists which was established agreed to these proposals. Unfortunately there was no way in which they could enforce them and few stage hypnotists today honour this Code. Hypnotism continues to be practised for entertainment and for treatment by lay therapists and so the problems continue to arise. Nevertheless, the debate continues also and doctors, dentists and psychologists pursue their efforts for effective legislation for restricting the use of hypnosis, as a therapy and in the experimental laboratory, to those properly qualified.

Support is obtained from the fact that hypnosis is totally banned from the stage in several countries in the world. These include Sweden, Norway, Brazil and Israel, also in three provinces of Australia, in Ontario and in eight states in the USA. Only members of the medical profession and psychologists are permitted to use hypnosis in Eastern Europe.

We may conclude this section with a further reference to Clagett Harding[7]. 'Authorities' he said, 'should be reminded that Bedlam was once a place for the amusement of the public, and that nitrous oxide inhalation was a popular parlour game at the turn of the century. Individuals exposed to this anaesthetic engaged in compulsive laughter and related absurd kinds of behaviour. Stage hypnosis is being used at this time in an analogous fashion.'

More widespread and sorely needed restraints are most certainly required.

REFERENCES

1. Kleinsorge H., 1964. Contraindications and dangers of hypnotherapy. In: *Psychiatrie, Neurologie und Medizinische Psychologie* (ed. Muller-Hegemann). Hirzel, Leipzig.
2. Hilgard J.R., Hilgard E.R. and Newman M., 1961. Sequelae to hypnotic induction with special reference to earlier chemical anaesthesia. *J. Nerv. Ment. Dis.,* **133,** 461–478.
3. Erickson M.H., 1962. Stage hypnotists back syndrome. *Am. J. Clin. Hypnosis,* **5,** 141–142.
4. Nesbitt W.R., 1964. The dangers of hypnotherapy. *Medical Times,* **92,** 597–602.
5. West L.J., and Deckert G.H., 1965. Dangers of hypnosis, *J. Am. Med. Assoc.,* **192,** 95–98.
6. Perry C., 1979. Hypnotic coercion and compliance to it: a review of evidence presented in a legal case. *Int. J. Clin. Exp. Hypnosis,* **XXVII,** 3, 187–218.
7. Harding H.C., 1978. Complications arising from hypnosis for entertainment. In: *Hypnosis at its Bicentennial* (eds Frankel and Zamansky). Plenum, New York.
8. Nelson R.A., 1965. *A Complete Course in Stage Hypnotism.* Nelson Enterprises, Columbus, OH.
9. Kleinhauz M., Dreyfuss D.A., Beran B. *et al.,* 1979. Some after-effects of stage hypnosis: a case study of psychopathological manifestations. *Int. J. Clin. Exp. Hypnosis,* **XXVII,** 219–226.
10. Singleton Lord Justice., 1952. Rains-Bath v Slater, Action Against Hypnotist: Retrial Ordered, Law Report (Court of Appeal), July 30.
11. Hypnotism Act, 1952. *An Act to Regulate the Demonstration of Hypnotic Phenomena for Purposes of Public Entertainment.* H.M.S.O., London.
12. British Medical Association, 1955. Medical use of hypnotism, psychological medicine group committee. *Br. Med. J.* (suppl.), 190–193.
13. Waxman D., 1978. Misuse of hypnosis. *Br. Med. J.,* **ii,** 571.
14. The Law Society, 1979. Hypnotism—therapy or entertainment? *Ga-*

zette, **76,** 1.
15. Kinnoull The Earl of, 1979. Hypnotism Bill (H L), Second Reading. House of Lords Official Report, 1541. H.M.S.O., London.
16. Crouch D., 1980. Hypnotism (Stage Performances). Question to the Secretary of State for the Home Department. *Hansard,* **6,** 490. London.
17. Whitelaw W., 1980. Hypnotism (Stage Performances). House of Commons. *Hansard,* **6,** 490, London.

Guidelines for the Use of Hypnosis for Beginners

It is of course tempting and it is indeed desirable that after some initial instruction and when one or two techniques of induction have been acquired, actually to use hypnosis in the treatment of a real patient.

With the enthusiasm of most new students, first attempts at treatment are frequently successful and this seems to whet the appetite, so that the doctor will tend to enlarge his sphere of activities and select more difficult subjects. Often the first few failures will then occur, the honeymoon period will come to an abrupt end and disillusionment will set in.

Patients must be chosen with particular care. The doctor, perhaps until now accustomed only to prescribing drugs and dispensing the wisdom of his experience, must continue to select the necessary treatment with equal painstaking judgement and as has already been indicated, must be equally cautious in the application of his newly acquired skill. He must be warned against attempting to treat every case with hypnosis. As we are all aware, there is nothing more discouraging than failed treatment—especially for the patient.

With this in mind therefore, a few basic guidelines have been drawn up which summarize the points already made and which it is hoped, will prevent the occurrence of many of the pitfalls which are so common. These are as follows:

1. Never treat any patient without taking a comprehensive medical and psychiatric history. Any investigation which may be indicated should be carried out before commencing treatment. For example, the diagnosis of cardiac pain, even if assessed as psychosomatic should always be confirmed by electrocardiogram, etc. This is frequently necessary in order to convince the patient of the absence of organic disease.

2. Hypnosis is not the panacea. It has specific uses. Apply selectively and with care. Be eclectic in your choice of treatment.

3. It should be remembered that hypnosis is not merely a pleasant form of relaxation.

4. A very particular relationship is established between patient and therapist and the latter must be prepared to recognize and to deal with any emotional difficulties which may arise therefrom.

5. A firm diagnosis must always be made before commencing treatment.

6. No condition should ever be treated with which one is unfamiliar or which one would be unable to handle without hypnosis.

7. Remember—an anxious patient may become more anxious, a depressed patient may become more depressed, or a psychotic patient even if in remission, but especially if presented with visual imagery, may have an exacerbation of symptoms if inappropriate treatment is applied.

8. Prescribe antidepressants if required. Do not treat by hypnosis, the patient who suffers from any psychosis, who is a psychopathic personality or who is mentally subnormal.

9. The process of hypnosis must be fully explained to the patient and he must be reassured of the safety of the procedure. He must know that he will never lose control or be made to do anything that he would normally not wish to do.

10. The patient must be well motivated and willing to undergo hypnosis.

11. Never 'try' to see if hypnosis works. Be certain in your mind that it is the treatment of choice—or you will fail.

12. If any patient is taking *any* drugs be sure you are aware of

what they are. If tranquillizers—tail off *slowly* as the condition improves. If taking antidepressants—handle with especial care.

13. Tranquillizers and antidepressants are perfectly safe if properly used. Ask yourself—does the patient need either, will they help? If so—*why not prescribe?* Antidepressants in particular should never be withheld and it might be safer to prescribe than to be in doubt.

14. If the patient fails to make progress after a reasonable number of treatment sessions then reassess the problem. Perhaps the patient is in fact depressed and this has been overlooked.

15. Never use hypnoanalysis unless this can be followed up, giving the patient the essential interpretation, understanding and insight-directed psychotherapy.

16. If regression is used, remember that what the patient says is not necessarily the truth. He may lie, confabulate or fantasize. But he may also say what he thinks to be the truth or wishes you to believe is the truth—and it is that which is important in therapy.

17. Never attempt symptom removal by direct suggestion unless you are absolutely sure of your ground. If you fail, you lose credibility, the technique is degraded and the patient's problem may become reinforced. If you succeed, this may well result in symptom substitution. In spite of some strenuous denials, this certainly does occur, especially in the highly anxious or hysterical personality.

18. Don't attempt any suggestions, for example, of rigidity or catalepsy, which might fail. Once again you will lose credibility, the technique is degraded and the problem you are attempting to treat may become more resistant.

19. Never suggest to a patient that he will do something which convention, or his beliefs would normally prevent him from doing, or that you will *make* him do something which really he simply does not wish to do. In fact you can never *make* your patient do anything which he does not wish. Not even stop smoking or give up his bad habit—or even go into hypnosis—if he does not wish to do so.

20. Never challenge or command a patient to do something nor say anything which could arouse conflict (unless deliberate use is

being made of some confusional technique).

21. Once you have learned to apply hypnotherapy you will gain a skill which will considerably enhance your professional standing. Use it with dignity, *for medical or dental reasons only and never for entertainment or as a party piece.*

22. Never treat by hypnosis any patient who is not your own, without the specific request or approval of that patient's medical practitioner or the responsible physician.

23. Always use hypnosis for that form of treatment which is within your own professional discipline. Never be too proud to refer the patient to the appropriate specialist if necessary.

24. Always arouse the patient with suggestions of well being, of calmness and composure and that he will be wide awake, alert and ready to get on with the day.

25. Once you have acquired the skill, do tell as many people as you wish about hypnosis but never demonstrate hypnosis to a lay audience and *never train any lay person to hypnotize.*

Index